Frontiers in Cardiovascular Drug Discovery

(Volume 3)

Edited by

Atta-ur-Rahman, *FRS*

Kings College

University of Cambridge

Cambridge

UK

&

M. Iqbal Choudhary

H.E.J. Research Institute of Chemistry

International Center for Chemical and Biological Sciences

University of Karachi

Karachi

Pakistan

Bentham Science Publishers Ltd.
Executive Suite Y - 2
PO Box 7917, Saif Zone
Sharjah, U.A.E.
Email: subscriptions@benthamscience.org

BENTHAM
SCIENCE

CONTENTS

PREFACE

Cardiovascular diseases are the major cause of morbidly and mortality in humans. Despite major advancements in cardiovascular drug discovery and development, heart diseases and stroke remain the leading public health concern and primary causes of death globally. The development of effective and safe medicines that control blood pressure and cholesterol has significantly reduced the death rate from heart diseases. However, with global rise in metabolic disorders and aging populations, the prevalence of hypertension, high cholesterol, and diabetes is increasing. Heart diseases and stroke are becoming a worldwide pandemic as developing nations are witnessing the increasing health burden caused by them. To tackle this problem, tremendous research work has been conducted to understand the cause of cardiovascular diseases at molecular levels. This has led to the identification of new drug targets which are now vigorously studied.

The 3rd volume of the ebook series, "*Frontiers in Cardiovascular Drug Discovery*" comprises six comprehensive reviews, contributed by leading experts in these fields. Each review is focused on a certain important aspect of cardiovascular drug discovery and development, including the identification of new molecular targets and the outcome of clinical studies.

Boukhris *et al.* have contributed a review on $P2Y_{12}$ receptor antagonists as efficient treatment of platelet dysfunctions, including platelet aggregation and thrombus formation. The authors have comprehensively reviewed the role of $P2Y_{12}$ receptors in thrombus formation, and the mechanism of action of various classes of $P2Y_{12}$ receptor antagonists as anti-platelets agents. They also present the literature pertaining to the clinical outcome of efficacy and safety of various new generation of anti-platelet drugs, as well as prospects of tailored or individualized anti-platelet therapy for improving the clinical outcome.

Various forms of acute heart failures are heterogeneous in nature. They are difficult to manage and the conditions are often difficult to treat. The development of pharmacotherapy of acute heart failures has been comprehensively reviewed by Panjrath *et al.* in Chapter 2. The authors review the various classes of drugs and their contributions in reducing the mortality due to acute heart failure. The development of new therapeutic agents under the new regulatory requirements is also discussed, along with potential future developments in heart failure management and treatment.

Amit Agrawal reviews the role of vasopressin (arginine vasopressin) in cardiovascular health. Vasopressin is an anti-diuretic hormone which performs many essential functions in the body including maintaining plasma osmolality and volume. It has a direct impact on cardiovascular functions. A key function of AVP in the body is to regulate the extracellular fluid volume by regulating the renal handling of water. Vasopressin acts on renal collecting ducts *via* V_2 receptors to increase water permeability (cAMP-dependent mechanism), which leads to decreased urine formation and thus increases the blood volume, cardiac output, and arterial pressures. Over the years, synthetic vasopressin has emerged as an important drug for the treatment of various shock states. The author has elegantly reviewed various uses of vasopressin in critical care, especially in the treatment of vasodilatory shock. The commentary on mechanism of action of vasopressin at molecular and receptor levels provides insight into the action of this smart drug which is finding new uses with every passing day.

Cerebral small vessel disease (CSVD) or microangiopathy is a group of diseases involving microangiopathy and unspecific arteriopathy. This is a common risk factor for cognitive impairment, characterized by hypertrophy, vascular modification, and endothelial dysfunction that alter cerebrovascular functions, and auto-regulation of cerebral blood flow. CSVDs increase the risk of ischemia and tissue bleeding and may be categorized into six classes, based on the tissue types that they affect. The review by Alvarez-Parez focuses on type 1 CSVD, which is among the most common conditions, also called arteriolosclerosis. It is associated with aging, arterial hypertension, and diabetes. The author reviews the literature on the etiology and treatment of type 1 CSVD. Various classes of anti-aggregant drugs (aspirin, ticlopidine, and aspirin plus other drugs) have shown efficacy in this condition. The results of clinical studies on various classes of drugs have been discussed in this excellent review.

Shagdarsuren *et al.* have contributed a review on recent developments on a novel class of therapeutic agents which block and disable the complement blocking system. The complement cascade is an integral component of the body's innate immune system, which boosts the capacity of antibodies and phagocytic cells to clear the invading microorganisms and damaged cells from the body. The complement system is involved in promoting inflammation in various pathological conditions. Most importantly, the complement cascade is known to be involved in obesity, fatty liver, diabetes and cardiovascular diseases (CVD). The complement system comprising several complex small proteins and their receptors, is known to be activated in cardiovascular diseases. This has attracted major scientific interests in various complement molecules /components as new therapeutic targets. The authors present an excellent commentary on various complement molecules, their primary and secondary receptors, and their functional roles in the onset and progression of CVDs. They have also summarized the beneficial results observed in various pre-clinical studies conducted on targeting of specific components of the complement system in CVD animal models. This new class of drugs which includes gene targeting agents, neutralizing antibodies, and small molecular inhibitors, holds great promise for the treatment of CVDs in future.

Antiplatelet and anticoagulant therapies are essential parts of cardiovascular and cerebrovascular diseases prevention and management. They are among the most difficult classes of therapies, where balancing the benefits of antiplatelet and anticoagulant drugs with the risk of gastrointestinal and other bleedings is a major challenge. Aspirin and warfarin have been the most frequently used medicines for this purpose, with high risks of bleeding, and other therapeutic limitations. Recently, several novel classes of antiplatelet and anticoagulant agents have been developed which specifically target the mechanism of coagulation pathways, and thus have improved therapeutic efficacy. These new drugs are also associated with the occurrence of bleedings, including gastrointestinal bleeding. Johnson *et al.* have reviewed the recent literature on the pharmacology of available antiplatelet and anticoagulant drugs, particularly with reference to the associated risks, such as gastrointestinal bleeding and toxicity. They have also provided data about currently available and in pipeline anticoagulant reversal agents. This review is therefore an excellent source of information about the merits and demerits of new antiplatelet and anticoagulant agents, as well as development of agents which can reverse the bleeding episodes as a result of anticoagulant therapies.

The editors wish to express profound gratitude to all the contributors for the timely submission of their review articles for the 3rd volume of the eBook series. We also appreciate the efforts of the entire team of Bentham Science Publishers for efficient processing. The efforts of Mr. Omer Shafi (Assistant Manager Publications), Mr. Shehzad Naqvi (Manager Publications) and team leader Mr. Mahmood Alam (Director Publications) for their assistance in putting together an excellent compilation of well written articles in this important field of biomedical research. We sincerely hope that this volume will receive wide appreciation from readers.

Dr. Atta-ur-Rahman
Kings College
University of Cambridge
Cambridge
UK
&
Dr. M. Iqbal Choudhary
H.E.J. Research Institute of Chemistry
International Center for Chemical and Biological Sciences
University of Karachi
Karachi
Pakistan

List of Contributors

Alfredo R. Galassi	Department of Medical Sciences and Pediatrics, Catheterization Laboratory and Cardiovascular Interventional Unit, Division of Cardiology, Cannizzaro Hospital, University of Catania, Italy
Amit Agrawal	Gandhi Medical College & Hamidia Hospital, Bhopal, MP, India
David A. Johnson	Department of Internal Medicine, Division of Gastroenterology and Hepatology, Eastern Virginia Medical School, Norfolk, USA
Edward C. Oldfield	Department of Internal Medicine, Eastern Virginia Medical School, Norfolk, USA
Erdenechimeg Shagdarsuren	Institute for Molecular Cardiovascular Research (IMCAR), University Hospital, RWTH Aachen, Germany
Francisco José Álvarez-Pérez	Medicine Department, Health Sciences Research Center, Sciences Faculty, Beira Interior University, Stroke Unit, Hospital of Covilha, Covilha, Portugal
Gansuvd Shagdarsuren	Department of Internal Medicine, School of Medicine, Mongolian National University of Medical Sciences, Ulaanbaatar, Mongolia
Gurpreet Sodhi	Department of Medicine (Cardiology) and Heart and Vascular Institute, The George Washington University School of Medicine and Health Sciences, Washington D.C., USA
Gurusher Panjrath	Department of Medicine (Cardiology) and Heart and Vascular Institute, The George Washington University School of Medicine and Health Sciences, Washington D.C., USA
Ju Kim	Department of Medicine (Cardiology) and Heart and Vascular Institute, The George Washington University School of Medicine and Health Sciences, Washington D.C., USA
Marouane Boukhris	Department of Medical Sciences and Pediatrics, Catheterization Laboratory and Cardiovascular Interventional Unit, Division of Cardiology, Cannizzaro Hospital, University of Catania, Italy Faculty of Medicine of Tunis, University of Tunis El Manar, Tunisia
Parth J. Parekh	Department of Internal Medicine, Division of Gastroenterology and Hepatology, Tulane University, New Orleans, USA
Salvatore D. Tomasello	Department of Medical Sciences and Pediatrics, Catheterization Laboratory and Cardiovascular Interventional Unit, Division of Cardiology, Cannizzaro Hospital, University of Catania, Italy
Santosh Vijayan	Institute for Translational Immunology, University Hospital, Johannes Gutenberg-University Mainz, Germany

Stephen Robie	Department of Medicine (Cardiology) and Heart and Vascular Institute, The George Washington University School of Medicine and Health Sciences, Washington D.C., USA
Yaw Asare	Institute for Stroke and Dementia Research, Klinikum der Universität München, Ludwig-Maximilians University, Munich, Germany
Zied Ibn Elhadj	Faculty of Medicine of Tunis, University of Tunis El Manar, Tunisia

Frontiers in Cardiovascular Drug Discovery

(Volume 3)

2

Frontiers in Cardiovascular Drug Discovery

Volume # 3

Editors: Atta-ur-Rahman and M. Iqbal Choudhary

ISSN (Online): 1879-6648

ISSN (Print): 2452-3267

ISBN (eBook): 978-1-68108-163-2

ISBN (Print): 978-1-68108-164-9

CHAPTER 1

P2Y12-Receptor Antagonists and the Concept of Tailored Strategy

Marouane Boukhris[1,2,*], **Salvatore D. Tomasello**[1], **Zied Ibn Elhadj**[2] and **Alfredo R. Galassi**[1]

[1] *Department of Medical Sciences and Pediatrics, Catheterization Laboratory and Cardiovascular Interventional Unit, Division of Cardiology, Cannizzaro Hospital, University of Catania, Italy*

[2] *Faculty of Medicine of Tunis, University of Tunis El Manar, Tunisia*

Abstract: Platelet represents the cornerstone of both physiologic hemostasis and thrombosis acting *via* different pathways. Adenosine diphosphate (ADP) plays a crucial role in platelet activation and thrombus formation through its interaction with platelet P2Y12 receptor, making therefore this receptor an interesting therapeutic target for anti-thrombotic agents.

Around the world, millions of people affected by coronary artery disease are treated with anti-platelet agents. Indeed, dual anti-platelet therapy, consisting of a combination of aspirin and a P2Y12 receptor antagonist, is the recommended strategy in patients with acute coronary syndrome and those who underwent percutaneous coronary intervention with stent implantation. Furthermore, the introduction of different generations of P2Y12 receptor antagonists has immensely improved the clinical outcome, as well established through literature.

Although the concept to replace "one size fits all" paradigm to a more individualized approach in anti-platelet therapy seems to be rational, in the area of based evidence medicine, a clear prognostic impact of such a strategy is not yet clearly demonstrated.

In the current chapter, we tried to summarize the mechanisms of P2Y12 receptor antagonists anti-platelet action, to report clinical proofs regarding the efficacy/safety of

* **Corresponding Auhor Marouane Boukhris:** Department of Medical Sciences and Pediatrics Catheterization Laboratory and Cardiovascular Interventional Unit Cannizzaro Hospital, University of Catania *Via* Messina 829, 95126, Catania, Italy; Tel: 0039-095-7263122-3623; Fax: +39-095-72631-4-3633; E-mail: mar1bou@hotmail.com

Atta-ur-Rahman and M. Iqbal Choudhary (Eds.)

new generations of this class of drugs, and to discuss the place of a tailored strategy and its impact on improving clinical outcome.

Keywords: Anti-aggregation therapy, Bleeding, Cangrelor, Clinical outcome, Clopidogrel, Coronary artery disease, Dual anti-platelet therapy, Elinogrel, Genetic testing, High on-treatment platelet reactivity, Ischemic event, Low on-treatment platelet reactivity, Percutaneous coronary intervention, Platelet aggregation, Platelet reactivity, Prasugrel, P2Y12 receptor, P2Y12 receptor inhibitors, Stent implantation, Ticagrelor.

INTRODUCTION

The primary function of platelets is to preserve vascular integrity and hemostasis; however, in presence of vascular disease, particularly atherosclerosis, this normal process can become excessive, leading to thrombotic events. The role of platelets in the pathophysiology of arterial thrombosis has been investigated over the past decades and established as crucial [1 - 3]. Platelet-dependent thrombotic events such as myocardial infarction (MI), stroke and even sudden cardiac death, often started by an acute plaque destabilization followed by platelet adhesion, activation and aggregation, which represented the key processes. Indeed, differently from normal endothelium platelets only adhere to disrupted endothelial surfaces. Thereafter, platelets undergo shape change, secrete the contents of their granules, transform endogenous arachidonic acid into thromboxane A2, and aggregate with one another, resulting in a platelet-dependent thrombus [2, 3].

Aspirin represents the first effective platelet inhibitor drug used in humans. It results in an irreversible modification of the enzyme cyclo-oxygenase preventing it to convert arachidonic acid into thromboxane A2 [4].

On the other hand, adenosine diphosphate (ADP) also plays a capital role in platelet activation. Originating from platelet dense granules, red blood cells and damaged endothelium, its interaction with platelet receptors (particularly P2Y12 receptors), leads to an activation-amplification cascade resulting in thrombus formation [5]. This capital role of ADP makes it an appropriate therapeutic target for anti-platelet agents acting differently from aspirin. In this respect, P2Y12 receptor antagonists had been introduced in cardiovascular diseases (Fig. **1**).

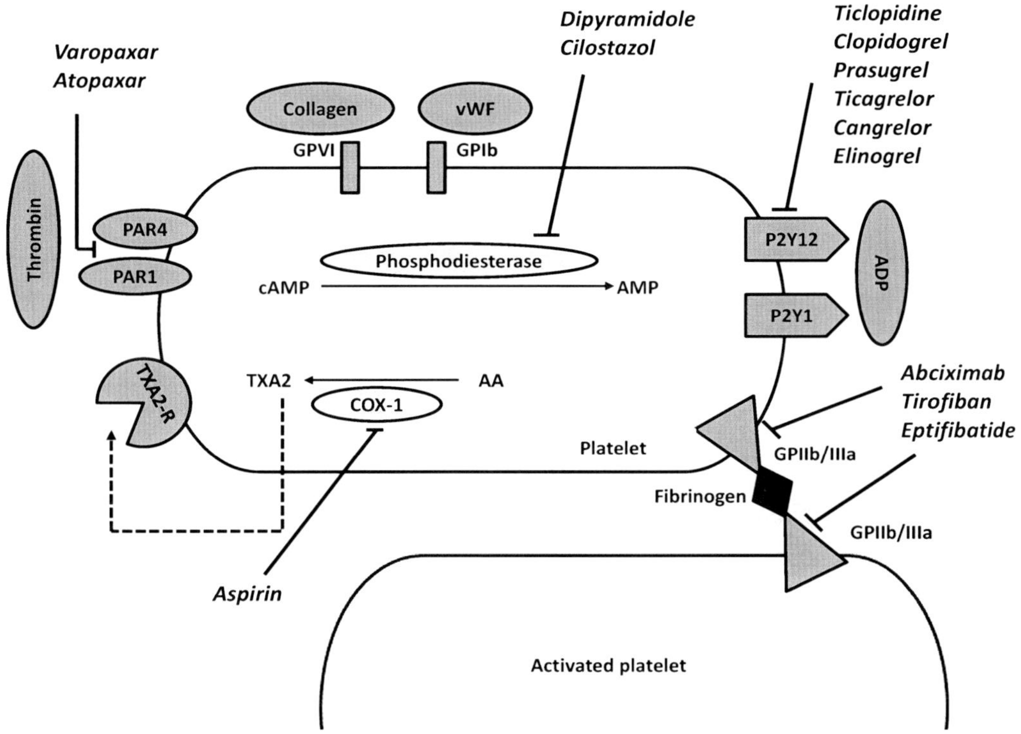

Fig. (1). Platelet activation and the mechanism of action of different anti-platelet agents.

Nowadays, around the world, millions of people affected by coronary artery disease (CAD), are treated with antiplatelet agents. Indeed, dual anti-platelet therapy (DAPT), consisting of a combination of aspirin and a P2Y12 receptor antagonist is the recommended strategy in patients with acute coronary syndrome (ACS) and those who underwent percutaneous coronary intervention (PCI) with stent implantation [6]. Furthermore, the introduction of new generations of P2Y12 receptor antagonists has immensely improved the clinical outcome,

During the last decade, the interest in platelet reactivity testing has grown, with the aim to obtain a tailored and personalized anti-aggregation strategy. However, the prognostic impact of such an approach remains not yet clearly demonstrated.

In the current chapter, we tried to summarize the mechanisms of P2Y12 receptor antagonists anti-platelet action, to report clinical proofs regarding the efficacy/safety of new generations of this class of drugs, and to discuss the place of a tailored strategy and its impact on improving clinical outcome.

ADP RECEPTORS

Platelets represent the cornerstone of both normal hemostasis maintenance and pathological thrombus formation. A vascular injury results in platelets translocation and adhesion to exposed subendothelium through the interaction between matrix components, such as von Willebrand factor (vWF) and collagen, and platelets receptors [3]. Platelet membrane GPIbα and GPVI recognize the activated conformation of vWF and collagen respectively, resulting in platelet activation involving integrin αIIbβ3 activation, which leads to platelet shape change, stable platelet adhesion, and release of granules contents. The thromboxane A2 generated within platelets, and ADP released from platelet granules, contribute to other platelets activation and recruitment [1 - 3, 7].

Table 1. P2Y receptor subtypes.

P2Y Receptor	Distribution	Pharmacological Ligand	Functional Coupling
P2Y1	platelets and neural cells	adenine nucleotide sensitive receptor	Gq-coupled
P2Y2	epithelia	mixed sensitive receptor	Gq-coupled
P2Y4	epithelia and placenta	uracil nucleotide sensitive receptor	Gq-coupled
P2Y6	blood vessels and brain	uracil nucleotide sensitive receptor	Gq-coupled
P2Y11	immunocytes	adenine nucleotide sensitive receptor	Gq-coupled
P2Y12	platelets and neural cells	adenine nucleotide sensitive receptor	Gi-coupled
P2Y13	ubiquitous	adenine nucleotide sensitive receptor	Gi-coupled
P2Y14	ubiquitous	UDP-glucose sensitive receptor	Gi-coupled

P2 receptors belong to nucleotide receptor family, mediating the actions of extracellular nucleotides to intercellular signaling [5, 8, 9]. Membrane-bound P2-receptors consist of two classes: P2X ligand-gated cation channels and G protein-coupled P2Y receptors. Mammalian P2X receptors are classified into 7 distinct subtypes (P2X1-P2X7) that are expressed abundantly in the nervous system playing important roles in nervous system and peripheral diseases. Eight subtypes of P2Y receptor (P2Y1, P2Y2, P2Y4, P2Y6, P2Y11, P2Y12 and P2Y13, P2Y14) have been described [5, 8]. Table **1** summarizes the distribution and the functional coupling of P2Y receptors.

The role of ADP in platelet aggregation passes through two G protein-coupled receptors, the Gq-coupled P2Y1 receptor and the Gi-coupled P2Y12 receptor [9]. The P2Y1 receptor participates in ADP-induced platelet shape change, while the P2Y12-coupled Gi signaling is important for potentiation of dense granule secretion, thromboxane A2 generation, irreversible aggregation and stabilization of a platelet thrombus [5, 10]. Despite its presence in platelets, the function of P2Y14 and its eventual contribution in platelet aggregation receptor remain unknowns.

P2Y12 RECEPTOR

The P2Y12 receptor was cloned and characterized in 2001, and is highly expressed in human platelets and to a smaller extent in brain. Its essential roles are platelet aggregation in addition to inhibition of neural cells [5].

The P2Y12 receptor structure contains the specific features of G protein-coupled receptors including 7 hydrophobic transmembrane regions connected by 3 extracellular loops and 3 intracellular loops [8]. Guanine nucleotide-binding regulatory proteins, or G proteins, mediate the interaction between cell surface receptors and intracellular enzyme, generating second messenger molecules during platelet activation. The G proteins are multimers, consisting of three distinct subunits including α, β and γ co-existing in different forms [11].

The P2Y12 receptor is coupled to αi2 subunit of G protein. The stimulation of the heterotrimeric G protein by ADP, leads to the dissociation of Gα and Gβγ subunits, activating thereafter various signaling pathways (Fig. **2**). The Gαi2 inhibits production of adenyl cyclase which results in reduction of cytosolic cyclic adenosine monophosphate (cAMP) concentrations [12, 13]. This decrease in cAMP reduces the activation of cAMP-dependent protein kinase (PKA) which is responsible for phosphorylation of the vasodilator-stimulated phosphoprotein (VASP) [14]. VASP is an actin regulatory protein that inhibits the integrin αIIbβ3 activation, and its phosphorylation plays an essential role in fibrinogen receptor activation in response to ADP and platelet aggregation [15].

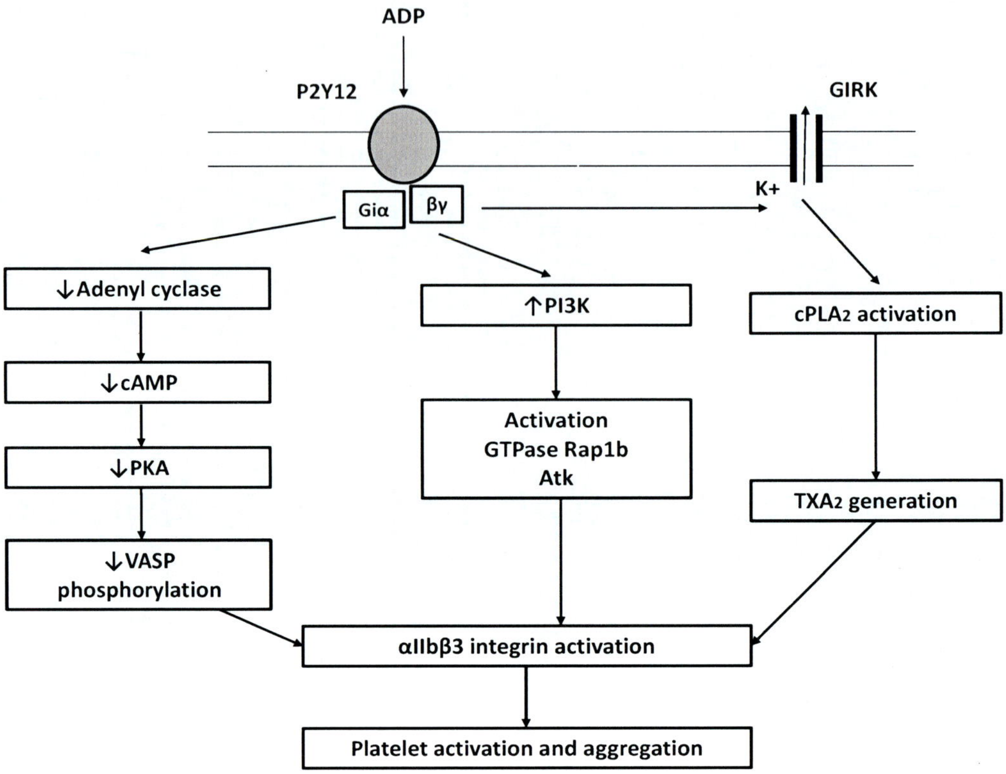

Fig. (2). P2Y12 receptor signaling pathways in platelet.

On the other hand, it has been shown that stimulation of P2Y12 by ADP, through Gβγ subunits, stimulates phosphatidyl inositol-3 kinase (PI3K) activity, leading to GTPase Rap1b activation [16]; this latter resulting in activation of integrin αIIbβ3 and platelet aggregation [16, 17]. Furthermore, PI3K initiates phosphorylation of protein kinase B, also known as Akt. This Akt activation in a PI3K-dependent pathway, after thromboxane A2 or thrombin stimulation, promotes ADP release from platelets dense granules that stimulate P2Y12 receptor signaling pathways resulting in enhancement of integrin αIIbβ3-mediated platelet aggregates and stabilization [18]. It was also reported that βγ dimers might activate the G-protein gated inwardly rectifying potassium channel (GIRK) *via* binding to their cytosolic regions mediating activation of Src tyrosine kinases downstream, which could play a role in ADP-induced cytosolic phospholipase A2 (cPLA2) phosphorylation *via* extracellular signal-regulated kinase (ERK), resulting in thromboxane A2 generation and platelet aggregation [19, 20].

Due to the complexity of the involved mechanisms, the P2Y12 signaling pathways which remained not yet completely elucidated. As P2Y12 receptor has a very selective distribution on tissues and plays a capital role in the thrombus formation and stabilization, it represents an optimal candidate for antiplatelet therapy.

P2Y12 INHIBITORS

The ideal antithrombotic agent is characterized by its predictable pharmacodynamics profile (avoid monitoring), rapid onset, rapid offset (and/or available antidote), compatible with adjunctive medicine, potent efficacy, low risk, low cost and easy administration. Current available inhibitors of P2Y12 receptor are categorized into indirect acting irreversible inhibitors (thienopyridines: ticlopidine, clopidogrel and prasugrel), and direct acting reversible P2Y12 inhibitors (ticagrelor, cangrelor and elinogrel) (Fig. **3**). Tables **2** and **3** summarize the characteristics of different P2Y12 receptor blockers and their relevant phase III trials, respectively.

Table 2. Characteristics of P2Y12 receptor inhibitors.

	Clopidogrel	**Prasugrel**	**Ticagrelor**	**Cangrelor**	**Elinogrel**
Class	Thienopyridine	Thienopyridine	Triazolopyrimidine	Triazolopyrimidine	quinazolinediones
Activation	Prodrug	Prodrug	Active drug	Active drug	Active drug
P2Y12 Rc inhibition	Irreversible	Irreversible	Reversible	Reversible	Reversible
Route of administration	Oral	Oral	Oral	Intravenous	Oral & intravenous
Half-life (active metabolite)	0.5 h	7 h	9 h	3-4 min	11 h
Loading dose	300-600 mg	60 mg	180 mg	-	-
Pre-treatment	Yes	No	No	-	-
Peak effect	6 h	4 h	2 h	15-30 min	20 min
Maintenance dose	75 mg	10 mg*	90 mg b.i.d	-	-
Duration of effect	3-10 days	5-10 days	3-4 days	1-2 h	8-24h

(Table 2) contd.....

	Clopidogrel	Prasugrel	Ticagrelor	Cangrelor	Elinogrel
Recommended delay of withdrawal before surgery	5 days	7 days	5 days	-	-
Recommendation in ACS **	Yes (Class IC)	Yes(Class IB)	Yes(Class IB)	Not recommended	Not recommended
Recommendation in SCAD **	Yes (Class IA)	Not recommended	Not recommended	Not recommended	Not recommended

Abbreviations ACS=acute coronary syndrome; SCAD=stable coronary artery disease.

* For prasugrel, a maintenance dose of 5 mg can be prescribed in particular clinical conditions such as elderly patients (≥75 years).

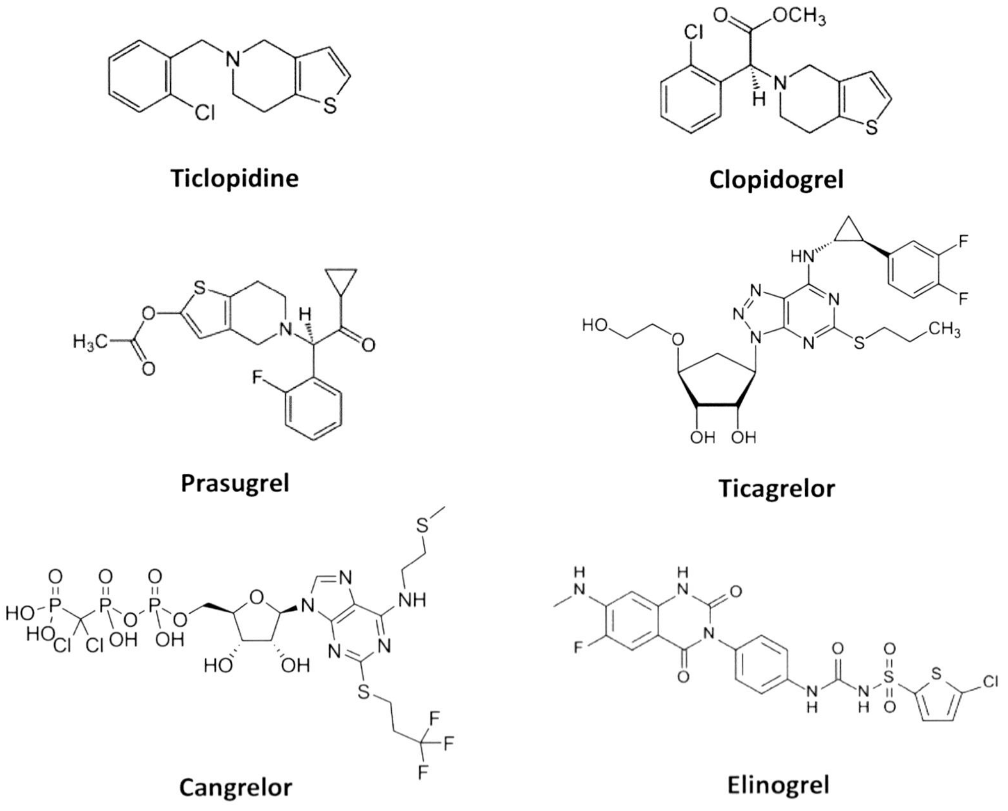

Fig. (3). P2Y12 receptors antagonists.

Table 3. Relevant clinical trials regarding P2Y12 receptor inhibitors.

Trial	Patients	Protocol	Primary Endpoints	Mortality	MI	Stroke	Stent Thrombosis	Bleeding
CAPRIE [1] (1996) [30]	19,185 Recent ischemic stroke, recent MI (17%), symptomatic PAD	Clopidogrel 75 mg *vs.* Aspirin 325 mg	*CV death, MI, stroke* Clopidogrel 5.32% *vs.* Aspirin 5.83% (p=0.043)	*CV causes* Clopidogrel 1.90% *vs.* Aspirin 2.06% (p=0.29)	Clopidogrel 5.03% *vs.* Aspirin 4.84% (p=0.66)	Clopidogrel 7.15% *vs.* 7.71% (p=0.26)	N/A	*Severe bleeding* Clopidogrel 1.38% *vs.* Aspirin 1.55% (p NS)
CURE [1] (2001) [31]	12,562 NSTEMI-ACS	Clopidogrel 75 mg (300 mg LD) *vs.* Placebo	*CV death, MI, stroke* Clopidogrel 9.3% *vs.* Placebo 11.4% (p<0.001)	*CV causes* Clopidogrel 5.1% *vs.* Placebo 5.5% (p=NS)	Clopidogrel 5.2% *vs.* Placebo 6.7% (p N/A)	Clopidogrel 1.2% *vs.* Placebo 1.4% (p N/A)	N/A	*Major bleeding* Clopidogrel 3.7% *vs.* Placebo 2.7% (p=0.001)
CLARITY [1] (2005) [33]	3,491 STEMI	Clopidogrel 75 mg (300 mg LD) *vs.* Placebo	*occluded artery, death, MI* Clopidogrel 15.0% *vs.* Placebo 21.7%	Clopidogrel 2.6% *vs.* Placebo 2.2% (p=0.49)	Clopidogrel 2.5% *vs.* Placebo 3.6% (p=0.08)	*At 30 days Clopidogrel 0.9% vs.* Placebo 1.7 (p NS)	N/A	*Major bleeding* Clopidogrel 1.3% *vs.* Placebo 1.0% (p=0.64)
HORIZONS AMI[1] (2009) [35]	3,311 STEMI undergoing primary PCI	Clopidogrel 600 mg LD *vs.* 300 mg LD2	*Any cause death, MI, stroke, unplanned revascularization* 600 mg 4.3% *vs.*300 mg 7.0 (p=0 .001)	*Cardiac death* 600 mg 1.9% *vs.* 300 mg 2.7% (p=0.11) *Any cause death* 600 mg 2.0% *vs.* 300 mg 3.1% (p=0.03)	600 mg 1.6% *vs.* 300 mg 2.4% (p=0.01)	600 mg 0.5% *vs.* 300 mg 1.0% (p=0.13)	600 mg 2.0% *vs.* 300 mg 3.1% (p=0.05)	*All major bleeding* 600 mg 7.5% *vs.* 300 mg 11.4% (p<0.001) *Non-CABG related major bleeding* 600 mg 6.1% *vs.* 300 mg 9.4% (p<0.001)
TRITON [2] (2007) [46]	13,608 undergoing PCI NSTE-ACS (74%) STEMI (26%)	Prasugrel 10 mg (60 mg LD) *vs.* Clopidogrel 75 mg (300 mg)	*CV death, MI, stroke* Prasugrel 9.9% *vs.* Clopidogrel 12.1% (p<0.001)	*CV death* Clopidogrel 5.1% *vs.* Placebo 5.5% (p=0.31) *Any cause* Prasugrel 3.0% *vs.* Clopidogrel 3.2% (p=0.64)	Prasugrel 7.3% *vs.* Clopidogrel 9.5% (p<0.001)	Prasugrel 1.0% *vs.* Clopidogrel 1.0% (p=0.93)	Prasugrel 1.1% *vs.* Clopidogrel 2.4% (p<0.001)	*Non-CABG related major bleeding* Prasugrel 2.4% *vs.* Clopidogrel 1.8% (p=0.03) *CABG-related bleeding* Prasugrel 13.4% *vs.* Clopidogrel 3.2% (p<0.001)

(Table 3) contd.....

Trial	Patients	Protocol	Primary Endpoints	Mortality	MI	Stroke	Stent Thrombosis	Bleeding
TRILOGY ACS[2](2012) [48]	7,243 NSTEMI-ACS	<75 years Prasugrel (10 mg) *vs.* Clopidogrel (75 mg) ≥75 years Prasugrel (5 mg) *vs.* Clopidogrel (75 mg)	*CV death, MI, stroke* Prasugrel 13.3% *vs.* Clopidogrel 13.9% (p=0.45)	CV death Prasugrel 6.6% *vs.* Clopidogrel 7.1% (p=0.38%) *Any cause* Prasugrel 8.3% *vs.* Clopidogrel 8.8% (p=0.40)	Prasugrel 7.7% *vs.* Clopidogrel 8.1% (p=0.58)	Prasugrel 1.3% *vs.* Clopidogrel 1.5% (p=0.52)	N/A	**TIMI criteria** Major bleeding Prasugrel 1.3% *vs.* Clopidogrel 1.0% (p=0.29) **Gusto criteria** Major bleeding Prasugrel 0.5% *vs.* Clopidogrel 0.6% (p=0.53)
ACCOAST [2] (2013) [49]	4,033 NSTEMI undergoing invasive strategy	Prasugrel pretreat 30 mg *vs.* No pretreat	*CV death, MI, emergency revascularization, need for GIIb/IIIa Pretreat 10.0% vs.* No pretreat 9.8% (p=0.81)	*CV death Pretreat 10.0% vs.* No pretreat 9.8% (p=0.81) *Any cause death Pretreat 0.4% vs.* No pretreat 0.5% (p=0.61)	*Pretreat 5.8% vs.* No pretreat 5.5% (p=0.60)	*Pretreat 0.4% vs.* No pretreat 0.5% (p=0.60)	N/A	**TIMI criteria** *Non-CABG related major bleeding* Pretreat 1.3% *vs.* No pretreat 0.5 (p=0.005)
PLATO [3] (2009) [58]	18,624 NSTEMI-ACS (59%) STEMI (38%) (invasive & non invasive)	Ticagrelor 90 mg b.i.d (180 mg LD) *vs.* Clopidogrel 75 mg (300-600 mg LD)	*Death from vascular causes, MI, stroke* Ticagrelor 9.0% *vs.* Clopidogrel 10.7% (p=0.0025)	*Vascular causes* Ticagrelor 4.0% *vs.* Clopidogrel 5.1% (p=0.001) *Any cause* Ticagrelor 3.9% *vs.* Clopidogrel 5.9% (p<0.001)	Ticagrelor 5.8% *vs.* Clopidogrel 6.9% (p=0.005)	Ticagrelor 1.5% *vs.* Clopidogrel 1.3% (p=0.22)	Ticagrelor 2.2% *vs.* Clopidogrel 3.0% (p=0.014)	**Plato criteria** *Major bleeding* Ticagrelor 11.6% *vs.* 11.2% (p=0.42) *Non-CABG major bleeding* Ticagrelor 4.5% *vs* .Clopidogrel 3.8% (p=0.03)
ATLANTIC [3] (2014) [60]	1,862 STEMI	Ticagrelor pretreat *vs.* No pretreatment	*ST resolution <70%, TIMI flow <3* Pretreat 72.7% *vs.* No pretreat 73.5% (p=0.73)	*Any cause death* Pretreat 3.3% *vs.* No pretreat 2.0% (p=0.08)	Pretreat 0.8% *vs.* No pretreat 1.1% (p=0.53)	Pretreat 0.4% *vs.* No pretreat 0.2% (p=0.39)	Pretreat 0% *vs.* No pretreat 0.8% (p=0.008)	**Plato criteria** *Non-CABG major bleeding* Pretreat 1.8% *vs.* No pretreat 1.6% (p=0.76)

(Table 3) contd.....

Trial	Patients	Protocol	Primary Endpoints	Mortality	MI	Stroke	Stent Thrombosis	Bleeding
CHAMPION PLATFORM [4] (2009) [65]	5,362 NSTEMI-ACS (95%)	Cangrelor (30µg/kg or 4µg/kg/mn) *vs.* Placebo	*Death,MI, emergency revascularization* Cangrelor 7.0% *vs.* Placebo 8.0% (p=0.14)	*Any cause* Cangrelor 0.3% *vs.* Placebo 0.7% (p=0.03)	Cangrelor 6.6% *vs.* Placebo 7.3% (p=0.33)	Cangrelor 0.3% *vs.* Placebo 0.2% (p=0.57)	Cangrelor 0.2% *vs.* Placebo 0.6% (p=0.02)	**ACUITY criteria** *Major bleeding* Cangrelor 5.5% *vs.* Placebo 3.5% (p<0.001) **TIMI criteria** *Major bleeding* Cangrelor 0.2% *vs.* Placebo 0.3% (p=0.17)
CHAMPION PCI [4] (2009) [66]	8,877 MI (49.1%)	Cangrelor (30µg/kg or 4µg/kg/mn) *vs.* Placebo	*Death MI, emergency revascularization* Cangrelor 7.5% *vs.* Placebo 7.1% (p=0.59)	*Any cause* Cangrelor 0.2% *vs.* Placebo 0.1% (p=0.42)	Cangrelor 7.1% *vs.* Placebo 6.6% (p=0.36)	Cangrelor 0.2% *vs.* Placebo 0.2% (p=0.77)	Cangrelor 0.2% *vs.* Placebo 0.3% (p=0.34)	**ACUITY criteria** *Major bleeding* Cangrelor 3.6% *vs.* Placebo 2.9% (p=0.06) **TIMI criteria** *Major bleeding* Cangrelor 0.4% *vs.* Placebo 0.3% (p=0.39)
CHAMPION PHOENIX [4] (2013) [67]	11,145 Undergoing PCI NSTEMI-ACS 25.4% STEMI 17.6%	Cangrelor (30µg/kg or 4µg/kg/mn) *vs.* Clopidogrel (300 mg or 600 mg LD)	*Death, MI, emergency revascularization, stent thrombosis Cangrelor 4.7%* *vs.* Clopidogrel 5.9% (0.005)	*CV death* Cangrelor 0.3% *vs.* Clopidogrel 0.3% (p>0.999) *Any cause* Cangrelor 0.3% *vs.* Clopidogrel 0.3% (p>0.999)	Cangrelor 3.8% *vs.* Clopidogrel 4.7% (p=0.02)	N/A	Cangrelor 0.8% *vs.* Clopidogrel 1.4% (p=0.01)	**GUSTO criteria** Cangrelor 0.2% *vs.* Clopidogrel 0.1% (p=0.44) **TIMI Criteria** Cangrelor 0.1% *vs.* Clopidogrel 0.1% (p>0.999)

[1]Clopidogrel; [2]Prasugrel; [3]Ticagrelor; [4]Cangrelor.

Abbreviations

ACS= acute coronary syndrome; CABG=coronary artery bypass grafting; CV=cardiovascular LD=loading dose; MI=myocardial infarction; N/A=not available; pretreat=preatreatment; STEMI= ST; NSTEMI= non-ST elevation myocardial infarction.

Thienopyridines

Thienopyridines are the first family of P2Y12 inhibitor. Being prodrugs, thienopyridines required to be metabolized to form active metabolite. The active metabolite then covalently and irreversibly binds to the P2Y12 receptor hence inhibiting it.

Ticlopidine

Ticlopidine is the first member of this class of antiplatelet agents. In 1972, Dr Eloy and coworkers, started to search for new anti-inflammatory drugs related to Tinoridine, a thienopyridine compound with anti-inflammatory and analgesic properties [21]. Several derivates had been synthesized to screen them on animal models mimicking human pathologies.

It appeared that none of the thienopyridine compounds synthesized had anti-inflammatory or analgesic effects; however, some of them displayed unexpected antiplatelet and antithrombotic activities after oral administration to rats [21]. It is worth mentioning that it was uncommon, at that time, to search for new antiplatelet agents. Indeed, the link between platelet aggregation, thrombosis and cardiovascular events was still ignored and at that time, vascular spasm was considered to be the major cause of the clinical complications of atherosclerosis.

One of the most active compounds discovered, ticlopidine, was rapidly selected for development and it was first evaluated in cardiac surgery for extracorporeal circulation, or in patients undergoing hemodialysis [21]. The drug was marketed in France, in 1978, for these restricted clinical indications, under the name Ticlid.

Pharmacokinetics & Pharmacodynamics

In the early 1990s, after Food and Drug Administration (FDA) approval, ticlopidine started to be prescribed in clinical practice. A single oral dose (250 mg dose) of ticlopidine is rapidly absorbed, and peak plasma concentration is achieved 1-3 h, with a half-life of 12 h; however, after repeated dosing at 250 mg bid, the elimination half-life rises to 4-5 days [22]. Hepatic biotransformation is necessary to obtain active metabolites. Although 13 metabolites have been distinguished, those responsible for the antiplatelet effect have not been identified.

The antiplatelet effect consists of irreversible alteration of the platelet surface of P2Y12 receptor, responsible for a reduction in ADP-induced platelet aggregation [23]. At 5 days, only 50% platelet aggregation inhibition is obtained with maintenance doses, while this percentage reached 60-70% at 8-11 days [24]. Ticlopidine metabolism passes through the cytochrome p450 system, and interactions with several drugs such as digoxin, theophylline and cimetidine have been reported [25]. Elimination of ticlopidine is mostly renal and gastrointestinal. Ticlopidine is dosed 250 mg twice daily, and the offset occurs after 11-13 days of discontinuation [22].

Efficacy & Safety

The Intracoronary Stenting and Antithrombotic Regimen trial was the first of the randomized trials and enrolled 517 patients in whom coronary stenting was performed (257 patients assigned to receive aspirin plus ticlopidine, and 260 patients assigned to receive anticoagulation with target international normalized ratio (INR) between 3.5 and 4.5 [26]. At 1 month, primary cardiac endpoints [defined as cardiac death, non fatal myocardial infarction (MI) and repeat revascularization] occurred in 6.2% in anticoagulant group *versus* 1.6% among patients receiving dual antiplatelet therapy, corresponding to 75% risk reduction ($p<0.001$) [26]. The benefit in patients receiving antiplatelet agent was only observed after the third days due to the delayed onset of action. The Stent Anticoagulation Restenosis Study enrolled 1653 patients undergoing emergency or elective percutaneous coronary interventions with stent placement, who were randomly to one of three regimen: ticlopidine 250 mg twice daily plus aspirin (100-325 mg daily), aspirin alone or aspirin 325 mg daily plus warfarin with an INR of 2.0-2.5 [27]. Therapy was continued for 30 days. Regarding cardiac events occurrence at 30 days, dual anti-platelet therapy was associated with 85% risk reduction as compared to aspirin alone, and 80% risk reduction as compared to aspirin plus warfarin [27]. In The Full Anticoagulation *versus* Aspirin and Ticlopidine (FANTASTIC) trial, ticlopidine plus aspirin group experienced less bleeding or vascular complications than aspirin plus anticoagulation group (13.5% *versus* 21%, respectively; $p=0.03$) [28]; however, this latter study also demonstrated the limitations of the slow onset of action of ticlopidine responsible for higher rate of acute stent thrombosis, and underlying the need for either pretreatment prior to the stent procedure or adjunctive anticoagulant therapy until ticlopidine exposure had been sufficient to inhibit platelet aggregation [28].

In addition to coronary artery disease, ticlopidine was also indicated in the setting of stroke or transient ischemic attack. In the Canadian American Ticlopidine Study, 1073 patients with ischemic stroke were randomized to ticlopidine 250 mg twice daily or placebo with a mean follow up of 2 years [29]. Stroke recurred less frequently in ticlopidine group as compared to placebo patients (18.6% *versus* 24.6%, respectively; p=0.017), similarly to the composite rate of myocardial infarction, stroke and vascular death which shows a relative reduction of 30.2% in ticlopidine group [29]. Furthermore, at 3-year follow up of the multicentre randomized Ticlopidine Aspirin Stroke Study (TASS) comparing ticlopidine (250 mg b.i.d) to aspirin (650 mg b.i.d) in patients with transient ischemic attack or minor stroke, a 21% reduction in fatal and non-fatal stroke was observed for ticlopidine (p=0.024) [30].

Serious, potentially life-threatening, hematological side-effects have been reported [27 - 31]. Neutropenia (defined as absolute neutrophil count<1200/ml) was observed in 2.4% of patients, while severe neutropenia (<450/ml) in 0.8%. In the majority of cases, the neutropenia was reversible. Aplastic anemia occurred in about one in 4000-8000 patients, while thrombotic thrombocytopenic purpura was observed in about one in 2000-4000 patients [31]. The peak of incidence was 3-6 weeks, while reactions were also reported few days after starting the ticlopidine. Gastrointestinal side-effects were common, rashes were noted in 5% of patients and ticlopidine was also associated with total serum cholesterol rise [31]. Moreover, severe liver dysfunction, hepatotoxicity mainly of cholestatic type, has been observed particularly in Japanese as compared to Caucasian patients that is associated with certain human leukocyte antigen subtypes (particularly HLA-A*3303) in the Japanese population [32]. These side effects are a drawback of using this medicine and encourage the development of a safer second-generation thienopyridine.

Clopidogrel

Clopidogrel emerged as a promising compound structurally similar to ticlopidine, but with fewer side-effects. Clopidogrel has since been shown to reduce thrombotic events stroke or established peripheral arterial disease, and for patients with ACS including those undergoing PCI.

Pharmacokinetics and Pharmacodynamics

Clopidogrel differs from ticlopidine by an additional carboxymethyl side group. It is rapidly absorbed *via* the oral route, and required to be metabolized by hepatic cytochrome (CYP) P-450 to form active metabolism. This process involves 2 steps: CYP2C19, CYP1A2 and CYP2B6 are responsible for the first metabolic step, whereas CYP2C19, CYP2C9, CYP2B6 and CYP3A are responsible for the second step [33]. Clopidogrel elimination is both renal and gastrointestinal. The mechanism of the antiplatelet effect is a permanent alteration of the platelet surface P2Y12 ADP receptor and inhibition of ADP-induced platelet activation and aggregation. The active metabolite half-life is around 1 h [34], and on maintenance doses a delay of 4-8 days is necessary to reach the peak of antiplatelet activity. However, significant advantage of clopidogrel is that loading doses (300 mg or 600 mg) are well tolerated and result in near-maximal platelet inhibition in 2-5 h [35]. Several pharmacokinetic interactions have been reported through literature and might explain, in addition to other factors, the huge variability in clopidogrel effects between individuals (see Table **5**, page 34).

Efficiency & Safety

The Clopidogrel *vs.* Aspirin in Patients at Risk of Ischemic Events (CAPRIE) trial was original by incorporating patients with three distinct indications into a single trial. The study aimed to compare clopidogrel 75 mg daily with aspirin 325 mg daily for prevention of vascular events in patients with recent stroke, MI, or peripheral vascular disease [36]. A total of 19,185 patients were enrolled with a mean follow-up of 1.9 years. The primary endpoint was a composite of stroke, MI or vascular death. The annualized event rates were 5.32% for clopidogrel and 5.83% for aspirin, corresponding to 8.7% relative reduction in favor of clopidogrel. The heterogeneity of benefits was significant (p=0.042) and most of the benefit seen in the peripheral arterial disease group was related to a reduction in MI [36]. The CURE trial was designed to compare the safety and efficacy of combined aspirin-clopidogrel therapy with aspirin alone in high-risk coronary disease patients [37]. The trial enrolled 12,562 patients with non-ST-elevation acute coronary syndromes. All patients received aspirin (75-325 mg daily) and were randomized to receive either clopidogrel (300 mg loading dose then 75 mg daily) or placebo for 3-12 months [37]. The composite endpoint, including cardiovascular death, nonfatal, MI and stroke was noticed in 11.4% of placebo group and in 9.3% of clopidogrel group, corresponding to a relative risk reduction of 20%.

The PCI-CURE trial included 2658 patients within the CURE trial who underwent elective PCI [38]. Patients received a median of 10 days of aspirin-clopidogrel or aspirin-placebo therapy prior to intervention and for 8 months thereafter. At 30 days, the composite endpoint occurrence was reduced by 30% (4.5% *versus* 6.4%; p=0:03) in favor of the clopidogrel-aspirin group [38]. Most patients in both the clopidogrel and placebo groups underwent stent implantation and therefore, received open-label thienopyridine, about 4 weeks after PCI. The clopidogrel pre-treatment was associated with 42% reduction in the primary outcome [38], suggesting that clopidogrel is likely to be useful not only in PCI capable centres, but also in those that do not have ready access to cardiac catheterisation facilities, because it allows time to stabilize the patient, before performing PCI or before transfer for invasive therapy.

The CLARITY TIMI 28 trial was designed to assess clopidogrel in the setting of ST elevation myocardial infarction (STEMI). A total of 3,491 patients were enrolled and randomly assigned to receive clopidogrel (300-mg loading dose, followed by 75 mg once daily) or placebo [39]. Primary efficacy endpoints (a composite of an occluded infarct-related artery on angiography or death or recurrent myocardial infarction before angiography) were encountered in 15.0% in the clopidogrel group *versus* 21.7% in the placebo group [odds ratio (OR) =0.64; 95% CI 0.53-0.76; p<0.001). At one month, clopidogrel therapy had reduced the odds of major cardiac events (MACE) by 20% (from 14.1% to 11.6% percent; p=0.03) [39]. Regarding bleeding, no difference was observed during in-hospital stay and at 30-day follow up [39]. In addition, the PCI CLARITY study confirmed the benefit of clopidogrel pretreatment, as early as possible, in reducing reduces the incidence of MACE both before and after PCI and without a significant increase in major or minor bleeding [40].

In HORIZONS AMI trial, the investigators sought to compare two regimen of clopidogrel loading dose (600 mg *versus* 300 mg) in STEMI patients (2,158 and 1,153 patients, respectively) undergoing primary PCI [41]. Patients who received a loading dose of 600 mg showed significantly lower 30-day unadjusted rates of mortality (1.9% *versus* 3.1%; p=0.03), reinfarction (1.3% *versus* 2.3%,p=0.02), and definite or probable stent thrombosis (1.7% *versus* 2.8%, p=0.04), without higher bleeding rates [41].

As compared with ticlopidine, the side-effect profile of clopidogrel is remarkably improved. Severe neutropenia (neutrophil count<450/ml) was observed in only 0.05% of patients [42]. Eleven cases of thrombotic thrombocytopenic purpura were only reported after more than 3 million patients had been exposed to clopidogrel. Hence, clopidogrel has a far safer profile than ticlopidine [43]. Gastrointestinal side-effects such as bloating, cramping and diarrhea are rare. Bleeding represents an extension of the antiplatelet effect and is significantly more common with clopidogrel plus aspirin than with aspirin alone. The optimal dose of aspirin is 100 mg daily, allowing reduction of major hemorrhage risk without compromising the efficacy of the dual anti-platelet therapy [37].

In early trials of ticlopidine after coronary interventions, drug therapy was restricted to 30 days due to hematological side-effects. The improved safety profile of clopidogrel has reduced the concern. The CREDO trial, similar to PCI-CURE, showed that both efficacy and safety of thienopyridine therapy could be extended to 12 months [40, 44].

Regarding its role in cerebrovascular disease, the CAPRIE trial showed a relative risk reduction of 5.2% for clopidogrel as compared with aspirin in stroke prevention [36]. Furthermore, as shown by the MATCH trial, clopidogrel alone is better tolerated than associated with aspirin [45]. Indeed, adding aspirin to clopidogrel in high-risk patients with recent ischaemic stroke or transient ischaemic attack is associated with a non-significant reduction in major vascular events; while, the risk of life-threatening or major bleeding increased significantly [45].

Prasugrel

Despite the proved efficacy of clopidogrel, this drug presented some limitations, particularly its high inter-variability (see below), encouraging the development of new molecules. On February 3, 2009, a new thienopyridine, prasugrel, was recommended for approval as an addition to aspirin for patients with ACS by the FDA Cardiovascular and Renal Drugs Advisory Committee.

Pharmacokinetics & Pharmacodynamics

Prasugrel is a third-generation member of oral thienopyridine. It is metabolized to the active platelet-inhibiting compound R-138727, which has specific affinity for the P2Y12 ADP receptor. Prasugrel is completely and rapidly absorbed and extensively metabolized in humans. The active metabolite is detectable in plasma after 15 min and reaches maximum concentration at 30 min [46]. The cytochrome isoenzymes that are responsible for the generation of the active metabolite are mainly CYP3A and CYP2B6 [47]. Furthermore, intestinal CYP3A contributes more in the generation of an active metabolite as compared to hepatic CYP3A; this fact might explain the rapid appearance of active metabolite in plasma [48]. Prasugrel has been demonstrated to be more rapid and potent in inhibition of platelet function than clopidogrel in different clinical settings, and is transformed into its active metabolite more efficiently as compared to clopidogrel [48]. The half life of its active metabolite is about 4 h and the maximal effect of prasugrel (60 mg loading dose) began to plateau approximately 1 h after administration compared to about 4 h for clopidogrel (300 mg loading dose) [48]. Moreover, it has been reported that active metabolite of prasugrel enhances the inhibitory effect on platelet aggregation of agents that acts *via* raising cAMP such as prostaglandin I2, adenosine and forskolin [49]. The antiaggregation effects of prasugrel last until 72 h after administration demonstrates a long duration of action of this drug [50].

Efficacy & Safety

JUMBO-TIMI 26 and PRINCIPLE-TIMI, two phase II studies, showed the safety and anti-platelet profile of prasugrel, allowing the feasibility of phase III studies [51, 52].

TRITON-TIMI 38, a phase III randomized trial, randomized 13,608 patients with an ACS undergoing PCI were to receive either clopidogrel or prasugrel (60 mg loading dose and 10 mg od maintenance dose) in addition to aspirin [53]. The primary efficacy endpoint was a composite of death from cardiovascular causes, non-fatal MI and non-fatal stroke, while the primary safety endpoints were TIMI life-threatening, major or minor bleeding not related to coronary artery bypass grafting. Endpoints were evaluated during in-hospital stay, at 30 days, 90 days and then every 3 months for up to a 15 months follow up period [53]. Prasugrel administration was associated with a significantly reduced rate of primary efficacy endpoint events (12.1% in the clopidogrel group *versus* 9.9% in the prasugrel group; hazard ratio 0.81; 95% CI 0.71 to 0.96; $p<0.001$), especially due to a reduction in MI. This represent a 2.2% absolute reduction and a 19% relative reduction of primary efficacy endpoints in patients receiving prasugrel. The rate of primary safety endpoints, however, was significantly higher in patients who received treatment with prasugrel (2.4% in the prasugrel group, *versus* 1.8% in the clopidogrel group; HR=1.32; 95% CI 1.03 to 1.68; $p=0.03$), particularly regarding fatal bleeding (0.4% *versus* 0.1%; $p=0.002$). The net clinical benefit including both efficacy and safety endpoints (death from any cause, non-fatal MI, non-fatal stroke, or non-CABG-related non-fatal TIMI major bleeding) was in favor of prasugrel (13.9% of patients in the clopidogrel group *versus* 12.2% in the prasugrel group; HR=0.87; 95% CI, 0.79 to 0.95; $p = 0.004$) [53]. Post-hoc analyses were performed to determine the subsets of patients who did not have a net clinical benefit from the use of prasugrel and those who had net clinical harm. A clinical history of stroke or transient ischemic attack was associated with a net worse outcome [53]. Patients ≥75 years of age and patients weighing <60 kg did not also have net clinical benefit; they did not have net clinical harm either. The bleeding rate in these two subgroups of patients was greater, despite being not statistically significant [53]. Among patients who did not fall in any of these three categories, prasugrel exhibited greater efficacy than clopidogrel, while the bleeding rates were comparable among the two groups.

In patients with STEMI undergoing PCI (n=3,534), Montalescot *et al.* [54] showed that prasugrel was more effective than clopidogrel for prevention of MACE (cardiac death, MI, target vessel revascularization) (OR=0.79, 95% CI

0.65-0.97; p=0.025) and stent thrombosis (OR= 0.58, 95% CI 0.36-0.93; p=0.0023), without an apparent excess in bleeding.

On the other hand, the TRILOGY ACS trial [55], which is a double blind randomized trial aimed to evaluate the efficacy/safety of prasugrel and clopidogrel in the setting of medically managed ACS. Two analyses were performed: a primary one involving 7243 patients <75 years receiving prasugrel (10 mg daily) or clopidogrel (75 mg daily); and a secondary one involving 2083 patients ≥75 years, on prasugrel (5 mg daily) or clopidogrel (75 mg daily). At a median follow-up of 17 months, the primary end point, defined as a composite of death from cardiovascular causes, MI, or stroke among patients under the age of 75 years occurred in 13.9% of the prasugrel group and 16.0% of the clopidogrel group (HR=0.91; CI 0.79 to 1.05; P=0.21) [55]. Similar results were observed in the overall population. Rates of severe and intracranial bleeding were similar in the two groups, regardless of the age [55]. Hence, patients undergoing invasive strategy in the setting of ACS, might take more benefit from prasugrel prescription than in whom non invasive approach is planned.

The ACCOAST trial was designed to assess the efficacy/safety of prasugrel in the setting of non ST elevation myocardial infarction (NSTEMI) [56]. A total of 4033 patients with a scheduled coronary angiography were enrolled. Patients were randomly assigned to receive prasugrel (30-mg loading dose) before the angiography (pretreatment group) or placebo (control group) [56]. When PCI was indicated, an additional 30 mg of prasugrel was given in the pretreatment group at the time of PCI and 60 mg of prasugrel was given in the control group [56]. No significant difference in primary efficacy endpoint was observed between the two groups. Furthermore, regarding safety, The rates of TIMI major bleeding and life-threatening bleeding not related to CABG were increased by a factor of 3 and 6, respectively in pretreatment group [56]. Thus, the investigators concluded to not recommend pretreatment with prasugrel, which should be administered once the coronary anatomy is known and PCI indicated.

Ticagrelor

Adenosine triphosphate (ATP) competitively antagonize ADP-induced platelet aggregation. However unfavourable properties of ATP, such as low potency and poor stability does not allow its use as P2Y12 receptor antagonist. Efforts were directed towards formulating ATP analogues with high potency and more stability. Subsequent modification of these compounds lead to discovery of selective and stable non-phosphate P2Y12 receptor antagonist AZD6140 (ticagrelor) [57].

Pharmacokinetics & Pharmacodynamics

Ticagrelor (AZD6140) is the first oral reversible ADP P2Y12 receptor antagonist and belongs to cyclopentyltriazolopyrimidine class [58]. Conversely to clopidogrel and prasugrel, ticagrelor mechanism is not competitive with ADP. Indeed, it acts *via* an allosteric modulation site, inhibiting receptor conformational change [59].

Iyu' *et al.* [60] have also revealed that ticagrelor mainly affects P2Y12 receptors with the ability to enhance the inhibitory effect of natural (*e.g.*, vascular prostaglandins I2, D2 and adenosine) and other (*e.g.*, forskolin) modulators of platelet functions which increase intracellular cAMP. Moreover, ticagrelor possesses a unique mechanism of inhibiting nonplatelet P2Y receptors located in vascular smooth muscle, reducing vasoconstriction and vasospasms, aiding in myocardial perfusion [61].

Ticagrelor was tested in healthy volunteers in dosage of 50-600 mg once daily or 50-300 mg twice daily [62]. Findings of phase I illustrated that the pharmacokinetics of ticagrelor is predictable and is associated with consistent inhibition of platelet activity. Ticagrelor is metabolized in the liver by CYP3A4 enzyme to produce active metabolite AR-C124910XX. Further metabolic conversion is not required for ticagrelor, as it directly and dose dependently inhibits P2Y12receptor with about 95% inhibition of platelet aggregation within 2-4 h [58]. Ticagrelor has an early onset of action within 2h [63]. Ticagrelor half life is around 9h and this drug requires to be administered twice daily (90 mg bid). Elimination of ticagrelor and AR-C124910XX occurs primarily *via* hepatic metabolism and biliary secretion; therefore, no dose adjustment is required for patients with renal failure [63]. Another advantage of ticagrelor is its shorter time for drug offset after withdrawal as compared to thienopyridines family [63, 64].

Efficiency & Safety

Platelet inhibition and patient outcome (PLATO) trial was designed to test the hypothesis that ticagrelor is superior to clopidogrel for prevention of recurrent thrombotic events in the setting of ACS population and this would be achieved with a clinically acceptable bleeding rate and overall safety profile. It was a phase III, randomized, double blind, double dummy, multicentre, multinational, event driven, parallel group study comparing efficacy and safety of ticagrelor *versus* clopidogrel in patients of ACS. The study enrolled 18,624 patients and the primary efficacy endpoint of PLATO was time to first occurrence of any event from the composite of death from vascular causes, MI or stroke [65]. At 1 year, ticagrelor significantly reduced the rate of the composite endpoint of CV death, MI, and stroke *versus* clopidogrel [relative risk reduction (RRR) 16%, absolute risk reduction 1.9%; p=0.0003] [65]. The Kaplan Meier curves separate early and continue to diverge over a period of 12 months, demonstrating the fact that ticagrelot benefit comes rapidly and grows with time. During the first month, there was an RRR of 12%, while from the second month thereafter, there was an RRR of 20%. In PLATO trial, for every 54 ACS patients treated with ticagrelor instead of clopidogrel one atherothrombotic event was prevented [65].

Analysis of secondary efficacy endpoints showed that ticagrelor treatment resulted in a statistically significant reduction in both cardiovascular mortality (4.0% *versus* 5.1%; HR=0.79; 95% CI: 0.69-0.91) and all-cause mortality (4.5% *vs.* 5.9%; HR=0.78; 95% CI: 0.69-0.98; p=0.001). Notably, the incidence of definite stent thrombosis was also reduced with ticagrelor as compared to clopidogrel (1.3% *versus* 1.9%; HR=0.68; 95% CI: 0.50-0.91; p=0.009) [65, 66].

Regarding safety, PLATO bleeding scale which was used in this trial takes into consideration both laboratory and clinical parameters for capturing bleeding events. There was no significant difference in the rate of major bleeding between ticagrelor and clopidogrel group (11.6% and 11.2%, respectively; p=0.43) [59]. There was also no significant difference in the rate of fatal/life threatening bleeding between two treatment groups (5.8% in both groups; p= 0.70) [59].

Although, there was noticed a higher rate of fatal intracranial bleeding with ticagrelor as compared to clopidogrel (0.1%] *versus* 0.01%; p=0.02), there were lower rates of fatal gastro intestinal and other fatal bleeding in the ticagrelor group than clopidogrel group (0.1%, *versus* 0.3%; p=0.03) [59]. No significant difference was observed regarding the rates of CABG-related major bleeding between two treatment groups; whereas, in the ticagrelor group, there was a higher rate of non-CABG-related major bleeding (4.5% *versus* 3.8%; p=0.03) [65].

In patients with ACS and planned invasive strategy (n=13,408) randomized in 1:1 manner to receive ticagrelor or clopidogrel, Cannon *et al.* [66] showed that those on ticagrelor experienced less primary endpoints (composite of vascular death, MI, stroke) at one-year follow-up (OR=0.84, 95% CI 0.75-0.94; p=0.0025), while no difference was observed in the rates of total major bleeding or severe bleeding.

The ATLANTIC trial, a randomized, double-blind study involving 1862 patients with ongoing STEMI, was designed to evaluate the benefit of pretreatment with ticagrelor [67]. Although prehospital administration of ticagrelor in the setting of STEMI appeared to be safe, it did not improve pre-PCI coronary reperfusion [67]. A median time difference between the two treatment strategies as short as 31 min might explain in part such a finding. However, The rates of definite stent thrombosis were lower in the prehospital group than in the in-hospital group (0% *versus* 0.8% in the first 24 hours; 0.2% *versus* 1.2% at 30 days) [67].

Regarding side effects, dyspnea occurred more frequently in ticagrelor group than clopidogrel group (13.8% *versus* 7.8%), corresponding to a calculated number needed to harm of 16 [65]. The precise mechanism for dyspnea seen with ticagrelor therapy is not yet clearly elucidated, and several theories have been postulated: 1) the suppression of adenosine deaminase activity, leading to increased adenosine concentrations; 2) the preferential affinity for adenosine receptor 1 (A1R) resulting in sustained placodal C-fiber activation; 3) direct release of ATP from red blood cells through pH alterations, and which acts as bronchial irritant; and 4) the structural similarity between ticagrelor and adenosine, and its probable role in the continuous stimulation of adenosine receptors [68]. In a dose-guiding trial, dose limitations were not related to bleeding events but rather intolerance to dyspnea and ventricular pauses [68]. Because dyspnea may be due to cardiac disease, one study evaluated patients with stable coronary artery disease for dyspnea related to ticagrelor therapy in a prespecified subanalysis excluding patients with significant lung disease such as chronic obstructive pulmonary disease and chronic or active asthma [69]. Dyspnea was reported by 38.6%, 9.3%, and 8.3% of patients in the ticagrelor, clopidogrel, and placebo groups, respectively [69]. In all cases, the dyspnea was considered to be mild to moderate; the duration of dyspnea lasted less than 24 hours for some patients, whereas others had experienced the side-effect during all the study duration [69]. Most of the cases of dyspnea in the study dissipated on medication cessation [58, 62]. Furthermore, the frequency of patient self-discontinuation of ticagrelor due to dyspneic events was reported to reach a concerning 6% in controlled trials [65]. Most importantly, mortality benefit of ticagrelor was maintained regardless dyspnea status [65]. Other side effects of ticagrelor, such as benign ventricular pauses and increased concentrations of uric acid and creatinine, have been also reported, but were unfrequent [65].

Cangrelor

Conversely to previous P2Y12 inhibitors which were orally prescribed, cangrelor represented an innovation and progress in anti-platelet therapy, as it provides the possibility of an intravenous administration.

Pharmacokinetics & Pharmacodynamics

Cangrelor (AR-C69931MX) is an ADP analog and is a direct-acting,reversible P2Y12 inhibitor liketicagrelor. Conversely to ticagrelor, cangrelor is administered by intravenous infusion. The platelet block from cangrelor has a rapid onset within minutes of infusion (15-30 min), rapidly achieving steady-state inhibition of platelet aggregation with a half life of approximately 2-5 min, and a rapid offset,with complete recovery of platelet function within 1 to 2 hours after stopping therapy [70]. In addition, cangrelor is not dependent on hepatic or renal mechanisms of activation or clearance [70].

Cangrelor is an analog of ATP, natural P2Y12 receptor antagonist, with a dose-dependent inhibitory effect [70]. It has been also reported that cangrelor enhances platelet cAMP level through unidentified platelet Gs protein-coupled receptor mediating inhibition of platelet function [71].

Efficacy & Safety

The phase III clinical evaluation of cangrelor was performed through 3 large randomized trials including patients undergoing PCI. In the first two trials, CHAMPION PLATFORM (n=5,362) and CHAMPION-PCI (n=8,877), cangrelor was not able to reach significant reduction of the primary outcome of peri-procedural ischaemic events [72, 73]. In May 2009, although 98% of the planned cohort for CHAMPION-PCI and 83% of the planned cohort of CHAMPION-PLATFORM had already been enrolled, both trials were stopped as they would not show the persuasive clinical efficacy needed for approval. However, cangrelor was not totally ineffective as it was able to reduce occurrence of stent thrombosis [72, 73]. The prognostic impact of cangrelor might be diluted because of the use of a periprocedural MI definition based on biomarkers elevation; indeed, this fact makes difficult to discriminate between events occurring after randomisation and those occurring before randomisation, particularly in patients presenting with elevated biomarkers at enrollment. In this respect, CHAMPION PHOENIX trial (n=11,145) used a more sensitive definition based on per-procedural angiographic complications and new ECG changes regardless biomarkers elevation [74]. Hence, the investigators of this latter study demonstrated significant reduction in the primary outcome favouring cangrelor administration [74]. In a meta-analysis combining the 3 CHAMPION trials, Steg *et al.* [75] demonstrated the efficiency of cangrelor active to reduce periprocedural ischaemic events, including stent thrombosis and MI. On the other hand, from a safety point of view, cangrelor increased the risk of bleeding [72 - 75]. Indeed, more major bleeding events with cangrelor were observed using the GUSTO and TIMI criteria and a significant increase using the ACUITY criteria [72 - 75]. Although the latter meta-analysis showed the efficacy of cangrelor, the reported benefits were only obtained when compared with a non-optimum antiplatelet prescription [75]. In fact, cangrelor was compared with placebo before PCI in most patients enrolled in the CHAMPION trials [72 - 74]; while pretreatment with clopidogrel is the gold standard and the common practice around the world. Moreover, a proportion of patients in the clopidogrel arm only received 300 mg as a loading dose of clopidogrel. Most importantly, reliable data for how cangrelor compares with either ticagrelor or prasugrel are not available.

Recently, Angiolillo *et al.* [76] compared the antiplatelet efficacy of cangrelor with placebo in patients undergoing CABG surgery who were being treated with a thienopyridine for secondary prevention of recurrent events following an ACS or coronary stent implantation. Cangrelor at an infusion dose of 0.75 I1/4g/kg per minute consistently achieved and maintained platelet inhibition at levels known to be associated with a low risk of thrombotic events compared with placebo [76]. Bridging with a prolonged infusion of Cangrelor (2-7 days) did not increase major bleeding prior to surgery, as defined according to several established classifications, although minor bleeding was numerically higher. The originality of the latter study is the fact that it attempts to address the lapse in thienopyridine therapy required for many surgical and invasive procedures. Indeed, the future of antiplatelet agents, particularly cangrelor, must also focus on bridging for high-risk patients undergoing CABG or other interventions.

Elinogrel

Like ticagrelor and cangrelor, elinogrel (PRT060128) is a direct-acting P2Y12 receptor inhibitors. It belongs to a unique anti-platelet drug class known as the quinazolinediones [77].

Pharmacocinetikcs & Pharmacodynamics

The originality of elinogrel comes from the fact that in addition to being reversible agent with fast onset and offset of action, it is the only P2Y12 receptor inhibitor which can be administered by both oral and intravenous route. Intravenous administration of elinogrel was shown to be well tolerated and safe, achieving immediate and high level of platelet inhibition. The average terminal half life at the 40 mg elinogrel administered intravenously was about 11 h, with a maximum platelet inhibition achieved at 20 min [78]. The inhibitory effect of platelet was completely reversible within 8-24 h of elinogrel administration [77]. Preliminary data on safety and tolerability of single dose intravenous loading doses (10-60 mg) of elinogrel have recommended this treatment as an adjunctive therapy for primary PCI in the setting of acute MI [79, 80]. Pharmacologically, the intravenous and oral forms of elinogrel are identical [80]. This fact might represent an advantage as it might prevent the potential the vulnerability associated with the transition from one intravenous to a different oral P2Y12 receptor inhibitor.

Efficacy & Safety

The ERASE MI trial was a pilot, phase II, randomized, double-blind, placebo-controlled, dose-escalation study designed to evaluate the safety and tolerability of escalating doses (10, 20, 40, and 60 mg) of elinogrel administered as a single intravenous bolus before the start of the diagnostic before primary PCI [79]. This study was prematurely terminated for administrative reasons and enrolled a limited number of patients. Seventy patients were randomly assigned to either elinogrel or placebo within each dosing group; and all patients received a 600-mg clopidogrel loading dose, followed by a second 300-mg clopidogrel loading dose 4 hours after PCI. The incidence of bleeding events was infrequent and appeared to be similar in patients treated with all doses of elinogrel *versus* placebo. No differences in serious adverse events, laboratory values, corrected TIMI frame count, or ST resolution were observed between elinogrel and placebo.

INNOVATE PCI trial, a randomized, double-blind, dose-ranging phase II trial, randomized 652 patients received either 300 or 600 mg of clopidogrel pre-PCI followed by 75 mg daily, or 80 or 120 mg of IV elinogrel, followed by 50, 100, or 150 mg oral elinogrel twice daily [80]. Regarding safety, TIMI combined bleeding was increased with elinogrel (HR=1.98; 95% CI 1.10 to 3.57), related largely to increased bleeding events requiring medical attention (elinogrel 11.5% *versus* clopidogrel 6.3%) and occurring primarily at the PCI access site [80]. Efficacy end points were similar, but there was a non significant higher frequency of peri-procedural MI in the elinogrel arms (OR, 1.59; 95% CI, 0.79 to 3.48) [80]. There was an increased incidence of dyspnea (elinogrel 12.3% *versus* clopidogrel 3.8%) and transaminase elevation (elinogrel 4.4% *versus* clopidogrel 1.0%) in the elinogrel arms [80].

Hence, despite the attractive pharmacological properties of elinogrel, data are scarcely reported in literature about its benefits and impact on patients' outcome;

in this respect, more extensive clinical investigations are required to determine the efficacy and safety of this drug.

BX 667

BX 667 is an orally active and reversible small-molecule P2Y12 receptor antagonist which is metabolized by esterases to the carboxylic acid active form, BX 048 [81]. Administration of BX 667 results in a rapid and sustained inhibition of platelet aggregation where the extent and duration of platelet inhibition is directly proportional to circulating plasma levels of both BX 667 and BX 048 [81]. Although first trials in rats and dogs were promising [81], data on humans are not available and further studies should be performed focusing on optimal dose selection, then clinical benefit from BX 667 prescription.

THE CONCEPT OF PERSONALIZED THERAPY

Differently from current ESC guidelines, which provide a class IB for both prasugrel and ticagrelor over clopidogrel (class IC) in the setting of ACS [82, 83], the ACC/AHA guidelines do not prefer one antiplatelet agent over other (recommendation IB for all three agents) [84].

Despite the onset of new more potent new anti-platelet agents and the inter-individuals variability of clopidogrel, this latter still have an important place in the armamentarium of cardiologists in CAD patients. Indeed, clopidogrel remains the only P2Y12 receptor blocker recommended in elective patients [85]. Furthermore, it also represents the P2Y12 receptor inhibitor of choice in patients with cerebrovascular disease or those with a high bleeding risk, as it is currently recommended in ACS patients with a need for oral anticoagulation. Moreover, many patients have contraindications for new P2Y12 inhibitors; thus, clopidogrel might represent the appropriate and even the only alternative in this patients' subset. In addition, many countries around the world have currently no access to ticagrelor or prasugrel at all because of their elevated cost, when many clopidogrel generics are available.

In this respect, the concept of personalized strategy might be considered as a rational approach and of interest in anti-platelet therapy prescription following each patient characteristics and response to treatment.

Factors Influencing Clopidogrel Variability

As a prodrug, clopidogrel needs to be metabolized to an active metabolite to exert its pharmacological effect. Several factors have been reported to be associated with active metabolite levels variability including clinical and genetic variables as well as drug-drug interactions (Table **4**).

Table 4. Characteristics of different platelet reactivity tests.

Test	Method	Sensitivity	Specificity	Ischemic Risk Cutoff	Bleeding Risk Cutoff	Advantages	Drawbacks
Light Transmission Aggregometry	optical aggregometry	60-80%	60-80%	>70%	<40%	historical gold standard, availability	large sample volumes, complex preparation, low reproducibility
Multiplate Analyzer	electric impedance	70-90%	85-100%	>46U	<19U	use of whole blood, small blood sample, short processing time, good reproducibility	requires pipetting
VerifyNow	turbidimetry: microbead agglutination	60-80%	60-90%	>208 PRU	<85PRU	automatic, use of whole blood, small blood sample, bedside use, good reproducibility	Limited by hematocrit and platelet count range
VASP phosphorylation	flow cytometry	85-100%	90-100%	>50%	<10%	most specific test	complex sample preparation, require flow cytometer and experienced technician

(Table 4) contd.....

Test	Method	Sensitivity	Specificity	Ischemic Risk Cutoff	Bleeding Risk Cutoff	Advantages	Drawbacks
PFA-100	shear-induced aggregation	90-100%	80-90%	≤72s	-	use of whole blood, small blood sample, short proceeding time,	dependent on vWF and hematocrit, does not correlate well with clopidogrel therapy, do not range of platelet response
Cone and platelet analyzer	shear-induced aggregation	90%	90%	-	-	use of whole blood, small blood sample, simple and rapid	not widely used, requires pipetting
Plateletworks	platelet counting	60-65%	<60%	-	-	use of whole blood, simple preparation	not well studied yet, requires pipetting
Thromboelastography	Thromboelastography	80%	75%	>47mm	<31mm	use of whole blood, global evaluation of hemostasis	low standardization, require pipetting

The relevant clinical factors contributing to response variability, are as follows: age [86, 87], diabetes mellitus [87, 88], ACS setting [89, 90], obesity [90], renal failure [91], impaired left ejection fraction [87, 89], inflammation [92], and smoking [93, 94]. The latter factor was shown to be less frequently associated with high-platelet on treatment (HPR), as tobacco stimulates CYP1A2 activity [93, 94].

On the hand, studies of genetic testing have identified individuals with genetic polymorphisms that may affect clopidogrel absorption, metabolism, and ultimately its pharmacodynamic effects. Loss-of-function (*e.g.* CYP2C19*2 and CYP2C19*3) and gain-of-function (*e.g.* CYP2C19*17) genotypes are associated with variable degrees of production of the active metabolite and, hence, of the pharmacodynamic response to the drug [95, 96]. Booman *et al.* [97] hypothesized that the impaired pharmacodynamic response to clopidogrel observed in CYP2C19*2 carriers could be due to an imbalance in the formation of pro-inflammatory and anti-inflammatory cytokines, which might contribute to alter platelet aggregability, rather than to impairment of clopidogrel metabolism.

In addition, intestinal absorption can be limited because of homozygous 3435C fiT mutation of ATP-binding cassette subfamily B member 1 (ABCB1), a gene encoding for the efflux pump P-glycoprotein, a key protein involved in thienopyridine absorption [98].

Interaction with other drugs, including some proton pump inhibitors (PPIs), calcium channel blockers (CCBs) and lipophilic statins, which are metabolized by CYP2C19 and CYP3A isoenzymes, might influence clopidogrel effects [99]. The competition for CYP 3A4 may explain why the antiplatelet effect of clopidogrel could be reduced when given concomitantly with atorvastatin or dihydropyridine calcium channel blockers (CCBs), Although, post-hoc analyses from 2 large clinical trials of clopidogrel did not report a worse outcome with atorvastatin, concomitant administration of CCBs and clopidogrel was reported to increase the risk of an adverse cardiovascular outcome (HR=3.5, 95% CI=1.4-8.6; p=0.005 *versus* patients not taking CCBs) [99]. On the other hand, exposure to PPIs, which are substrates for an inhibitor of CYP2C19, has also been shown to be associated with a significantly increased risk of acute MI among clopidogrel users in prescription database analyses (1.38% incidence of MI in 1 year in clopidogrel users not taking a PPI compared with 3.08% incidence in clopidogrel users with low PPI exposure based on prescription adherence and 5.03% in clopidogrel users with high PPI exposure; $p<0.05$) [100]. Compared with placebo, omeprazole but not pantoprazole or esomeprazole appears to reduce the antiplatelet effect of clopidogrel [100]. The CYP3A4 and CYP3A5 inhibition by ketoconazole also affects formation of clopidogrel and was demonstrated to reduce its platelet inhibition activity, while its association with rifampicin (a CYP3A4 and CYP2C19 inducer) leads to potentiation of clopidogrel active metabolite thus, consequently greater platelet inhibition [96, 101].

Finally, non-compliance needs to be considered an obvious and frequent cause of poor response to clopidogrel and should always be investigated.

Anti-Platelet Function Testing

The degree of platelet inhibition by clopidogrel can be detected by laboratory investigation and corresponds to the phenotype of its response. The objective of platelet function testing is to evaluate the degree of platelet inhibition by the respective antiplatelet drug and its impact on the risk of ischemic/bleeding events.

Numerous studies have shown that the level of platelet inhibition by clopidogrel varies considerably between patients. Platelet function measurements in clopidogrel-treated patients have shown that, on average, 25% of patients (up to 50%, dependent on the assay used) have HPR [101, 102].

The ideal test should be easy to perform, rapid, highly reproducible, cost-effective and able to provide prognostic information Nowadays, several test systems.characterizing some of the biological pathways of platelet activation are available, for monitoring the effect of anti-platelet function. Each test has its specific advantages and disadvantages, as summarized in Table **5**. The level of the anti-platelet action of P2Y12 inhibitors can be quantified through the following methods: platelet aggregometry, flow cytometry, shear-dependent assays, platelet counting, thrombelastography.

Table 5. Factors influencing clopidogrel variability.

Clinical Factors
Age Diabetes mellitus Acute coronary syndrome Obesity Renal failure Smoking Compliance
Genes Polymorphisms
CYP2C19*2 loss of function CYP2C19*3, *8 loss of function CYP2C19*17 gain of function ABCB1 gene variants ITGB3 gene variants
Drug Interactions
Calcium-channel blockers Proton-pump inhibitors (Omeprazole+++) Statins Ketoconazole Rifampicin

Platelet Aggregometry

Platelet aggregometry is a platelet function test based on the stimulation of platelet platelet aggregation with various agonists. Two different techniques are most commonly employed: optical and impedance aggregometry.

Light Transmission Aggregometry

LTA (optical, turbidimetric) is the mostly widely used platelet function test. To detect inhibition of the P2Y12 receptor, ADP is added, and the change in the light transmittance is then recorded. The parameters used are the maximal aggregation and the final aggregation responses, expressed as percentages [103 - 105].

Impedance Aggregometry (MEA)

MEA is an impedance aggregometer used for measurement of whole-blood platelet aggregation (Multiplate analyzer). For the detection of inhibitory effects at the P2Y12 receptor, ADP is used as an agonist, with or without the antagonist prostaglandin E1 (PGE1). A dilution of whole blood and 0.9% NaCl is stirred in the test cuvettes, ADPA3/4PGE1 or ADP alone is added, and the increase in electrical impedance is expressed as the AUC of the impedance tracing. The system detects the electrical impedance change caused by adhesion and aggregation of platelets on 2 independent electrode-set surfaces in the test cuvette, expressed as arbitrary aggregation units x minutes or as units (U) [106 - 108].

VerifyNow Assay

The VerifyNow assay is a citrated whole-blood optical detection system measuring agonist-induced activation of platelets, which bind to fibrinogen-coated polystyrene beads. When the platelet-bead complexes fall out of the solution, infrared light transmittance increases. The assay needs ADP and PGE1 as agonist/antagonist combination and the results are reported as P2Y12 reaction units [109, 110].

Flow Cytometry

VASP Phosphorylation

The VASP phosphorylation assay (BioCytex, Marseille, France) measures the inhibition of the P2Y12 receptor and 1 of its intracellular signaling pathways: phosphorylation of VASP (see below). Blood samples are incubated with ADP and/or PGE1 before fixation. Platelets are permeabilized, labeled with a monoclonal antibody against serine 239-phosphorylated VASP or its isotope, followed by a secondary fluorescein isothiocyanate-conjugated polyclonal goat anti-mouse antibody. Mean fluorescence intensity is determined using a flow cytometer. Platelet reactivity is expressed as the platelet reactivity index (PRI) [111, 112].

P-Selectin Method

The P-selectin is a glycoprotein rapidly translocated from α-granules of platelets and endothelial cells to the cell surface on stimulation [113]. It mediates rolling of platelets and neutrophils on activated endothelial cells as well as interactions of activated platelets with neutrophils and monocytes [114]. Furthermore, it was demonstrated to have a role in determining the size and stability of platelet aggregates [115]. Hence, p-selectin expression can be effectively used to assess platelet function. Platelets are stimulated in whole blood by adding the combination of ADP and the Thromboxane A2 mimetic U46619 (ADP/U4).The stimulated samples is then fixed using a fixative solution before measuring P-selectin by flow cytometry in order to monitor the anti-platelet effect of P2Y12 receptor antagonists [116].

Shear-Dependent Assay

Platelet Function Analyzer

The PFA-100 platelet function analyzer (Dade Behring, Marburg, Germany) measures the time required for occlusion of the aperture by platelet plugs (closure time) under high shear rates (5,000 to 6,000/s). A constant vacuum is maintained in the system that mimics the pressure of the capillary. The instrument aspirates a blood sample under constant vacuum from the sample reservoir through a capillary and a microscopic aperture cut into the membrane, which leads to high shear-induced platelet plug formation. For the detection of the effects of ADP antagonists, the membrane is coated with collagen/adenosine diphosphate (CADP) or CADP/PGE1 [117].

Cone and Platelet Analyzer

The cone and platelet analyzer (Impact-R, DiaMed, Cressier, Switzerland) tests whole-blood platelet adhesion and aggregation under flow conditions. Whole blood is pre-incubated with ADP, and a shear rate of 1,800/s is applied. The adherent platelets are stained, and the percentage of surface coverage and the average size of the objects are determined by an image analyzer [118].

Platelet Counting

Plateletworks

The Plateletworks test (Helena Laboratories, Beaumont, Texas) is based on single platelet disappearance.Whole-blood samples are collected in tubes containing Ethylenediaminetetraacetic acid (EDTA) and tubes containing ADP. Single platelet counts are performed on each sample. The ratio between the aggregated platelets in the agonist sample and the platelet count in the reference tube is used as the degree of platelet aggregation [119].

Thrombelastography

The thrombelastography (TEG) hemostasis analyzer (Haemoscope, Niles, Illinois) measures platelet-fibrin clot strength. The thrombin assay in its primary function is insensitive to P2Y12 inhibition and aspirin effect. Most of the studies used reptilase and factor XIIIa to generate a cross-linked fibrin clot. The contribution of P2Y12 receptor to the clot formation is measured by the addition ADP [120].

Anti-Platelet Function Testing & Clinical Impact

Several studies have investigated the association between HPR the occurrence of adverse ischemic events after PCI. In a meta-analysis of 6 prospective studies including 3,059 patients on clopidogrel undergoing PCI in whom platelet function was assessed with VerifyNow assay, Brar *et al.* [121] showed that HPR was associated with increasing rate of long-term MACE (death, MI, or stent thrombosis). Notably, the highest quartile of PRU values was also associated with a significant increase in the individual rates of nonfatal MI and stent thrombosis at 2 years. Furthermore, every 10-U increase in PRU was associated with a 4% greater rate of events, and a PRU cutoff of 230 appeared to best predict MACE occurrence, particularly stent thrombosis at follow up [121].

The investigators of ADAPT-DES sought to evaluate the associations between platelet reactivity according to the VerifyNow assay and both ischemic and bleeding events at 1-year follow-up in a large cohort of 8,583 patients undergoing PCI and receiving dual anti-aggregation therapy (aspirin and clopidogrel) [122]. Two cutoffs of HPR were employed: PRU>208 and PRU>230; and HPR rates were 42.7% and 35% according the 2 definitions, respectively. Although platelet reactivity >208 PRU did not predict mortality, it was associated with a higher rate of stent thrombosis (adjusted HR: 2.49; 95% CI: 1.43-4.31) and MI (adjusted HR: 1.42; 95% CI: 1.09-1.86) [122]. The same findings were observed with a cutoff of 230 PRU. Interestingly, in the latter registry, HPR was associated with a 27% reduction of bleeding (adjusted HR: 0.73; 95% CI: 0.61-0.89) [122].

On the other hand, the variability of platelet reactivity levels on clopidogrel treatment does not only lead to inadequate platelet inhibition and HPR. Indeed, on the other side of the spectrum, some patients' platelets appear to be excessively inhibited by standard doses of anti-platelet medication: the so called low on-treatment platelet reactivity (LPR) [123]. In a cohort of 346 PCI patients on clopidogrel, Mohktar *et al.* [124] showed that LPR on treatment as evaluated by VASP assay before PCI, is an independent predictor of non-CABG related TIMI major bleeding. In 2533 PCI patients treated with clopidogrel, Multiplate test was employed and LPR, defined as <188 AU/min, was significantly associated with post-procedural TIMI major bleeding in hospital (OR 2.6, 95% CI 1.3-5.2; p= 0.005) [90].

These findings assumed the presence of a A"therapeutic window A" that could provide an optimal prescription of P2Y12 inhibitors. Campo *et al.* [125] reported that reactivity of between 86 and 238 PRU, as assessed by VerifyNow assay, showed lower incidence of both ischemic (death, stroke, MI) and bleeding events at 1-year follow up. In 2,533 patients who received 600 mg of clopidogrel and underwent PCI, Sibbing *et al.* [90] found that lower risk for occurrence of both TIMI major bleeding and stent thrombosis platelet reactivity was observed in the range of 189-467 AU x min, as measured with the Multiplate analyzer. The POBA study evaluated platelet reactivity at 1 month for consecutive 1,542 patients undergoing PCI in the setting of ACS (on clopidogrel 75 mg, clopidogrel 150 mg, and prasugrel 10 mg) [126]. ROC curve analysis identified a PRI<10% as the strongest predictor of non-access site-related bleeding complications at 6 months. PRI in a range of 10-50% identified patients with the lowest event rate of combined bleeding and stent thrombosis (5.7%) when compared with patients classified as non-responder (8%) and hyper-responder (17.4%), respectively [126].

However, there are still some limitations to generalize platelet function testing in everyday practice. Indeed, the published studies have been conducted with different assays, different timing of platelet function measurement, different definition of HPR (even with the same assay), different definitions of bleeding and ischemic events, and heterogeneity in population risk profiles. Therefore, a consensus document was published in 2013 proposing cutoff values for the different platelet function tests [127]. Since platelet inhibition varies over time, and particularly during the first month of DAPT, differences in timing can lead to significant variability in test results [128]. Furthermore, the therapeutic window of on-treatment platelet reactivity is likely patient-specific, as it may vary according to the patient phenotype, such as clinical presentation (ACS or stable patients), presence of diabetes mellitus, renal function, age, and genotype [129].

For all these reasons, the current ESC and ACCF/AHA/ SCAI guidelines provide a Class IIb recommendation for platelet function testing to facilitate the choice of P2Y12 inhibitor in selected patients with high risk for thrombotic events following PCI, while routine testing is not recommended (Class III) [82, 84].

Genotype Testing

Several genes involved in thienopyridin metabolism and action, have been shown to contribute in its variability. Because its involvement in both oxidative steps, CYP2C19 plays a crucial role in clopidogrel metabolism. CYP2C19*2 (loss-o--function allele) represents a frequent condition observed in both Asian and Caucasian populations where 30% and 15% of them, respectively are carriers of at least 1 of these alleles [130]. Therefore, during the last decade, many investigators focused on CYP2C19 polymorphism, with the ambition to identify patients who might take less benefit from clopidogrel therapy. Platelet function testing has demonstrated a gene-dose effect for this allelic variant: ADP-induced platelet aggregation increases from wild-type homozygous patients (*1/*1) through heterozygous (*1/*2) and over to homozygous (*2/*2) allele carriers [131]. However the impact of CYP2C19 loss of function on clopidogrel action and patients' outcome is still controversial. Indeed, although some studies have reported that CYP2C19*2 allele was associated with a reduced anti-platelet effect of clopidogrel and increased risk for adverse cardiovascular events [132, 133], other authors have shown no difference between patients who were heterozygous or homozygous for loss-of-function alleles and those who were not carriers of the alleles [134, 135]. Such findings could be due to the fact that the CYP2C19*2 allele carriage contributes in only 5% to 12% of the variation of ADP-induced aggregation [136]. Other CYP2C19 variants (*3 to *8) have also been identified [137]. Although they have a low allele frequency in Caucasians (<1%), contributing thereby only to a minor extent to HPR, in East Asian population up to 17% of patients are carriers of the CYP2C19*3 allele, which also plays a role as a predictor of HPR [137, 138].

Conversely, the gain-of-function mutation (CYP2C19*17) results in increased enzyme activity thus, exaggerated bioactivation of clopidogrel [139]. However, the real impact of such a mutation regarding bleeding risk is also conflicting. Although some authors reported an association of the CYP2C19*17 allele with LPR and hemorrhagic events occurrence [139], other studies failed to confirm such an association [135, 140].

Being involved in different steps of clopidogrel metabolism, other genes have been investigated, such as ABCB1 (clopidogrel intestinal efflux), PON-1(involved in clopidogrel activation), ITGB3 (intracellular signaling), and P2Y12 (gene encoding the receptor) [97, 141]. Their implication in patients' cardiovascular prognosis is still not yet well established, requiring further studies.

In addition to DNA sequencing, two assays for CYP2C19*2 are actually available the Spartan RX system (Spartan Bioscience, Ottawa, Ontario, Canada) and the Verigene XP system (Nanosphere, Northbrook, Illinois). The Verigene system uses whole blood, the Spartan system uses a buccal swab. The Verigene system is based on gold nanoparticle techniques, whereas the Spartan system uses polymerase chain reaction. The Verigene system detects several CYP2C19 allelic variants, while the Spartan system detects only CYP2C19*2. The necessary time to get results for the Spartan and the Verigene systems is 1h and 3 h, respectively [142].

Genetic Testing & Clinical Impact

In healthy volunteers, the presence of CYP2C19 reduced function allele was associated with a 32.4% relative reduction ($p<0.001$) of serum active clopidogrel metabolites a relative reduction of about 25% in mean platelet aggregation ($p<0.001$) [133, 137, 141]. Accordingly, among patients with ACS undergoing stenting and treated with clopidogrel in the TRITON-TIMI 38 trial, CYP2C19 reduced function-allele carriers had a higher rate of major adverse cardiac events (HR: 1.53; $p=0.01$), including stent thrombosis (HR: 3.09; $p=0.02$), compared with noncarriers [141]. Similarly, Sibbing *et al.* [143] reported that CYP2C19*2 carriers had a significantly higher cumulative 30-day incidence of stent thrombosis compared with CYP2C19 wild-type homozygotes (HR: 3.81; $p<0.007$). Otherwise, the *17 gain-of function alleles was recognized to be associated with significantly lower ADP-induced platelet aggregation after clopidogrel intake ($p=0.039$) [144]. Importantly, *17 carriers have an approximately twofold increase in the risk of TIMI major and minor bleeding [144].

To date, it was shown that genetic polymorphism of CYP2C19 only accounts for a small part of HPR (<12%) [137]. Furthermore, the sensitivity of the *2-carrier state to detect HPR was as low as 56% [132], and several genes testing would be too complex and too expensive to be performed in practice. Thus, it is probable that platelet reactivity assessment, which takes into account external and internal factors responsible for HPR, would be more appropriate and practical.

Inter-Individual Variability of New P2Y12 Inhibitors

The deacetylation of prasugrel by intestinal esterases leads to the formation of an inactive thiolactone metabolite. Then, this latter undergoes oxidative metabolism; the CYP isoenzymes mainly involved are CYP3A and CYP2B6. This latter fact might explain that, conversely to clopidogrel, the common genetic functional CYP polymorphism does not affect the active metabolite serum levels, inhibition of platelet aggregation, nor the clinical outcome of prasugrel-treated patients [145]. Despite being already an active drug, the major metabolite of ticagreolor (AR-C124910XX) which also has anti-platelet properties, requires for its formation a passage through CYP3A4 [146]. Conversely to clopidogrel, no relevant interactions have been reported for new P2Y12 inhibitors neither with CCBs, statins nor PPIs during the different phases studies. However, ketoconazole, rifampicin, clarithromycin or dexamethasone have been described to have an impact on ticagrelor pharmacokinetics [146]. Interestingly, concomitant use of morphine was a strong predictor of HPR in patients treated with clopidogrel, prasugrel and ticagrelor, indicating that impaired or delayed absorption of those drugs induced by morphine might be the underlying mechanism of slower action onset in STEMI patients [147].

Through literature, HPR was even reported with prasugrel and ticagrelor in certain clinical settings, resulting in higher rates of ischemic events. Indeed, 12% to 19% of patients on chronic hemodialysis and who were clopidogrel nonresponders, showed HPR with prasugrel [148]. Furthermore, neither prasugrel nor ticagrelor showed a consistent effect in reducing platelet function during or shortly after primary percutaneous coronary PCI in STEMI patients [142]. Indeed, Alexopoulos *et al.* reported non-responders rates as high as 34.6% and 46.2%, respectively, 2 h after the respective loading doses [149].

Needless to say, new more potent P2Y12 inhibitors are responsible for higher rate of LPR, thus, resulting in more bleeding events.

Personalized Therapy

Based on the large body of evidence demonstrating that HPR is associated with a higher risk of thrombotic events, various therapeutic options have been tested to decrease ischemic risk in patients with HPR including: 1) increasing clopidogrel dose or tailoring therapy according to PR monitoring; 2) novel P2Y12-receptor inhibitors such as prasugrel, ticagrelor; and 3) the addition of cilostazol.

Increasing clopidogrel dose may accelerate the time course and enhance the magnitude of subsequent platelet inhibition. However it may require high doses of up to 2400 mg (>32 pills), and about 10% of patients remained with HPR (<50% or less using the VASP index) [150]. Furthermore, while the majority of heterozygote carriers of CYP2C19*2 had a sufficient level of platelet inhibition by increased clopidogrel dosage, a much higher proportion of homozygotes failed to respond despite daily doses of 300 mg (4 pills) of clopidogrel [151].

In a small study, Bonello *et al.* [150] showed that a tailored P2Y12 prescription according to platelet reactivity monitoring was associated with an improvement of clinical outcome by reducing the rate of stent thrombosis. The GRAVITAS trial was the first large-scale clinical trial to test the clinical impact of high- *versus* standard-dose clopidogrel in HPR patients [152]. In this trial, platelet function was measured in patients (n=5,429) with stable CAD or NSTEMI, on DAPT with aspirin and clopidogrel, 12-24 hours after successful PCI with drug-eluting stent [152]. HPR, defined as PRU≥230 with Verify Now assay, was observed in 2,214 patients (40.8%), who were thereafter randomized to receive clopidogrel 75 mg or 150 mg for 6 months. Although, double-dose clopidogrel reached to achieve a 22% absolute reduction in the rate of HPR at 1 month, it did not improved the primary endpoint (cardiovascular death, nonfatal MI, or stent thrombosis) (2.3% *versus* 2.3%; HR=1.01; 95% CI: 0.58-1.76; p=0.97) [152]. However, the latter study had some major limitations including the inadequacy of high-dose clopidogrel to modify platelet reactivity, timing of platelet reactivity evaluation, the cutoff value used, the exclusion of periprocedural events and a low risk profile cohort. Although RECLOSE 2-ACS registry included higher risk cohort of all-comers ACS, with a MACE rate as high as 14.6% at 2 years among HPR patients, the use of high-dose clopidogrel or switching to ticlopidine in this patients subset did not affect the outcomes [153].

The MADONNA study aimed to compare two cohorts of patients with CAD undergoing PCI (guided and non-guided treatment) during follow-up of 30 days [154]. Responsiveness to clopidogrel was assessed by the Multiplate analyzer, and the clopidogrel non-responders in the guided group received repeated loading doses of clopidogrel or prasugrel. The primary endpoint (stent thrombosis) was significantly reduced in the guided cohort (0.2% *versus* 1.9%; p=0.027) [154].The TRIGGER PCI trial enrolled stable patients who underwent successful PCI with drug-eluting stents. Platelet function testing with Verify Now assay was performed 2-7 hours after a maintenance dose of clopidogrel 75 mg the day after the index procedure [154]. Patients (n=423) showing HPR (PRU>208) were randomized to receive either prasugrel 10 mg daily or clopidogrel 75 mg daily. Although prasugrel significantly decreased platelet reactivity and rate of HPR as compared with clopidogrel, it was not possible to evaluate its impact on outcome [155]. Indeed, the study was terminated prematurely (423 patients were randomized and 273 completed 6 months of follow up) for futility because only 1 patient (on clopidogrel) in the entire cohort experienced the primary efficacy endpoint at 6 months [155].

In the ARCTIC trial, the investigators randomly assigned 2,440 patients scheduled for PCI with drug-eluting stent implantation to either a conventional strategy or a tailored strategy based on systematic assessment of the biological response to both aspirin and clopidogrel (VerifyNow assay) before PCI and at day 7-14, with adjustment of anti-aggregation therapy in suboptimal responders [156]. HPR on clopidogrel was defined as PRU>235 or inhibition <15%. Patients with on-clopidogrel HPR received either glycoprotein IIb/IIIa inhibitors and an additional loading dose of clopidogrel (≥600 mg), or a loading dose of prasugrel (60 mg) before PCI, followed by a maintenance dose of clopidogrel 150 mg or prasugrel 10 mg [156]. At 14-30 days after the index procedure, patients with HPR on clopidogrel were switched to prasugrel 10 mg or received a 75-mg increase in the maintenance dose of clopidogrel; those with LPR (>90% inhibition) were switched to clopidogrel 75 mg. At 1 year, the tailored strategy failed to reduce the primary endpoint occurrence (composite of death, MI, stent thrombosis, stroke, or urgent revascularization) compared to conventional strategy (34.6% *versus* 31.1%; HR=1.13; 95% CI: 0.98-1.29; p=0.10) [156]. The primary endpoint was driven by incidence of MI (30.3% *vs*. 28.4%; p=0.32) [156]. The rate of major bleeding was similar between groups. However, one of the major limitations of this trial was a low percentage of patients on prasugrel therapy; indeed, 3.3% were switched to prasugrel at the time of the index procedure and 17% at 14-30-days, while the majority received high-dose of clopidogrel. Regarding ticagrelor use as an alternative to HPR, we are still waiting for the results of some ongoing trials such as MATTIS-D (NCT01643031), TAILOR-PCI (NCT01742117), to better appreciate the impact of such a strategy on patients' prognosis. It has also been suggested that one single 60 mg oral dose of elinogrel overcomes, reversibly, the high platelet reactivity due to CYP2C19*2 genotype on standard dual anti-platelet therapy with aspirin and clopidogrel [157].

Cilostazol, a quinolinone-derivative medication, which reversibly inhibits platelet aggregation *via* its selective inhibition of phosphodiesterase type 3, resulting in increased

cAMP (Fig. **1**). Some authors reported study that addition of cilostazol to dual antiplatelet therapy (triple antiplatelet therapy) might lead to greater ADP-induced platelet inhibition compared with conventional dual antiplatelet therapy. Woo *et al.* [158] sought to assess the functional impact of cilostazol in chronic kidney disease (CKD) patients on hemodialysis, a setting associated with low response to clopidogrel. Seventy-four patients with CKD undergoing hemodialysis and percutaneous coronary intervention were enrolled. Patients were randomly assigned to receive clopidogrel (75 mg/d [group 1, n = 24]), high-maintenance dose of clopidogrel [150 mg/d (group 2, n = 25)], or clopidogrel (75 mg/d) with cilostazol [200 mg/d (group 3, n = 25)] for 14 days. Another 50 patients with normal renal function undergoing PCI were treated with 75 mg of clopidogrel and served as the control group. the CKD groups had significantly higher platelet aggregation activity compared with the control groups. The rate of HPR was significantly lower in group 3 than in groups 1 and 2 (10% *versus* 43% *vs*. 32%, respectively; p<0.05) [158]. Capranzano *et al.* [159] showed that cilostazol reduces platelet reactivity both in HPR and non-HPR patients, and its effects are enhanced in HPR patients with diabetes mellitus. In a recent meta-analysis, Bengalore *et al.* [160] showed that as compared to DAPT, the adjunction of cilostazol led to a 60% reduction in the risk of HPR (RR=0.40; 95% CI 0.30 to 0.53), the risk of MACE (incident rate ratio (IRR)=0.68; 95% CI 0.60 to 0.78), target lesion revascularization (IRR=0.57; 95% CI 0.44 to 0.73), target vessel revascularization (IRR=0.69; 95% CI 0.59 to 0.81) and stent thrombosis (IRR=0.63; 95% CI 0.40 to 0.98) with no difference for other outcomes including bleeding [160].

CONCLUSION

In patients with ACS or undergoing elective PCI, inhibition of the platelet P2Y12 receptor is standard of care. In literature, the efficacy/safety of clopidogrel, prasugrel and ticagrelor are well recognized, while the benefit of cangrelor and elinogrel in clinical practice is still not yet established, requiring further investigations.

Tailoring treatments based on biomarkers and genes is an emerging field in multiple areas of medicine, and seems to be a rational and A"fashionable A" way to treat patients. Some recent findings encouraged the cardiology community to think about replacing the "one size fits all" paradigm to the potential benefit of individualized antiplatelet regimen. However, in the area of evidence based medicine, a clear prognostic impact of an anti-platelet strategy based on genetic and platelet reactivity function is not yet proved. Therefore, although it can be useful in some cases and particular conditions it is too early to generalize it in common practice. Furthermore randomized trials should be performed to assess the best protocol and the best patients population to take benefit from tailored anti-platelet prescription.

ABBREVIATIONS

ADP = adenosine diphosphate;

cAMP = cyclic adenosine monophosphate;

GIRK = G-protein gated inwardly rectifying potassium channel;

PI3K = phosphatidyl inositol-3 kinase;

PKA = cAMP-dependent protein kinase;

cPLA2 = ADP-induced cytosolic phospholipase A2;

TXA2 = thromboxane A2;

VASP = vasodilator-stimulated phosphoprotein

CONFLICT OF INTEREST

The authors confirm that they have no conflict of interest to declare for this publication.

ACKNOWLEDGEMENTS

We would thank Dr. Francesco Marzà and Mrs. Stella Seminara for their support and collaboration.

REFERENCES

[1] DavA G, Patrono C. Platelet activation and atherothrombosis. N Engl J Med 2007; 357(24): 2482-94. [http://dx.doi.org/10.1056/NEJMra071014] [PMID: 18077812]

[2] Vorchheimer DA, Becker R. Platelets in atherothrombosis. Mayo Clin Proc 2006; 81(1): 59-68. [http://dx.doi.org/10.4065/81.1.59] [PMID: 16438480]

[3] Savage B, Almus-Jacobs F, Ruggeri ZM. Specific synergy of multiple substrate-receptor interactions in platelet thrombus formation under flow. Cell 1998; 94(5): 657-66. [http://dx.doi.org/10.1016/S0092-8674(00)81607-4] [PMID: 9741630]

[4] Nitelius E, Brantmark B, Fredholm B, *et al.* Actions and interactions of acetylsalicylic acid, salicylic acid and diflunisal on platelet aggregation. Eur J Clin Pharmacol 1984; 27(2): 165-8. [http://dx.doi.org/10.1007/BF00544040] [PMID: 6499897]

[5] Dorsam RT, Kunapuli SP. Central role of the P2Y12 receptor in platelet activation. J Clin Invest 2004; 113(3): 340-5. [http://dx.doi.org/10.1172/JCI20986] [PMID: 14755328]

[6] Windecker S, Kolh P, Alfonso F, *et al.* Authors/Task Force members. 2014 ESC/EACTS guidelines on myocardial revascularization: The task force on Myocardial revascularization of the European society of cardiology (ESC) and the European association for cardio-Thoracic surgery (EACTS) developed with the special contribution of the European association of percutaneous cardiovascular interventions (EAPCI). Eur Heart J 2014; 35(37): 2541-619. [http://dx.doi.org/10.1093/eurheartj/ehu278] [PMID: 25173339]

[7] Nieswandt B, Watson SP. Platelet-collagen interaction: is GPVI the central receptor? Blood 2003; 102(2): 449-61. [http://dx.doi.org/10.1182/blood-2002-12-3882] [PMID: 12649139]

[8] von KA1/4gelgen I. Pharmacological profiles of cloned mammalian P2Y-receptor subtypes.

Pharmacol Ther 2006; 110(3): 415-32.
[http://dx.doi.org/10.1016/j.pharmthera.2005.08.014] [PMID: 16257449]

[9] Communi D, Janssens R, Suarez-Huerta N, Robaye B, Boeynaems JM. Advances in signalling by extracellular nucleotides. The role and transduction mechanisms of P2Y receptors. Cell Signal 2000; 12(6): 351-60.
[http://dx.doi.org/10.1016/S0898-6568(00)00083-8] [PMID: 10889463]

[10] Kahner BN, Shankar H, Murugappan S, Prasad GL, Kunapuli SP. Nucleotide receptor signaling in platelets. J Thromb Haemost 2006; 4(11): 2317-26.
[http://dx.doi.org/10.1111/j.1538-7836.2006.02192.x] [PMID: 17059469]

[11] Gilman AG. G proteins: transducers of receptor-generated signals. Annu Rev Biochem 1987; 56: 615-49.
[http://dx.doi.org/10.1146/annurev.bi.56.070187.003151] [PMID: 3113327]

[12] Ohlmann P, Laugwitz KL, NA1/4rnberg B, *et al.* The human platelet ADP receptor activates Gi2 proteins. Biochem J 1995; 312(Pt 3): 775-9.
[PMID: 8554519]

[13] Jantzen HM, Milstone DS, Gousset L, Conley PB, Mortensen RM. Impaired activation of murine platelets lacking G alpha(i2). J Clin Invest 2001; 108(3): 477-83.
[http://dx.doi.org/10.1172/JCI12818] [PMID: 11489941]

[14] Gachet C. The platelet P2 receptors as molecular targets for old and new antiplatelet drugs. Pharmacol Ther 2005; 108(2): 180-92.
[http://dx.doi.org/10.1016/j.pharmthera.2005.03.009] [PMID: 15955565]

[15] Waldmann R, Nieberding M, Walter U. Vasodilator-stimulated protein phosphorylation in platelets is mediated by cAMP- and cGMP-dependent protein kinases. Eur J Biochem 1987; 167(3): 441-8.
[http://dx.doi.org/10.1111/j.1432-1033.1987.tb13357.x] [PMID: 2820726]

[16] Lova P, Paganini S, Hirsch E, *et al.* A selective role for phosphatidylinositol 3,4,5-trisphosphate in the Gi-dependent activation of platelet Rap1B. J Biol Chem 2003; 278(1): 131-8.
[http://dx.doi.org/10.1074/jbc.M204821200] [PMID: 12407113]

[17] Lova P, Paganini S, Sinigaglia F, Balduini C, Torti M. A Gi-dependent pathway is required for activation of the small GTPase Rap1B in human platelets. J Biol Chem 2002; 277(14): 12009-15.
[http://dx.doi.org/10.1074/jbc.M111803200] [PMID: 11815620]

[18] Kim S, Jin J, Kunapuli SP. Akt activation in platelets depends on Gi signaling pathways. J Biol Chem 2004; 279(6): 4186-95.
[http://dx.doi.org/10.1074/jbc.M306162200] [PMID: 14623889]

[19] Shankar H, Kahner BN, Prabhakar J, Lakhani P, Kim S, Kunapuli SP. G-protein-gated inwardly rectifying potassium channels regulate ADP-induced cPLA2 activity in platelets through Src family kinases. Blood 2006; 108(9): 3027-34.
[http://dx.doi.org/10.1182/blood-2006-03-010330] [PMID: 16857990]

[20] Shankar H, Murugappan S, Kim S, *et al.* Role of G protein-gated inwardly rectifying potassium channels in P2Y12 receptor-mediated platelet functional responses. Blood 2004; 104(5): 1335-43.
[http://dx.doi.org/10.1182/blood-2004-01-0069] [PMID: 15142872]

[21] Maffrand JP. The story of clopidogrel and its predecessor, ticlopidine: Could these major antiplatelet and antithrombotic drugs be discovered and developed today? C R Chim 2012; 15: 737-43. [http://dx.doi.org/10.1016/j.crci.2012.05.006]

[22] Quinn MJ, Fitzgerald DJ. Ticlopidine and clopidogrel. Circulation 1999; 100(15): 1667-72. [http://dx.doi.org/10.1161/01.CIR.100.15.1667] [PMID: 10517740]

[23] Di Minno G, Cerbone AM, Mattioli PL, Turco S, Iovine C, Mancini M. Functionally thrombasthenic state in normal platelets following the administration of ticlopidine. J Clin Invest 1985; 75(2): 328-38. [http://dx.doi.org/10.1172/JCI111705] [PMID: 3156146]

[24] Puri RN, Colman RW. ADP-induced platelet activation. Crit Rev Biochem Mol Biol 1997; 32(6): 437-502. [http://dx.doi.org/10.3109/10409239709082000] [PMID: 9444477]

[25] Desager JP. Clinical pharmacokinetics of ticlopidine. Clin Pharmacokinet 1994; 26(5): 347-55. [http://dx.doi.org/10.2165/00003088-199426050-00003] [PMID: 8055680]

[26] Schömig A, Neumann FJ, Kastrati A, *et al.* A randomized comparison of antiplatelet and anticoagulant therapy after the placement of coronary-artery stents. N Engl J Med 1996; 334(17): 1084-9. [http://dx.doi.org/10.1056/NEJM199604253341702] [PMID: 8598866]

[27] Leon MB, Baim DS, Popma JJ, *et al.* A clinical trial comparing three antithrombotic-drug regimens after coronary-artery stenting. N Engl J Med 1998; 339(23): 1665-71. [http://dx.doi.org/10.1056/NEJM199812033392303] [PMID: 9834303]

[28] Bertrand ME, Legrand V, Boland J, *et al.* Randomized multicenter comparison of conventional anticoagulation *versus* antiplatelet therapy in unplanned and elective coronary stenting. The full anticoagulation *versus* aspirin and ticlopidine (fantastic) study. Circulation 1998; 98(16): 1597-603. [http://dx.doi.org/10.1161/01.CIR.98.16.1597] [PMID: 9778323]

[29] Gent M, Blakely JA, Easton JD, *et al.* The Canadian American Ticlopidine Study (CATS) in thromboembolic stroke. Lancet 1989; 1(8649): 1215-20. [http://dx.doi.org/10.1016/S0140-6736(89)92327-1] [PMID: 2566778]

[30] Hass WK, Easton JD, Adams HP Jr, *et al.* A randomized trial comparing ticlopidine hydrochloride with aspirin for the prevention of stroke in high-risk patients. N Engl J Med 1989; 321(8): 501-7. [http://dx.doi.org/10.1056/NEJM198908243210804] [PMID: 2761587]

[31] Jacobson AK. Platelet ADP receptor antagonists: ticlopidine and clopidogrel. Best Pract Res Clin Haematol 2004; 17(1): 55-64. [http://dx.doi.org/10.1016/j.beha.2004.03.002] [PMID: 15171957]

[32] Hirata K, Takagi H, Yamamoto M, *et al.* Ticlopidine-induced hepatotoxicity is associated with specific human leukocyte antigen genomic subtypes in Japanese patients: a preliminary case-control study. Pharmacogenomics J 2008; 8(1): 29-33. [http://dx.doi.org/10.1038/sj.tpj.6500442] [PMID: 17339877]

[33] Miao J, Liu R, Li Z. Cytochrome P-450 polymorphisms and response to clopidogrel. N Engl J Med 2009; 360(21): 2250-1. [PMID: 19469033]

[34] Easton JD. Clinical aspects of the use of clopidogrel, a new antiplatelet agent. Semin Thromb Hemost 1999; 25 (Suppl. 2): 77-82.
[PMID: 10440429]

[35] Pache J, Kastrati A, Mehilli J, *et al.* Clopidogrel therapy in patients undergoing coronary stenting: value of a high-loading-dose regimen. Catheter Cardiovasc Interv 2002; 55(4): 436-41.
[http://dx.doi.org/10.1002/ccd.10092] [PMID: 11948888]

[36] A randomised, blinded, trial of clopidogrel *versus* aspirin in patients at risk of ischaemic events (CAPRIE). Lancet 1996; 348(9038): 1329-39.
[http://dx.doi.org/10.1016/S0140-6736(96)09457-3] [PMID: 8918275]

[37] Peters RJ, Mehta SR, Fox KA, *et al.* Effects of aspirin dose when used alone or in combination with clopidogrel in patients with acute coronary syndromes: observations from the Clopidogrel in Unstable angina to prevent Recurrent Events (CURE) study. Circulation 2003; 108(14): 1682-7.
[http://dx.doi.org/10.1161/01.CIR.0000091201.39590.CB] [PMID: 14504182]

[38] Mehta SR, Yusuf S, Peters RJ, *et al.* Effects of pretreatment with clopidogrel and aspirin followed by long-term therapy in patients undergoing percutaneous coronary intervention: the PCI-CURE study. Lancet 2001; 358(9281): 527-33.
[http://dx.doi.org/10.1016/S0140-6736(01)05701-4] [PMID: 11520521]

[39] Sabatine MS, Cannon CP, Gibson CM, *et al.* Addition of clopidogrel to aspirin and fibrinolytic therapy for myocardial infarction with ST-segment elevation. N Engl J Med 2005; 352(12): 1179-89.
[http://dx.doi.org/10.1056/NEJMoa050522] [PMID: 15758000]

[40] Sabatine MS, Cannon CP, Gibson CM, *et al.* Effect of clopidogrel pretreatment before percutaneous coronary intervention in patients with ST-elevation myocardial infarction treated with fibrinolytics: the PCI-CLARITY study. JAMA 2005; 294(10): 1224-32.
[http://dx.doi.org/10.1001/jama.294.10.1224] [PMID: 16143698]

[41] Dangas G, Mehran R, Guagliumi G, *et al.* Role of clopidogrel loading dose in patients with ST-segment elevation myocardial infarction undergoing primary angioplasty: results from the HORIZONS-AMI (harmonizing outcomes with revascularization and stents in acute myocardial infarction) trial. J Am Coll Cardiol 2009; 54(15): 1438-46.
[http://dx.doi.org/10.1016/j.jacc.2009.06.021] [PMID: 19796737]

[42] Schrör K. Antiplatelet drugs. A comparative review. Drugs 1995; 50(1): 7-28.
[http://dx.doi.org/10.2165/00003495-199550010-00002] [PMID: 7588091]

[43] Bennett CL, Connors JM, Carwile JM, *et al.* Thrombotic thrombocytopenic purpura associated with clopidogrel. N Engl J Med 2000; 342(24): 1773-7.
[http://dx.doi.org/10.1056/NEJM200006153422402] [PMID: 10852999]

[44] Best PJ, Steinhubl SR, Berger PB, *et al.* The efficacy and safety of short- and long-term dual antiplatelet therapy in patients with mild or moderate chronic kidney disease: results from the Clopidogrel for the Reduction of Events During Observation (CREDO) trial. Am Heart J 2008; 155(4): 687-93.
[http://dx.doi.org/10.1016/j.ahj.2007.10.046] [PMID: 18371477]

[45] Diener HC, Bogousslavsky J, Brass LM, *et al.* Aspirin and clopidogrel compared with clopidogrel

alone after recent ischaemic stroke or transient ischaemic attack in high-risk patients (MATCH): randomised, double-blind, placebo-controlled trial. Lancet 2004; 364(9431): 331-7. [http://dx.doi.org/10.1016/S0140-6736(04)16721-4] [PMID: 15276392]

[46] Farid NA, Smith RL, Gillespie TA, *et al.* The disposition of prasugrel, a novel thienopyridine, in humans. Drug Metab Dispos 2007; 35(7): 1096-104. [http://dx.doi.org/10.1124/dmd.106.014522] [PMID: 17403916]

[47] Rehmel JL, Eckstein JA, Farid NA, *et al.* Interactions of two major metabolites of prasugrel, a thienopyridine antiplatelet agent, with the cytochromes P450. Drug Metab Dispos 2006; 34(4): 600-7. [http://dx.doi.org/10.1124/dmd.105.007989] [PMID: 16415119]

[48] Brandt JT, Payne CD, Wiviott SD, *et al.* A comparison of prasugrel and clopidogrel loading doses on platelet function: magnitude of platelet inhibition is related to active metabolite formation Am Heart J 2007; 153(1): 66-e9-16. [http://dx.doi.org/10.1016/j.ahj.2006.10.010]

[49] IyA D, Glenn JR, White AE, Fox SC, Dovlatova N, Heptinstall S. $P2Y_{12}$ and EP3 antagonists promote the inhibitory effects of natural modulators of platelet aggregation that act *via* cAMP. Platelets 2011; 22(7): 504-15. [http://dx.doi.org/10.3109/09537104.2011.576284] [PMID: 21591981]

[50] Angiolillo DJ. ADP receptor antagonism: what's in the pipeline? Am J Cardiovasc Drugs 2007; 7(6): 423-32. [http://dx.doi.org/10.2165/00129784-200707060-00005] [PMID: 18076209]

[51] Wiviott SD, Antman EM, Winters KJ, *et al.* Randomized comparison of prasugrel (CS-747, LY640315), a novel thienopyridine P2Y12 antagonist, with clopidogrel in percutaneous coronary intervention: results of the Joint Utilization of Medications to Block Platelets Optimally (JUMBO)-TIMI 26 trial. Circulation 2005; 111(25): 3366-73. [http://dx.doi.org/10.1161/CIRCULATIONAHA.104.502815] [PMID: 15967851]

[52] Wiviott SD, Trenk D, Frelinger AL, *et al.* Prasugrel compared with high loading- and maintenance-dose clopidogrel in patients with planned percutaneous coronary intervention: the Prasugrel in Comparison to Clopidogrel for Inhibition of Platelet Activation and Aggregation-Thrombolysis in Myocardial Infarction 44 trial. Circulation 2007; 116(25): 2923-32. [http://dx.doi.org/10.1161/CIRCULATIONAHA.107.740324] [PMID: 18056526]

[53] Antman EM, Wiviott SD, Murphy SA, *et al.* Early and late benefits of prasugrel in patients with acute coronary syndromes undergoing percutaneous coronary intervention: a TRITON-TIMI 38 (TRial to Assess Improvement in Therapeutic Outcomes by Optimizing Platelet InhibitioN with Prasugrel-Thrombolysis In Myocardial Infarction) analysis. J Am Coll Cardiol 2008; 51(21): 2028-33. [http://dx.doi.org/10.1016/j.jacc.2008.04.002] [PMID: 18498956]

[54] Montalescot G, Wiviott SD, Braunwald E, *et al.* Prasugrel compared with clopidogrel in patients undergoing percutaneous coronary intervention for ST-elevation myocardial infarction (TRITON-TIMI 38): double-blind, randomised controlled trial. Lancet 2009; 373(9665): 723-31. [http://dx.doi.org/10.1016/S0140-6736(09)60441-4] [PMID: 19249633]

[55] Roe MT, Armstrong PW, Fox KA, *et al.* Prasugrel *versus* clopidogrel for acute coronary syndromes without revascularization. N Engl J Med 2012; 367(14): 1297-309.

[http://dx.doi.org/10.1056/NEJMoa1205512] [PMID: 22920930]

[56] Montalescot G, Bolognese L, Dudek D, *et al.* Pretreatment with prasugrel in non-ST-segment elevation acute coronary syndromes. N Engl J Med 2013; 369(11): 999-1010. [http://dx.doi.org/10.1056/NEJMoa1308075] [PMID: 23991622]

[57] Springthorpe B, Bailey A, Barton P, *et al.* From ATP to AZD6140: the discovery of an orally active reversible P2Y12 receptor antagonist for the prevention of thrombosis. Bioorg Med Chem Lett 2007; 17(21): 6013-8. [http://dx.doi.org/10.1016/j.bmcl.2007.07.057] [PMID: 17827008]

[58] Teng R, Butler K. Pharmacokinetics, pharmacodynamics, tolerability and safety of single ascending doses of ticagrelor, a reversibly binding oral P2Y(12) receptor antagonist, in healthy subjects. Eur J Clin Pharmacol 2010; 66(5): 487-96. [http://dx.doi.org/10.1007/s00228-009-0778-5] [PMID: 20091161]

[59] VAN Giezen JJ, Nilsson L, Berntsson P, *et al.* Ticagrelor binds to human P2Y(12) independently from ADP but antagonizes ADP-induced receptor signaling and platelet aggregation. J Thromb Haemost 2009; 7(9): 1556-65. [http://dx.doi.org/10.1111/j.1538-7836.2009.03527.x] [PMID: 19552634]

[60] IyA D, Glenn JR, White AE, *et al.* Mode of action of P2Y(12) antagonists as inhibitors of platelet function. Thromb Haemost 2011; 105(1): 96-106. [http://dx.doi.org/10.1160/TH10-07-0482] [PMID: 20941457]

[61] Cattaneo M, Schulz R, Nylander S. Adenosine-mediated effects of ticagrelor: evidence and potential clinical relevance. J Am Coll Cardiol 2014; 63(23): 2503-9. [http://dx.doi.org/10.1016/j.jacc.2014.03.031] [PMID: 24768873]

[62] Butler K, Teng R. Pharmacokinetics, pharmacodynamics, safety and tolerability of multiple ascending doses of ticagrelor in healthy volunteers. Br J Clin Pharmacol 2010; 70(1): 65-77. [http://dx.doi.org/10.1111/j.1365-2125.2010.03669.x] [PMID: 20642549]

[63] Husted S, Emanuelsson H, Heptinstall S, Sandset PM, Wickens M, Peters G. Pharmacodynamics, pharmacokinetics, and safety of the oral reversible P2Y12 antagonist AZD6140 with aspirin in patients with atherosclerosis: a double-blind comparison to clopidogrel with aspirin. Eur Heart J 2006; 27(9): 1038-47. [http://dx.doi.org/10.1093/eurheartj/ehi754] [PMID: 16476694]

[64] Storey RF, Husted S, Harrington RA, *et al.* Inhibition of platelet aggregation by AZD6140, a reversible oral P2Y12 receptor antagonist, compared with clopidogrel in patients with acute coronary syndromes. J Am Coll Cardiol 2007; 50(19): 1852-6. [http://dx.doi.org/10.1016/j.jacc.2007.07.058] [PMID: 17980251]

[65] Wallentin L, Becker RC, Budaj A, *et al.* Ticagrelor *versus* clopidogrel in patients with acute coronary syndromes. N Engl J Med 2009; 361(11): 1045-57. [http://dx.doi.org/10.1056/NEJMoa0904327] [PMID: 19717846]

[66] Cannon CP, Harrington RA, James S, *et al.* Comparison of ticagrelor with clopidogrel in patients with a planned invasive strategy for acute coronary syndromes (PLATO): a randomised double-blind study. Lancet 2010; 375(9711): 283-93. [http://dx.doi.org/10.1016/S0140-6736(09)62191-7] [PMID: 20079528]

[67] Montalescot G, van 't Hof AW, Lapostolle F, *et al.* Prehospital ticagrelor in ST-segment elevation myocardial infarction. N Engl J Med 2014; 371(11): 1016-27. [http://dx.doi.org/10.1056/NEJMoa1407024] [PMID: 25175921]

[68] Belchikov YG, Koenig SJ, Dipasquale EM. Potential role of endogenous adenosine in ticagrelor-induced dyspnea. Pharmacotherapy 2013; 33(8): 882-7. [http://dx.doi.org/10.1002/phar.1293] [PMID: 23712633]

[69] Storey RF, Bliden KP, Patil SB, *et al.* Incidence of dyspnea and assessment of cardiac and pulmonary function in patients with stable coronary artery disease receiving ticagrelor, clopidogrel, or placebo in the ONSET/OFFSET study. J Am Coll Cardiol 2010; 56(3): 185-93. [http://dx.doi.org/10.1016/j.jacc.2010.01.062] [PMID: 20620737]

[70] Greenbaum AB, Grines CL, Bittl JA, *et al.* Initial experience with an intravenous P2Y12 platelet receptor antagonist in patients undergoing percutaneous coronary intervention: results from a 2-part, phase II, multicenter, randomized, placebo- and active-controlled trial. Am Heart J 2006; 151(3): e1-689-0.

[71] Srinivasan S, Mir F, Huang JS, Khasawneh FT, Lam SC, Le Breton GC. The P2Y12 antagonists, 2-methylthioadenosine 5'-monophosphate triethylammonium salt and cangrelor (ARC69931MX), can inhibit human platelet aggregation through a Gi-independent increase in cAMP levels. J Biol Chem 2009; 284(24): 16108-17. [http://dx.doi.org/10.1074/jbc.M809780200] [PMID: 19346255]

[72] Bhatt DL, Lincoff AM, Gibson CM, *et al.* Intravenous platelet blockade with cangrelor during PCI. N Engl J Med 2009; 361(24): 2330-41. [http://dx.doi.org/10.1056/NEJMoa0908629] [PMID: 19915222]

[73] Harrington RA, Stone GW, McNulty S, *et al.* Platelet inhibition with cangrelor in patients undergoing PCI. N Engl J Med 2009; 361(24): 2318-29. [http://dx.doi.org/10.1056/NEJMoa0908628] [PMID: 19915221]

[74] Bhatt DL, Stone GW, Mahaffey KW, *et al.* Effect of platelet inhibition with cangrelor during PCI on ischemic events. N Engl J Med 2013; 368(14): 1303-13. [http://dx.doi.org/10.1056/NEJMoa1300815] [PMID: 23473369]

[75] Steg PG, Bhatt DL, Hamm CW, *et al.* Effect of cangrelor on periprocedural outcomes in percutaneous coronary interventions: a pooled analysis of patient-level data. Lancet 2013; 382(9909): 1981-92. [http://dx.doi.org/10.1016/S0140-6736(13)61615-3] [PMID: 24011551]

[76] Angiolillo DJ, Firstenberg MS, Price MJ, *et al.* Bridging antiplatelet therapy with cangrelor in patients undergoing cardiac surgery: a randomized controlled trial. JAMA 2012; 307(3): 265-74. [http://dx.doi.org/10.1001/jama.2011.2002] [PMID: 22253393]

[77] Ueno M, Rao SV, Angiolillo DJ. Elinogrel: pharmacological principles, preclinical and early phase clinical testing. Future Cardiol 2010; 6(4): 445-53. [http://dx.doi.org/10.2217/fca.10.67] [PMID: 20608816]

[78] Lieu H, Conley PB, Andre P, *et al.* Initial intravenous experience with PRT060128 (PRT128), an orally available, direct-acting, and reversible P2Y12 inhibitor. J Thromb Haemost 2007; 5: 292. [http://dx.doi.org/10.1111/j.1538-7836.2007.tb02050.x] [PMID: 17635739]

[79] Berger JS, Roe MT, Gibson CM, *et al.* Safety and feasibility of adjunctive antiplatelet therapy with intravenous elinogrel, a direct-acting and reversible P2Y12 ADP-receptor antagonist, before primary percutaneous intervention in patients with ST-elevation myocardial infarction: the Early Rapid ReversAl of platelet thromboSis with intravenous Elinogrel before PCI to optimize reperfusion in acute Myocardial Infarction (ERASE MI) pilot trial. Am Heart J 2009; 158(6): 998-1004.e1. [http://dx.doi.org/10.1016/j.ahj.2009.10.010] [PMID: 19958867]

[80] Welsh RC, Rao SV, Zeymer U, *et al.* A randomized, double-blind, active-controlled phase 2 trial to evaluate a novel selective and reversible intravenous and oral P2Y12 inhibitor elinogrel *versus* clopidogrel in patients undergoing nonurgent percutaneous coronary intervention: the INNOVATE-PCI trial. Circ Cardiovasc Interv 2012; 5(3): 336-46. [http://dx.doi.org/10.1161/CIRCINTERVENTIONS.111.964197] [PMID: 22647518]

[81] Wang YX, Vincelette J, da Cunha V, *et al.* A novel P2Y(12) adenosine diphosphate receptor antagonist that inhibits platelet aggregation and thrombus formation in rat and dog models. Thromb Haemost 2007; 97(5): 847-55. [PMID: 17479197]

[82] Hamm CW, Bassand JP, Agewall S, *et al.* ESC Guidelines for the management of acute coronary syndromes in patients presenting without persistent ST-segment elevation: The Task Force for the management of acute coronary syndromes (ACS) in patients presenting without persistent ST-segment elevation of the European Society of Cardiology (ESC). Eur Heart J 2011; 32(23): 2999-3054. [http://dx.doi.org/10.1093/eurheartj/ehr236] [PMID: 21873419]

[83] Steg PG, James SK, Atar D, *et al.* ESC Guidelines for the management of acute myocardial infarction in patients presenting with ST-segment elevation. Eur Heart J 2012; 33(20): 2569-619. [http://dx.doi.org/10.1093/eurheartj/ehs215] [PMID: 22922416]

[84] O'Gara PT, Kushner FG, Ascheim DD, *et al.* 2013 ACCF/AHA guideline for the management of ST-elevation myocardial infarction: executive summary: a report of the American College ofCardiology Foundation/American Heart Association Task Force on Practice Guidelines: developed in collaboration with the American College of Emergency Physicians and Society for Cardiovascular Angiography and Interventions. Catheter Cardiovasc Interv 2013; 82(1): E1-E27. [http://dx.doi.org/10.1002/ccd.24776] [PMID: 23299937]

[85] Montalescot G, Sechtem U, Achenbach S, *et al.* 2013 ESC guidelines on the management of stable coronary artery disease: the Task Force on the management of stable coronary artery disease of the European Society of Cardiology. Eur Heart J 2013; 34(38): 2949-3003. [http://dx.doi.org/10.1093/eurheartj/eht296] [PMID: 23996286]

[86] Capranzano P, Tamburino C, Capodanno D, *et al.* Platelet function profiles in the elderly: results of a pharmacodynamic study in patients on clopidogrel therapy and effects of switching to prasugrel 5 mg in patients with high platelet reactivity. Thromb Haemost 2011; 106(6): 1149-57. [http://dx.doi.org/10.1160/TH11-05-0346] [PMID: 22011914]

[87] Geisler T, Grass D, Bigalke B, *et al.* The residual platelet aggregation after deployment of intracoronary stent (PREDICT) score. J Thromb Haemost 2008; 6(1): 54-61. [http://dx.doi.org/10.1111/j.1538-7836.2007.02812.x] [PMID: 17949474]

[88] Angiolillo DJ, Bernardo E, Sabaté M, *et al.* Impact of platelet reactivity on cardiovascular outcomes in

patients with type 2 diabetes mellitus and coronary artery disease. J Am Coll Cardiol 2007; 50(16): 1541-7.
[http://dx.doi.org/10.1016/j.jacc.2007.05.049] [PMID: 17936152]

[89] Cayla G, Hulot JS, O'Connor SA, *et al.* Clinical, angiographic, and genetic factors associated with early coronary stent thrombosis. JAMA 2011; 306(16): 1765-74.
[http://dx.doi.org/10.1001/jama.2011.1529] [PMID: 22028352]

[90] Sibbing D, Schulz S, Braun S, *et al.* Antiplatelet effects of clopidogrel and bleeding in patients undergoing coronary stent placement. J Thromb Haemost 2010; 8(2): 250-6.
[http://dx.doi.org/10.1111/j.1538-7836.2009.03709.x] [PMID: 19943882]

[91] Park SH, Kim W, Park CS, Kang WY, Hwang SH, Kim W. A comparison of clopidogrel responsiveness in patients with *versus* without chronic renal failure. Am J Cardiol 2009; 104(9): 1292-5.
[http://dx.doi.org/10.1016/j.amjcard.2009.06.049] [PMID: 19840579]

[92] Geisler T, Mueller K, Aichele S, *et al.* Impact of inflammatory state and metabolic control on responsiveness to dual antiplatelet therapy in type 2 diabetics after PCI: prognostic relevance of residual platelet aggregability in diabetics undergoing coronary interventions. Clin Res Cardiol 2010; 99(11): 743-52.
[http://dx.doi.org/10.1007/s00392-010-0179-x] [PMID: 20526607]

[93] Bliden KP, Dichiara J, Lawal L, *et al.* The association of cigarette smoking with enhanced platelet inhibition by clopidogrel. J Am Coll Cardiol 2008; 52(7): 531-3.
[http://dx.doi.org/10.1016/j.jacc.2008.04.045] [PMID: 18687246]

[94] Jeong YH, Cho JH, Kang MK, *et al.* Smoking at least 10 cigarettes per day increases platelet inhibition by clopidogrel in patients with ST-segment-elevation myocardial infarction. Thromb Res 2010; 126(4): e334-8.
[http://dx.doi.org/10.1016/j.thromres.2010.03.020] [PMID: 20451242]

[95] Jeong YH, Kim IS, Park Y, *et al.* Carriage of cytochrome 2C19 polymorphism is associated with risk of high post-treatment platelet reactivity on high maintenance-dose clopidogrel of 150 mg/day: results of the ACCEL-DOUBLE (Accelerated Platelet Inhibition by a Double Dose of Clopidogrel According to Gene Polymorphism) study. JACC Cardiovasc Interv 2010; 3(7): 731-41.
[http://dx.doi.org/10.1016/j.jcin.2010.05.007] [PMID: 20650435]

[96] Cattaneo M. New P2Y(12) inhibitors. Circulation 2010; 121(1): 171-9.
[http://dx.doi.org/10.1161/CIRCULATIONAHA.109.853069] [PMID: 20048234]

[97] Bouman HJ, SchoA"mig E, van Werkum JW, *et al.* Paraoxonase-1 and clopidogrel efficacy. Nat Med 2011; 17: 1042-4. [reply].
[http://dx.doi.org/10.1038/nm.2469] [PMID: 21170047]

[98] Mega JL, Close SL, Wiviott SD, *et al.* Genetic variants in ABCB1 and CYP2C19 and cardiovascular outcomes after treatment with clopidogrel and prasugrel in the TRITON-TIMI 38 trial: a pharmacogenetic analysis. Lancet 2010; 376(9749): 1312-9.
[http://dx.doi.org/10.1016/S0140-6736(10)61273-1] [PMID: 20801494]

[99] Cattaneo M. Response variability to clopidogrel: is tailored treatment, based on laboratory testing, the right solution? J Thromb Haemost 2012; 10(3): 327-36.

[http://dx.doi.org/10.1111/j.1538-7836.2011.04602.x] [PMID: 22221409]

[100] Bhatt DL. Clopidogrel and proton pump inhibitors. CMAJ 2014; 186(3): 213. [http://dx.doi.org/10.1503/cmaj.114-0015] [PMID: 24549709]

[101] Matetzky S, Shenkman B, Guetta V, *et al.* Clopidogrel resistance is associated with increased risk of recurrent atherothrombotic events in patients with acute myocardial infarction. Circulation 2004; 109(25): 3171-5. [http://dx.doi.org/10.1161/01.CIR.0000130846.46168.03] [PMID: 15184279]

[102] Gurbel PA, Bliden KP, Hiatt BL, O'Connor CM. Clopidogrel for coronary stenting: response variability, drug resistance, and the effect of pretreatment platelet reactivity. Circulation 2003; 107(23): 2908-13. [http://dx.doi.org/10.1161/01.CIR.0000072771.11429.83] [PMID: 12796140]

[103] Gurbel PA, Antonino MJ, Bliden KP, *et al.* Platelet reactivity to adenosine diphosphate and long-term ischemic event occurrence following percutaneous coronary intervention: a potential antiplatelet therapeutic target. Platelets 2008; 19(8): 595-604. [http://dx.doi.org/10.1080/09537100802351065] [PMID: 19012177]

[104] Bliden KP, DiChiara J, Tantry US, Bassi AK, Chaganti SK, Gurbel PA. Increased risk in patients with high platelet aggregation receiving chronic clopidogrel therapy undergoing percutaneous coronary intervention: is the current antiplatelet therapy adequate? J Am Coll Cardiol 2007; 49(6): 657-66. [http://dx.doi.org/10.1016/j.jacc.2006.10.050] [PMID: 17291930]

[105] Chen L, Bracey AW, Radovancevic R, *et al.* Clopidogrel and bleeding in patients undergoing elective coronary artery bypass grafting. J Thorac Cardiovasc Surg 2004; 128(3): 425-31. [http://dx.doi.org/10.1016/j.jtcvs.2004.02.019] [PMID: 15354103]

[106] Siller-Matula JM, Christ G, Lang IM, Delle-Karth G, Huber K, Jilma B. Multiple electrode aggregometry predicts stent thrombosis better than the vasodilator-stimulated phosphoprotein phosphorylation assay. J Thromb Haemost 2010; 8(2): 351-9. [http://dx.doi.org/10.1111/j.1538-7836.2009.03699.x] [PMID: 19943879]

[107] Rahe-Meyer N, Winterhalter M, Boden A, *et al.* Platelet concentrates transfusion in cardiac surgery and platelet function assessment by multiple electrode aggregometry. Acta Anaesthesiol Scand 2009; 53(2): 168-75. [http://dx.doi.org/10.1111/j.1399-6576.2008.01845.x] [PMID: 19175576]

[108] Ranucci M, Baryshnikova E, Soro G, Ballotta A, De Benedetti D, Conti D. Multiple electrode whole-blood aggregometry and bleeding in cardiac surgery patients receiving thienopyridines. Ann Thorac Surg 2011; 91(1): 123-9. [http://dx.doi.org/10.1016/j.athoracsur.2010.09.022] [PMID: 21172499]

[109] Jakubowski JA, Payne CD, Li YG, *et al.* The use of the Verify now P2Y12 point-of-care device to monitor platelet function across a range of P2Y12 inhibition levels following prasugrel and clopidogrel administration. Thromb Haemost 2008; 99(2): 409-15. [PMID: 18278193]

[110] Cuisset T, Hamilos M, Sarma J, *et al.* Relation of low response to clopidogrel assessed with point-o--care assay to periprocedural myonecrosis in patients undergoing elective coronary stenting for stable angina pectoris. Am J Cardiol 2008; 101(12): 1700-3.

[http://dx.doi.org/10.1016/j.amjcard.2008.02.054] [PMID: 18549843]

[111] Siller-Matula JM, Panzer S, Jilma B. Reproducibility and standardized reporting of the vasodilator-stimulated phosphoprotein phosphorylation assay. Platelets 2008; 19(7): 551-4. [http://dx.doi.org/10.1080/09537100802272634] [PMID: 18979368]

[112] Aleil B, Ravanat C, Cazenave JP, Rochoux G, Heitz A, Gachet C. Flow cytometric analysis of intraplatelet VASP phosphorylation for the detection of clopidogrel resistance in patients with ischemic cardiovascular diseases. J Thromb Haemost 2005; 3(1): 85-92. [http://dx.doi.org/10.1111/j.1538-7836.2004.01063.x] [PMID: 15634270]

[113] Hsu-Lin S, Berman CL, Furie BC, August D, Furie B. A platelet membrane protein expressed during platelet activation and secretion. Studies using a monoclonal antibody specific for thrombin-activated platelets. J Biol Chem 1984; 259(14): 9121-6. [PMID: 6746643]

[114] Frenette PS, Johnson RC, Hynes RO, Wagner DD. Platelets roll on stimulated endothelium *in vivo*: an interaction mediated by endothelial P-selectin. Proc Natl Acad Sci USA 1995; 92(16): 7450-4. [http://dx.doi.org/10.1073/pnas.92.16.7450] [PMID: 7543682]

[115] Merten M, Thiagarajan P. P-selectin expression on platelets determines size and stability of platelet aggregates. Circulation 2000; 102(16): 1931-6. [http://dx.doi.org/10.1161/01.CIR.102.16.1931] [PMID: 11034941]

[116] Fox SC, May JA, Shah A, Neubert U, Heptinstall S. Measurement of platelet P-selectin for remote testing of platelet function during treatment with clopidogrel and/or aspirin. Platelets 2009; 20(4): 250-9. [http://dx.doi.org/10.1080/09537100902912451] [PMID: 19440925]

[117] Jilma B. Platelet function analyzer (PFA-100): a tool to quantify congenital or acquired platelet dysfunction. J Lab Clin Med 2001; 138(3): 152-63. [http://dx.doi.org/10.1067/mlc.2001.117406] [PMID: 11528368]

[118] Panzer S, Eichelberger B, Koren D, Kaufmann K, Male C. Monitoring survival and function of transfused platelets in Bernard-Soulier syndrome by flow cytometry and a cone and plate(let) analyzer (Impact-R). Transfusion 2007; 47(1): 103-6. [http://dx.doi.org/10.1111/j.1537-2995.2007.01070.x] [PMID: 17207237]

[119] Breet NJ, van Werkum JW, Bouman HJ, *et al.* Comparison of platelet function tests in predicting clinical outcome in patients undergoing coronary stent implantation. JAMA 2010; 303(8): 754-62. [http://dx.doi.org/10.1001/jama.2010.181] [PMID: 20179285]

[120] Scharbert G, Auer A, Kozek-Langenecker S. Evaluation of the platelet mapping assay on rotational thromboelastometry ROTEM. Platelets 2009; 20(2): 125-30. [http://dx.doi.org/10.1080/09537100802657735] [PMID: 19235055]

[121] Brar SS, ten Berg J, Marcucci R, *et al.* Impact of platelet reactivity on clinical outcomes after percutaneous coronary intervention. A collaborative meta-analysis of individual participant data. J Am Coll Cardiol 2011; 58(19): 1945-54. [http://dx.doi.org/10.1016/j.jacc.2011.06.059] [PMID: 22032704]

[122] Stone GW, Witzenbichler B, Weisz G, *et al.* Platelet reactivity and clinical outcomes after coronary

artery implantation of drug-eluting stents (ADAPT-DES): a prospective multicentre registry study. Lancet 2013; 382(9892): 614-23.
[http://dx.doi.org/10.1016/S0140-6736(13)61170-8] [PMID: 23890998]

[123] Janssen PW, ten Berg JM, Hackeng CM. The use of platelet function testing in PCI and CABG patients. Blood Rev 2014; 28(3): 109-21.
[http://dx.doi.org/10.1016/j.blre.2014.03.004] [PMID: 24745727]

[124] Mokhtar OA, Lemesle G, Armero S, *et al.* Relationship between platelet reactivity inhibition and non-CABG related major bleeding in patients undergoing percutaneous coronary intervention. Thromb Res 2010; 126(2): e147-9.
[http://dx.doi.org/10.1016/j.thromres.2010.01.013] [PMID: 20129650]

[125] Campo G, Parrinello G, Ferraresi P, *et al.* Prospective evaluation of on-clopidogrel platelet reactivity over time in patients treated with percutaneous coronary intervention relationship with gene polymorphisms and clinical outcome. J Am Coll Cardiol 2011; 57(25): 2474-83.
[http://dx.doi.org/10.1016/j.jacc.2010.12.047] [PMID: 21679849]

[126] Cuisset T, Grosdidier C, Loundou AD, *et al.* Clinical implications of very low on-treatment platelet reactivity in patients treated with thienopyridine: the POBA study (predictor of bleedings with antiplatelet drugs). JACC Cardiovasc Interv 2013; 6(8): 854-63.
[http://dx.doi.org/10.1016/j.jcin.2013.04.009] [PMID: 23968703]

[127] Tantry US, Bonello L, Aradi D, *et al.* Consensus and update on the definition of on-treatment platelet reactivity to adenosine diphosphate associated with ischemia and bleeding. J Am Coll Cardiol 2013; 62(24): 2261-73.
[http://dx.doi.org/10.1016/j.jacc.2013.07.101] [PMID: 24076493]

[128] Price MJ, Angiolillo DJ, Teirstein PS, *et al.* Platelet reactivity and cardiovascular outcomes after percutaneous coronary intervention: a time-dependent analysis of the Gauging Responsiveness with a VerifyNow P2Y12 assay: Impact on Thrombosis and Safety (GRAVITAS) trial. Circulation 2011; 124(10): 1132-7.
[http://dx.doi.org/10.1161/CIRCULATIONAHA.111.029165] [PMID: 21875913]

[129] Angiolillo DJ, Rollini F. Switching from prasugrel to clopidogrel: navigating in unknown waters. JACC Cardiovasc Interv 2013; 6(2): 166-8.
[http://dx.doi.org/10.1016/j.jcin.2012.12.001] [PMID: 23428008]

[130] Gurbel PA, Tantry US, Shuldiner AR, Kereiakes DJ. Genotyping: one piece of the puzzle to personalize antiplatelet therapy. J Am Coll Cardiol 2010; 56(2): 112-6.
[http://dx.doi.org/10.1016/j.jacc.2010.04.008] [PMID: 20471192]

[131] Gurbel PA, Shuldiner AR, Bliden KP, Ryan K, Pakyz RE, Tantry US. The relation between CYP2C19 genotype and phenotype in stented patients on maintenance dual antiplatelet therapy. Am Heart J 2011; 161(3): 598-604.
[http://dx.doi.org/10.1016/j.ahj.2010.12.011] [PMID: 21392617]

[132] Shuldiner AR, O'Connell JR, Bliden KP, *et al.* Association of cytochrome P450 2C19 genotype with the antiplatelet effect and clinical efficacy of clopidogrel therapy. JAMA 2009; 302(8): 849-57.
[http://dx.doi.org/10.1001/jama.2009.1232] [PMID: 19706858]

[133] Collet JP, Hulot JS, Pena A, *et al.* Cytochrome P450 2C19 polymorphism in young patients treated

with clopidogrel after myocardial infarction: a cohort study. Lancet 2009; 373(9660): 309-17. [http://dx.doi.org/10.1016/S0140-6736(08)61845-0] [PMID: 19108880]

[134] Wallentin L, James S, Storey RF, *et al.* Effect of CYP2C19 and ABCB1 single nucleotide polymorphisms on outcomes of treatment with ticagrelor *versus* clopidogrel for acute coronary syndromes: a genetic substudy of the PLATO trial. Lancet 2010; 376(9749): 1320-8. [http://dx.doi.org/10.1016/S0140-6736(10)61274-3] [PMID: 20801498]

[135] Bhatt DL, Paré G, Eikelboom JW, *et al.* The relationship between CYP2C19 polymorphisms and ischaemic and bleeding outcomes in stable outpatients: the CHARISMA genetics study. Eur Heart J 2012; 33(17): 2143-50. [http://dx.doi.org/10.1093/eurheartj/ehs059] [PMID: 22450429]

[136] Hochholzer W, Trenk D, Fromm MF, *et al.* Impact of cytochrome P450 2C19 loss-of-function polymorphism and of major demographic characteristics on residual platelet function after loading and maintenance treatment with clopidogrel in patients undergoing elective coronary stent placement. J Am Coll Cardiol 2010; 55(22): 2427-34. [http://dx.doi.org/10.1016/j.jacc.2010.02.031] [PMID: 20510210]

[137] Simon T, Verstuyft C, Mary-Krause M, *et al.* Genetic determinants of response to clopidogrel and cardiovascular events. N Engl J Med 2009; 360(4): 363-75. [http://dx.doi.org/10.1056/NEJMoa0808227] [PMID: 19106083]

[138] Harmsze AM, van Werkum JW, Ten Berg JM, *et al.* CYP2C19*2 and CYP2C9*3 alleles are associated with stent thrombosis: a case-control study. Eur Heart J 2010; 31(24): 3046-53. [http://dx.doi.org/10.1093/eurheartj/ehq321] [PMID: 20833683]

[139] Frére C, Cuisset T, Gaborit B, Alessi MC, Hulot JS. The CYP2C19*17 allele is associated with better platelet response to clopidogrel in patients admitted for non-ST acute coronary syndrome. J Thromb Haemost 2009; 7(8): 1409-11. [http://dx.doi.org/10.1111/j.1538-7836.2009.03500.x] [PMID: 19496924]

[140] Paré G, Mehta SR, Yusuf S, *et al.* Effects of CYP2C19 genotype on outcomes of clopidogrel treatment. N Engl J Med 2010; 363(18): 1704-14. [http://dx.doi.org/10.1056/NEJMoa1008410] [PMID: 20979470]

[141] Mega JL, Close SL, Wiviott SD, *et al.* Genetic variants in ABCB1 and CYP2C19 and cardiovascular outcomes after treatment with clopidogrel and prasugrel in the TRITON-TIMI 38 trial: a pharmacogenetic analysis. Lancet 2010; 376(9749): 1312-9. [http://dx.doi.org/10.1016/S0140-6736(10)61273-1] [PMID: 20801494]

[142] Siller-Matula JM, Trenk D, Schrör K, *et al.* Response variability to P2Y12 receptor inhibitors: expectations and reality. JACC Cardiovasc Interv 2013; 6(11): 1111-28. [http://dx.doi.org/10.1016/j.jcin.2013.06.011] [PMID: 24262612]

[143] Sibbing D, Stegherr J, Latz W, *et al.* Cytochrome P450 2C19 loss-of-function polymorphism and stent thrombosis following percutaneous coronary intervention. Eur Heart J 2009; 30(8): 916-22. [http://dx.doi.org/10.1093/eurheartj/ehp041] [PMID: 19193675]

[144] Sibbing D, Koch W, Gebhard D, *et al.* Cytochrome 2C19*17 allelic variant, platelet aggregation, bleeding events, and stent thrombosis in clopidogrel-treated patients with coronary stent placement. Circulation 2010; 121(4): 512-8.

[http://dx.doi.org/10.1161/CIRCULATIONAHA.109.885194] [PMID: 20083681]

[145] Schrör K, Siller-Matula JM, Huber K. Pharmacokinetic basis of the antiplatelet action of prasugrel. Fundam Clin Pharmacol 2012; 26(1): 39-46. [http://dx.doi.org/10.1111/j.1472-8206.2011.00986.x] [PMID: 21895761]

[146] Siller-Matula JM, Jilma B. Ticagrelor: from discovery to Phase III clinical trial. Future Cardiol 2010; 6(6): 753-64. [http://dx.doi.org/10.2217/fca.10.89] [PMID: 21142630]

[147] Hobl EL, Stimpfl T, Ebner J, *et al.* Morphine decreases clopidogrelA concentrations and effects: a randomized, double-blind, placebo-controlled trial. J Am Coll Cardiol 2014; 63(7): 630-5. [http://dx.doi.org/10.1016/j.jacc.2013.10.068] [PMID: 24315907]

[148] Alexopoulos D, Panagiotou A, Xanthopoulou I, *et al.* Antiplatelet effects of prasugrel *vs.* double clopidogrel in patients on hemodialysis and with high on-treatment platelet reactivity. J Thromb Haemost 2011; 9(12): 2379-85. [http://dx.doi.org/10.1111/j.1538-7836.2011.04531.x] [PMID: 21985070]

[149] Alexopoulos D, Xanthopoulou I, Gkizas V, *et al.* Randomized assessment of ticagrelor *versus* prasugrel antiplatelet effects in patients with ST-segment-elevation myocardial infarction. Circ Cardiovasc Interv 2012; 5(6): 797-804. [http://dx.doi.org/10.1161/CIRCINTERVENTIONS.112.972323] [PMID: 23169985]

[150] Bonello L, Camoin-Jau L, Armero S, *et al.* Tailored clopidogrel loading dose according to platelet reactivity monitoring to prevent acute and subacute stent thrombosis. Am J Cardiol 2009; 103(1): 5-10. [http://dx.doi.org/10.1016/j.amjcard.2008.08.048] [PMID: 19101221]

[151] Cook NR. Use and misuse of the receiver operating characteristic curve in risk prediction. Circulation 2007; 115(7): 928-35. [http://dx.doi.org/10.1161/CIRCULATIONAHA.106.672402] [PMID: 17309939]

[152] Price MJ, Angiolillo DJ, Teirstein PS, *et al.* Platelet reactivity and cardiovascular outcomes after percutaneous coronary intervention: a time-dependent analysis of the Gauging Responsiveness with a VerifyNow P2Y12 assay: Impact on Thrombosis and Safety (GRAVITAS) trial. Circulation 2011; 124(10): 1132-7. [http://dx.doi.org/10.1161/CIRCULATIONAHA.111.029165] [PMID: 21875913]

[153] Parodi G, Marcucci R, Valenti R, *et al.* High residual platelet reactivity after clopidogrel loading and long-term cardiovascular events among patients with acute coronary syndromes undergoing PCI. JAMA 2011; 306(11): 1215-23. [http://dx.doi.org/10.1001/jama.2011.1332] [PMID: 21934054]

[154] Siller-Matula JM, Francesconi M, Dechant C, *et al.* Personalized antiplatelet treatment after percutaneous coronary intervention: the MADONNA study. Int J Cardiol 2013; 167(5): 2018-23. [http://dx.doi.org/10.1016/j.ijcard.2012.05.040] [PMID: 22656044]

[155] Trenk D, Stone GW, Gawaz M, *et al.* A randomized trial of prasugrel *versus* clopidogrel in patients with high platelet reactivity on clopidogrel after elective percutaneous coronary intervention with implantation of drug-eluting stents: results of the TRIGGER-PCI (Testing Platelet Reactivity In Patients Undergoing Elective Stent Placement on Clopidogrel to Guide Alternative Therapy With

Prasugrel) study. J Am Coll Cardiol 2012; 59(24): 2159-64.
[http://dx.doi.org/10.1016/j.jacc.2012.02.026] [PMID: 22520250]

[156] Collet JP, Cuisset T, Rangé G, *et al.* Bedside monitoring to adjust antiplatelet therapy for coronary stenting. N Engl J Med 2012; 367(22): 2100-9.
[http://dx.doi.org/10.1056/NEJMoa1209979] [PMID: 23121439]

[157] Gurbel PA, Bliden KP, Antonino MJ, *et al.* The effect of elinogrel on high platelet reactivity during dual antiplatelet therapy and the relation to CYP2C19*2 genotype: first experience in patients. J Thromb Haemost 2010; 8(1): 43-53.
[http://dx.doi.org/10.1111/j.1538-7836.2009.03648.x] [PMID: 19817997]

[158] Woo JS, Kim W, Lee SR, *et al.* Platelet reactivity in patients with chronic kidney disease receiving adjunctive cilostazol compared with a high-maintenance dose of clopidogrel: results of the effect of platelet inhibition according to clopidogrel dose in patients with chronic kidney disease (PIANO-2 CKD) randomized study. Am Heart J 2011; 162(6): 1018-25.
[http://dx.doi.org/10.1016/j.ahj.2011.09.003] [PMID: 22137075]

[159] Capranzano P, Ferreiro JL, Ueno M, *et al.* Pharmacodynamic effects of adjunctive cilostazol therapy in patients with coronary artery disease on dual antiplatelet therapy: impact of high on-treatment platelet reactivity and diabetes mellitus status. Catheter Cardiovasc Interv 2013; 81(1): 42-9.
[http://dx.doi.org/10.1002/ccd.24416] [PMID: 22431415]

[160] Bangalore S, Singh A, Toklu B, *et al.* Efficacy of cilostazol on platelet reactivity and cardiovascular outcomes in patients undergoing percutaneous coronary intervention: insights from a meta-analysis of randomised trials. Open Heart 2014; 1(1): e000068.
[http://dx.doi.org/10.1136/openhrt-2014-000068] [PMID: 25332804]

CHAPTER 2

Evolution of Heart Failure Pharmacotherapy

Gurpreet Sodhi, Ju Kim, Stephen Robie and **Gurusher Panjrath***

Department of Medicine (Cardiology) and Heart and Vascular Institute, The George Washington University School of Medicine and Health Sciences, Washington D.C., USA

Abstract: Heart Failure is a chronic disease with increasing prevalence around the world. It is associated with significant mortality, morbidity, and healthcare costs. Over the past 2-3 decades, major advances in drug development have contributed significantly in decreasing mortality among those with chronic systolic heart failure. However, similar advances are missing in patients experiencing acute heart failure and heart failure with preserved ejection fraction. In the current chapter, we will review the historical development of pharmacotherapy in heart failure medical management. A comparative review of contribution of each class towards reducing mortality will be performed. More importantly, drugs which failed to succeed or impact significantly will be reviewed and an insight on why they may have failed will be provided. Development of new drugs is limited by regulatory requirements as well as disease heterogeneity. New agents under development will be summarized and mode of their action will be detailed. This chapter aims to serve as a comprehensive resource on strategies both past and current as well as provide discussion regarding potential future developments in heart failure pharmacotherapy.

Keywords: ACE inhibitors, Aldosterone antagonists, Beta blockers, BiDil, Diastolic dysfunction, Digoxin, Diuretics, Dobutamine, Heart decompensation, Heart failure, History, Ibopamine, Ivabradine, Milrinone, Natriuretic peptides, Novel therapies, Pharmacology, Statin, Systolic dysfunction, Vasodilator.

* **Corresponding Author Gurusher Panjrath:** Department of Medicine (Cardiology) and Heart and Vascular Institute, The George Washington University School of Medicine and Health Sciences, Washington D.C., USA; Tel: 202-74--2323; Fax: 202-741-2324; E-mail: gpanjrath@mfa.gwu.edu

Atta-ur-Rahman and M. Iqbal Choudhary (Eds.)

INTRODUCTION

The collection of symptoms that are regarded as the syndrome of 'congestive heart failure' have been reported since the era of Hippocrates, who made note of the physical signs of pulmonary congestion: 'When the ear is held to the chest, and one listens for some time, it may be heard to see the inside like the boiling of vinegar' [1]. From the beginning, disordered fluid balance was a key component to the clinical understanding of what would develop into congestive heart failure. As our understanding of heart failure and the complexity of the body's response has evolved, so has the development of pharmacologic treatment. To understand the evolution of therapeutic treatment options, one must appreciate the development of our understanding of the disease itself.

When viewing the progression of heart failure therapeutics retrospectively, one may successfully divide our understanding of the disease etiology into three general models: cardiorenal, cardiocirculatory, and neurohormonal [1]. Of course, these models came into play when it was clear that the heart was indeed the center of pathology. This concept was not entirely clear for several centuries [1]. Until Harvey's revelation regarding circulation, the physiologic function of the heart was not entirely well understood [1, 2]. Thus, the concept of disordered fluid balance, independent of the crucial role played by the heart and the cardiovascular system, with the accompanying symptoms of swelling and shortness of breath, dominated pathophysiologic understanding for several years [1].

As our initial understanding of the disease process focused upon the outward symptomatic manifestations of heart failure, symptomatic relief was focused on the management of anasarca or, as it was so commonly referred to, 'dropsy' [1]. Volume control at any cost was the predominate concentration of treatment. The focus on the volume sequelae of congestive heart failure is a predominant focus of the 'cardiorenal' model of heart failure. Hence, the earliest attempts at pharmacologic therapy would attempt to manipulate this pathophysiologic pathway [1]. Medications were primarily judged on their ability to reduce total body volume. This was often done with no clear understanding of the drugs' true mechanisms of action or effects. Treatments such as foxglove (modern day Digitalis) were uti-lized on the observation of their therapeutic effects with little appreciation for their underlying machinations [2]. Diuretics, in some primitive form or another, were utilized with great frequency. Prior to their advent, reduction in circulating volume, whether *via* diaphoretics, purgatives, or direct blood letting, were commonplace [1, 3]. Some attempts to reduce swelling even went so far as to utilize external mechanical measures such as 'congesting cuffs', the practice of applying tourniquets to the peripheral extremities, in an attempt to capture volume in the periphery and decrease pulmonary pressures [3]. These efforts were not necessarily due to poor scientific approach persay. Indeed, they often made sense given the limited understanding of pathophysiology at the time. However, work clearly needed to be done to move beyond the simplistic external observations that initially drove the cardiorenal era.

The concept of 'dropsy of the chest' came into view during the 17th century [3]. The heart's role was not widely regarded in the syndrome until vivisection became more prevalent and an understanding of structural heart disease developed in the 18th century [1, 3]. A clear differentiation of cardiac and renal etiologies were developed by John Blackall and Richard Bright during this time period [3]. Though there existed primitive manifestations of modern medications such as foxglove, therapies up to the advent of the second world war were frequently of limited therapeutic benefit and had a high index of toxicity [4, 5]. The earliest forms of diuretics had high toxic potential and commonly included the use of organic mercurials [4]. Primitive diuretics provided much needed symptom relief but the natural history and progression of heart failure, their mechanisms and existence not quite characterized at this time, were not impeded by these therapies [1, 3, 4]. As such, researchers continued to search for additional theoretical models that explained not only symptom development, but also disease progression.

In 1833, Bertin was one of the first to note that dilatation 'weakens the contractile power of the muscular substance', but the direct correlation with dropsy remained elusive [1]. Still, this focus on the structural consequences upon the heart in congestive heart failure was tantamount. With the prevalence of rheumatic heart disease and infectious valvulopathies like syphilis, the initial understandings of heart failure pathology were limited largely to structural heart disease [1, 6]. In the first half of the 20th century, nearly three quarters of all heart disease in

England was related to valvular heart disease [6]. This was even more striking in the United States, as nearly 70% of heart disease patients were noted to have a valvular disorder [7 - 9]. As surgical treatments advanced and valvular heart disease began to abate, the development of new pharmacologic techniques from the medical community remained stymied [6]. This was about to dramatically change with the development of advanced technologies that would allow for invasive and non-invasive assessments of cardiac function [1].

The advent of the cardiac catheterization dramatically shifted the comprehension of heart failure and its etiology [1, 10]. Starling had proposed a workable model of cardiac output in 1918, but its implications had yet to be fully appreciated until the demonstration of its effects *via* heart catheterization [1]. With this new technology, it was finally possible to measure internal pressures of the heart while it was functioning within the body. As such, there became an appreciation of hemodynamics. This was the genesis of the 'cardiocirculatory model' of heart failure. Though the augmentation of end-diastolic volume was identified early as a means to augment cardiac output along the Starling curve, the concept of myocardial contractility became a focal point for pharmacologic augmentation [1]. The initial emphasis that the heart operated solely on the descending limb of the Starling curve fell to the wayside as Sarnoff demonstrated multiple variations of Starling's mechanism which represented potentially tenable working states [11]. This variety of working states laid the groundwork for various pharmacologic pathways that may be exploited.

The concept of depressed myocardial contractility in heart failure was not entirely clear prior to the era of modern cardiology. The dilated heart was thought to be subject to loss of mass or working against an obstruction. Given the high prevalence of valvular heart disease, this does not seem overly outlandish. It was also felt to be in a state of energy starvation or a function of geometric retardation brought on by excessive dilatation [1]. The work of Braunwald et al in the 1950's and 60's made clear that a depression of inotropic function in the heart contributed greatly to the clinical deterioration of myocardial function [11, 12]. This discovery occurred parallel to the development of cellular physiology and the role of calcium in the function of myocardial contractility [13]. Thus the research base of the time shifted away from purely symptom control with diuresis and more to the manipulation of hemodynamics *via* the augmentation of forward flow with inotropic agents [11]. Though intuitive appearing, these treatments failed to show appreciable mortality reduction and, much to the surprise of experts, would infrequently increase mortality [1, 11]. It was becoming clear that heart failure in and of itself represented a generalized clinical syndrome involving multiple organ systems and a complex series of maladaptive mechanisms that were not readily apparent or quantifiable at the time. Further research into these mechanisms led to the next great advance in heart failure pharmacotherapeutics [1, 11].

At this point in development, treatments such as diuretics and cardiac glycosides provided symptomatic relief, but little in the way of reduction in adverse outcomes [1]. These tried and true treatments that had existed for centuries were not providing the necessary mortality reductions to alter the overall trajectory of heart failure as a clinical syndrome. The cardiocirculatory model provided the groundwork for the introduction of vasodilator therapies, including ACE inhibitors [14]. Much of the previous hemodynamic medications had focused on pre-load, but physiologic research revealed vasodilators provided the opportunity to reduce afterload, which had the opportunity to increase ejection fraction, decrease diastolic pressures, and improve energetics of the heart [1]. With the advent of invasive monitoring and technologies such as cardiac catheterization, an appreciation for the impact of hemodynamics developed [1]. This led to a movement toward augmentation of various hemodynamic factors such as peripheral vaso-constriction to augment cardiac function. Though treatments targeting renal driven fluid retention and hemodynamic augmentation provided symptom relief, mortality reduction had proved elusive [1, 15].

It had long been known that the body contains numerous homeostatic mechanisms that help to support cardiovascular function in times of duress [17]. It was also known that these mechanisms could, if inappropriately prolonged, add to the stress placed upon the heart [17]. The increase of peripheral vascular resistance and expansion of vascular volume secondary to depressed renal perfusion do well to support overall function in the setting of shock or hemorrhage, but can have dire consequences when inappropriately activated. In the early 1980s, researchers began to quantify the degree to which the sympathetic nervous system (SNS) and, specifically, the renin-angiotensin-aldosterone (RAAS) were activated in the setting of the heart failure syndrome [15 - 17]. The SNS and RAAS became a compelling target for pharmacologic therapy. It was suggested that persistently elevated levels of renin-aldosterone and continuous sympathetic nervous system activation may contribute to short-term benefit, but lead to potentially disastrous remodeling [1]. These suspicions would provide the theoretical basis for what would become the neurohormonal model of heart failure [1, 11, 16]. Additional therapies also began to appear on the horizon. Long thought to be contraindicated in the setting of congestive heart failure, case reports began to circulate showing potential survival benefits from beta blockade therapies [19]. However, their true potential was yet to be explored.

Studies based on this neurohormonal model yielded the first data that showed a mortality benefit with a class of medications. Vasodilators had been disparaged with the results of VHeFT. However, further investigation of vasodilatory agents in the class of ACE inhibitors would provide surprising and welcome results [19, 20]. The CONSENSUS and SOLVD trials both revealed that ACE inhibition had positive effects far beyond that which one would expect from hemodynamic alterations *via* vasodilatation alone could offer [19, 20]. These trials established, for the first time, a true mortality benefit [19, 20]. The further pursuit of this model of heart failure would produce further success in the 1990s and into the 21st century.

With the establishment of ACE inhibition as clearly providing mortality benefit, the potential of beta blockade was further investigated [18]. Beta blockers were initially developed as anti-anginal medications whose proposed mechanism of action was energy conservation through myocardial suppression [21]. To assume that such a medication would potentially be of use in a setting of pre-existing depressed cardiac function required a great leap of faith. However, there had been numerous case reports revealing positive effects of beta blockade medications in this setting [18]. This concept was finally put to the test in the Metoprolol in Dilated Cardiomyopathy (MDC) trial that attempted to establish the long-term benefits of beta blockade in heart failure [22]. Despite the negative hemodynamic effects, the suspected benefits of sympathetic suppression and the suspected prolonged deleterious remodeling effects would prove effective. Following MDS, the cardiac insufficiency bisoprolol study (CIBIS) established beta blockers as a potential mainstay of therapy [23]. Further trials solidified beta blockers as a cornerstone of therapy with ACE inhibitors [1].

Following the success of ACE inhibitors and beta blockers, aldosterone became the next target as it is an integral element of the body's response to cardiovascular insult [1, 11]. Spironolactone, an aldosterone blockade agent, had long been utilized as an anti-hypertensive agent developed in the 1950s. It had fallen out of favor due to a high degree of side-effects related to androgen blockade including gynecomastia and sexual dysfunction [24]. With the revelations of the neurohormonal model; however, interest with this mechanism of action was renewed. A series of clinical trials showed that aldosterone antagonism, in conjunction with ACE inhibition and beta blockade, had added mortality benefit [25 - 27]. With the introduction of eplerenone, the side effect profile that was once prohibitive with the use of spironolactone became less prevalent [27]. With this new addition, the armamentarium of congestive heart failure medications expanded even more.

The advancement of pharmacologic therapies over the course of medical history is varied and fraught with both successes and failures [1]. Heart failure as a clinical entity has proven to be vastly more complex than a simple reduction in heart function. It is a complex, multi-faceted syndrome that involves multiple compensatory mechanisms with both beneficial and devastating effects. The specific targeting of these varied mechanisms has opened the door to additional and further nuanced therapies. As the general understanding of the pathophysiologic models of heart failure as a clinical entity have evolved, so have the therapies at our disposal. For several generations, there were therapies that provided symptomatic relief, but no proven mortality benefit. In the last 30 years, there has been a profound expansion in the number of pharmacologic therapies that provide proven mortality benefit [1]. Though treatment has progressed greatly from modest beginnings, there proves to be opportunity for expansion on the horizon. Heart failure with preserved ejection fraction remains an elusive target with its own peculiarities requiring specialized pharmacologic intervention. Additionally, target cell therapies, potential regenerative treatments, and treatments that attack specific cytokine pathways are in the development at various stages [28]. Heart failure pharmacology will continue to expand as our understanding of the clinical syndrome continues to develop. What follows is a generalized review of the current treatments available for chronic and acute systolic heart failure syndromes, as well as those attributed to heart failure with preserved ejection fraction. An impressive amount of advancement has been made in pharm-acotherapy for heart failure; however a great deal of additional research remains.

CHRONIC SYSTOLIC HEART FAILURE

Heart failure is one of the leading diagnoses in hospitalized patients. It is endemic amongst all age groups and is rapidly rising to affect close to 5.1 million Americans greater than 20 years old. It is projected that by 2030, the prevalence of heart failure will increase by 25% from the 2013 estimates [29]. Similar increases are expected worldwide, though the underlying etiology of heart failure may vary based on geography and genetics. The foundation of pharmacotherapy of chronic systolic heart failure has been neurohormonal antagonism through the inhibition of the renin-angiotensin-aldosterone (RAA) axis and sympathetic nervous system (SNS). In addition, there has been a focus on therapies that target vasoconstriction and impaired nitric oxide metabolism, inflammation, and poor pump function [30].

β-Blockers

Elevated levels of sympathetic activity are central to the progression of chronic systolic heart failure. Elevated levels of norepinephrine saturate beta-receptors, which can be reversed with β-blockers and therefore improve myocardial contractility and chronotropic response. Treatment with β-blockers has also been shown to improve not only left ventricular systolic function but also a patient's symptoms, clinical status, and risk of death and hospitalization [31].

These benefits have been seen across gender and racial lines, with or without comorbidities such as coronary artery disease and diabetes mellitus. There is added benefit if β-blockers are combined with ACE inhibitors. β-blockers should be given to all patients with chronic systolic heart failure, unless there are contraindications or if the patients are not able to tolerate the medication. β-blockers should be started in patients with stable heart failure with reduced ejection fraction (HF*r*EF) - with mild or no symptoms of heart failure.

Table 1. Major trials that studied β-blockers for systolic heart failure patients.

Intervention	Clinical Trial	Patients	Follow-up	Results
Bucindolol *vs.* placebo Dose utilized: 100 mg qd (<75kg) 200 mg qd (>75kg)	BEST [35]	N=1354; NYHA III-IV; EF ≤ 35%	(mean) 2 years	stopped prematurely as it failed to show overall mortality benefit; there was a greater reduction in cardiac mortality in treatment group, but a subgroup analysis did not show benefit in the African American group
Bisoprolol *vs.* placebo Dose utilized: Most common achieved: 10 mg qd	CIBIS II [43]	N=2622; NYHA III-IV; EF ≤ 35%; receiving diuretic and ACE inhibitor; renal impairment	(mean) 1.3 years	stopped prematurely as there was a significant reduction in all-cause mortality
Carvedilol *vs.* placebo Mean dose achieved: 20 mg bid	COPERNICUS [50]	N=2289; NYHAIII-IV; EF ≤ 25%; receiving diuretic and ACE inhibitor; exclusion - ICU patients	(mean) 10.4 years	stopped early due to significant mortality benefit in carvedilol group
Metoprolol XL *vs.* placebo	MERIT-HF [42]	N=3991; NYHA II-IV; EF ≤ 40%; receiving diuretics, ACE inhibitor/ARB, hydralazine, nitrate, and/or digoxin	(mean) 1 year	stopped early as all-cause mortality was lower in metoprolol group

EF = Ejection fraction; NYHA = New York Heart Association; ACE = Angiotensin converting enzyme; ARB = Angiotensin receptor blocker.

Three β-blockers have been studied extensively, and have been shown to have a mortality benefit in stable, chronic HF*r*EF patients - carvedilol, metoprolol succinate, and bisoprolol [32] (Table **1**). Carvedilol and metoprolol tartrate have been shown to have similar hemodynamic profiles, but when compared head to head in the COMET (Carvedilol or Metoprolol European Trial) Trial, carvedilol showed superiority. This trial studied over 3,000 patients with NYHA class II-IV heart failure symptoms and had evidence of chronic systolic heart failure with an ejection fraction < 35% and randomized them to carvedilol or metoprolol tartrate.

After nearly 5 year follow up, there was a significant morality benefit with carvedilol [33]. It should be noted, however, that the predominate trials establishing efficacy of metoprolol utilized the succinate formulation of metoprolol.

Although these three β-blockers have significant impact towards improving the progression of chronic systolic heart failure and reducing mortality, this does not appear to be a class effect. For example, nebivolol is a selective beta-1 blocker that was studied in elderly heart failure patients with impaired and preserved left ventricular ejection fraction in the SENIORS (Study of Effects of Nebivolol Intervention on Outcomes and Rehospitalization in Seniors With Heart Failure) study. This revealed there was no difference in mortality and hospitalizations when nebivolol was administered to elderly patients with impaired ejection fraction (≤35%) and preserved ejection fraction (>35%) [34].

Bucindolol is another non-selective β-antagonist with α-1 blocker properties and mild intrinsic sympatholytic activity that was studied in the BEST (Beta-Blocker Evaluation of Survival Trial). Although this was a large clinical trial of bucindolol in patients with heart failure, it was stopped prematurely as it failed to show overall mortality benefit. The benefits on cardiac mortality and re-hospitalization rates were observed in the trial, but it did not extend to all groups, including African Americans, those with severely reduced ejection fraction, and with patients with NYHA class IV heart failure [35]. There is some retrospective data that suggests atenolol may have utility in chronic systolic heart failure [36]; however, further prospective trials, need to be done to better elucidate the effectiveness of atenolol in chronic systolic heart failure.

The initiation of any of these β-blockers should be at low doses and titrated up depending on the patient's hemodynamics. In general, most patients will tolerate gradual increments in the doses of any of these β-blockers. If adverse effects are seen at any given point, increasing the dose of the β-blocker should be avoided. In some occasions, the β-blocker may need to be discontinued. Although it is not good practice to initiate medications immediately prior to discharge, there is evidence to suggest β-blockers, particularly carvedilol can be safely started prior to discharge [37].

An evidence-based approach should be used during the maintenance therapy of β-blockers. In general, the aim should be to titrate the β-blockers to the target doses studied in the clinical trials [31]. Younger patients and those weighing more than 70 kg may be able to tolerate higher doses. The magnitude of heart rate reduction is more clinically significant than rapid up-titration of the β-blockers to the target doses in clinical trials [38]. This was exemplified in a study that retrospectively evaluated thirty-five trials analyzing all-cause mortality, left ventricular ejection fraction, and heart rates. There was a major contribution of β-blockers towards mortality benefit with reduction of heart rate and not so much achieving a target heart rate. In addition, abrupt withdrawal of β-blockers can have detrimental effects on left ventricular function, left atrial size, and heart rate over a several month period. After re-administration of β-blockers in a small trial in patients with dilated cardiomyopathy, there was a subsequent improvement in ejection fraction [39]. It is possible that long-term treatment with β-blockers can cause an up regulation of ventricular beta-adrenergic receptors which allows a more normal physiological response to sympathetic stimulation.

It is important to monitor for side effects during administration of β-blockers, particularly in the first 30 days following initiation. Common side effects include: worsening heart failure symptoms, profound bradycardia or hypotension, and different degrees of heart block. Even with mild heart failure symptoms, β-blockers should be continued. There are several benefits that can be achieved with the addition of β-blockers to conventional therapy, including reduction of heart rate, long-term physiological adaption towards sympathetic levels, and improvement of left ventricular ejection fraction. Cardiogenic shock requiring inotropic or vasopressor therapy, significant heart block, and/or bradycardia are contraindications to the initiation of β-blockers. Usually, the slowing of heart rate or the development of first-degree heart block is well tolerated. It is important to consider other causes of heart failure that can produce similar side effects. Initiating various heart failure medications at different times of the day or different days of the week to observe a patient's response may be warranted. It can be difficult to ascertain whether the observed effects are secondary to the medications, the patient's heart failure, or to an additional co-morbidity. For example, fatigue experienced by patients with chronic systolic heart failure may be due to medications or the condition itself. It is important to weigh the risk and benefits of the heart failure medications and be attentive to the timing of the medication and its relationship to the development of the potential side effects.

Beta Blockers and Special Populations

There are special populations of heart failure patients that make practitioners hesitant to initiate β-blockers or skeptical whether β-blockers make any difference. For example, several studies have surfaced over the last decade that addressed the role of β-blockers in patients who are elderly, with diabetes, renal disease, or right ventricular dysfunction. Renal failure is a frequent co-morbidity in patients with chronic systolic heart failure. When present, it increases the risk of worse outcomes. β-blocker initiation has a theoretical risk of reducing cardiac output and subsequently decreasing renal blood flow, thereby worsening renal function. There have been trends of decreased prescription rates of β-blockers because of fear of this adverse potential. Several recent retrospective and prospective studies have sought to answer this dilemma [40]. Prior to these studies, the majority of large clinical trials evaluated beta blockers had excluded those patients with significant renal disease. Ito and colleagues studied the effects of metoprolol tartrate and carvedilol on renal function in patients with heart failure and found that β-blockers improve systolic function and either improve or maintain renal function in those with renal dysfunction [41]. Furthermore, two prospective trials (MERIT-HF and CIBIS-II) showed a reduction in 1-year mortality rate in patients with heart failure and renal dysfunction. However, because these studies included patients with both systolic dysfunction and renal dysfunction, it is difficult to differentiate the true impact of β-blockers on clinical outcomes. Post-hoc analyses in each of these two trials showed a reduced risk of hospitalization due to heart failure or combined endpoint of all-cause mortality/ heart failure in patients with stage III chronic kidney disease when compared to patients with normal renal function [42 - 44]. Both renal dysfunction and heart failure are associated with high sympathetic tone. The beneficial impact β-blockers have on these combined co-morbidities may be secondary to reducing this sympathetic activity. Further studies are needed to identify whether an optimal agent and target dose of β-blockers exists that provides the maximum benefit. At this point, it is clear that β-blockers should be administered to patients with chronic systolic heart failure with any degree of renal dysfunction.

Right ventricular dysfunction has become increasingly important in the study of chronic heart failure as it is associated with poor outcomes [45]. The BEST (Beta-Blocker Evaluation of Survival Trial) study is one of the largest clinical prospective trials that examined the effect of β-blockers on low right ventricular ejection fraction. BEST showed a negative impact of bucindolol, in addition to other standard heart failure therapies, on mortality in stable chronic systolic heart failure [46]. Given that the most common cause of right ventricular systolic dysfunction is left ventricular dysfunction, one possible explanation for this is that the combined poor outcomes of right and left ventricular systolic function are too significant for bucindolol, or any β-blocker, to make a significant impact on mortality and outcomes.

It is also possible that the choice of the β-blocker impacts the outcome of patients with right ventricular systolic dysfunction. This was proven in a recent trial performed in Turkey by Tatli and colleagues who studied the effects of carvedilol on right ventricular ejection fraction and inflammatory markers in patients with systolic heart failure. In a small, single center trial, 74 patients were prospectively followed with a left ventricular ejection fraction less than 40%, on standard heart failure treatment randomized to either carvedilol or placebo. Carvedilol clearly had a great improvement in left and right ventricular ejection fraction and added benefit of reduction of inflammation levels [47]. Despite the small number of patients in this study, it speaks to the role of β-blockers, specifically carvedilol, on right ventricular dysfunction. Improvement of left ventricular dysfunction itself may have a large role in improvement of right ventricular function. These effects are explained by the reduction in pulmonary capillary wedge pressure leading to reduced right ventricular afterload, which in turn would improve right ventricular function. The study also showed a reduction in TNF-alpha and IL-6 levels. Larger trials are needed to corroborate these findings, though it is clear that carvedilol may have a positive impact on right ventricular and left ventricular dysfunction.

Many trials do not address elderly patients with chronic systolic heart failure. As therapies have improved, the prevalence of heart failure among elderly populations has steadily increased. As a result, further studies into the effects of commonly utilized therapies in this population has become essential. In general, standard therapies for chronic systolic heart failure patients need to be started more gradually than if started in younger patients. More vigilance for side effects needs to be taken for therapies in elderly patients. Clinical data on β-blockers as well as other therapies in chronic systolic heart failure in elderly patients are limited as most trials excluded patients over the age of 65 years. As supported in the ACC/AHA guidelines, these agents should used with clinical judgment in all elderly patients. Future trials should focus on the effects of guideline directed medical therapy on patients greater than 65 years old to delineate its impact on morbidity and mortality [48]. There is one prospective, randomized control trial which studied nebivolol and its impact on outcomes and re-hospitalization in seniors with heart failure (SENIORS). This study showed that nebivolol reduced the risk of all-cause mortality or admission rates in elderly patients (age greater than 70) with heart failure and reduced left ventricular ejection fraction [49]. The majority of elderly patients will tolerate the effects of β-blockers, but only at approximately half the target dose achieved in major trials. Regardless, elderly patients tend to tolerate the effects of β-blockers, and therefore should not be denied this therapy.

Diabetes is a common co-morbid condition associated with systolic heart failure and is associated with worse outcomes. Only a paucity of studies had sought to define the mortality benefits of β-blockers in diabetics with chronic systolic heart failure until a meta-analysis in 2003 sought to answer this question. Trials that included more than 100 patients were in the analysis, including the ANZ-Carvedilol, BEST, Carvedilol-US Trials, CIBIS-II, COPERNICUS, and MERIT-HF trials. It appears there is mortality benefit with the treatment of β-blockers in diabetic heart failure patients, including diastolic and chronic systolic heart failure patients. However, the benefit is not as substantial as seen in those without diabetes [50]. However, the benefit of metoprolol succinate in chronic systolic heart failure patients extends to the subgroup of diabetics as well. In addition, analysis of combined data from the CIBIS-II, MERIT-HF, and COPERNICUS trials showed no evidence of increased risks of hypo- and hyperglycemia commonly thought to be associated with the use of β-blockers [51]. Therefore, β-blockers should not be withheld in those with diabetes and chronic systolic heart failure.

Controversies exist regarding the impact of β-blockers on outcomes between men and women. There are no large clinical trials to date addressing this question; however, one single center prospective trial that included approximately 600 patients with chronic systolic heart failure showed no gender difference on survival. A significant limitation of this study was that more men had ischemic cardiomyopathy and there was not an equal balance of women and men enrolled in the study [52]. Future trials should be conducted on a larger scale with a better balance of women and men to answer this question.

At times, chronic systolic heart failure patients may exhibit physical exam signs of poor perfusion to the extremities. Peripheral vasoconstriction is the assumed physiological response in a patient who has a compromised cardiac output. Concern exists that with the use of β-blockers, critical limb ischemia may develop due to β_2 blockage. Therefore, using β_1 selective agents in heart patients, who also suffer from severe peripheral vascular disease, is advised. Alternatively, agents such as carvedilol can also be used given its α_1 blocking effects. The use of specific β-blockers will help the patients tolerate claudication better as well treat their underlying chronic heart failure.

There is clear evidence showing significant mortality benefit with β-blockers in patients with chronic systolic heart failure. Either carvedilol or metoprolol succinate are preferred agents and the choice of one over another may depend on other factors such as their relative effect on blood pressure and heart rate. Metoprolol succinate offers the advantage of once daily dosing and is recommended for heart failure treatment by the American College of Cardiology, American Heart Association, and European Society of Intensive Care Medicine [31]. Metoprolol tartrate is not US Food and Drug Administration (FDA) approved for chronic systolic heart failure. Furthermore, it is the succinate formulation, rather than the tartrate formulation, that has been studied in trials showing mortality benefit. When starting and titrating β-blockers, the initial doses should be low and increased slowly, especially in elderly patients [32]. It is important to educate the patient and continue to monitor for side effects. Side effects are mostly well tolerated and more recent evidence suggests the benefits often outweigh the risks. In fact, approximately one-third of COPD patients have heart failure. Recent evidence suggests that COPD and asthma patients can tolerate cardio-selective β-blockers. Even in less severe pulmonary disease, most patients can tolerate non-selective β-blockers [53].

Angiotensin-Converting Enzyme (ACE) Inhibitors/Angiotensin Receptor Blockers (ARBs)

In chronic systolic heart failure, the renin angiotensin aldosterone system (RAAS) system is overactive, leading to pathological results. In the early stages of chronic systolic heart failure, the role of the RAAS system is to maintain hemodynamic stability. This is through up-regulation of ACE (angiotensin converting enzyme) and conversion of angiotensin I to angiotensin II, a potent vasoconstrictor that leads to salt retention, and downstream neurohormonal activation. Long-term consequences of continuous activation include worsening heart failure symptoms, increased blood pressure, cardiac fibrosis, and left ventricular hypertrophy. In addition, ACE causes degradation of potent vasodilators bradykinin and substance P [54]. Over time, the cycle continues and worsens the progression of chronic systolic heart failure. In addition, hypertension ensues, increasing afterload and hindering any chance of improvement of left ventricular dysfunction. With long-standing chronic systolic failure, renal dysfunction also ensues. Inhibition of ACE can halt this cycle, help remodel the left ventricle, improve cardiac output, induce vasodilation to relieve hypertension, and help promote natriuresis [55]. There have been many clinical trials in the last two decades that have shown ACE inhibitors significantly decrease mortality, myocardial infarction, and hospitalizations in heart failure [54]. Despite maximal doses of ACE inhibitors in the treatment of chronic systolic heart failure, studies have suggested angiotensin II is also produced through non-ACE dependent pathways. As a consequence, over the last decade, angiotensin II receptor blockers (ARBs) have been studied both in conjunction with and in comparison with ACE inhibitors to evaluate the effects on outcomes in chronic systolic heart failure [56].

Various heart failure guidelines around the world recommend ACE inhibitors for patients with chronic systolic heart failure, unless contraindicated, due to its clear contribution to morbidity and mortality reduction. ARBs are recommended as an alternative if ACE inhibitors can not be tolerated [31]. The benefits of ACE inhibitors have been seen in both symptomatic as well as asymptomatic chronic systolic heart failure, regardless of whether coronary artery disease was present. ACE inhibitors are recommended in combination with β-blockers as they provide incremental benefit on reduction of all-cause and cardiovascular mortality. In patients who have more than mild heart failure symptoms, it may be prudent to start an ACE inhibitor or ARB first. Once the patient approaches euvolemic clinical status, β-blockers may then be added.

The results from large clinical trials over the last two decades have clearly shown a large benefit of ACE inhibitors towards long term and short term morbidity and mortality in the treatment of asymptomatic and symptomatic patients with left ventricular systolic dysfunction from either ischemic or non-ischemic etiology [54]. The CONSENSUS (Cooperative North Scandinavian EnaLapril Survival Study) trial evaluated enalapril in patients with significant heart failure symptoms. A significant mortality benefit was observed with enalapril when compared to placebo. Enalapril also showed two other added benefits of improving NYHA functional class and halting the progression of left ventricular dysfunction [57]. These findings support the short-term benefits over a six month period. At the end of the trial, the patients were offered open-label enalapril, and were followed for an additional 10 years. A 30% mortality risk reduction was found, which affirmed the long-term benefit of ACE inhibitors [58]. The SOLVD (Studies of Left Ventricular Dysfunction) Prevention Trial studied the effects of enalapril on asymptomatic patients with left ventricular ejection fraction ≤35%. This three-year trial demonstrated a reduction in heart failure symptoms and hospitalizations for heart failure [59]. SOLVD-TREATMENT sought to establish the effects of enalapril on similar patients, but with symptoms of heart failure and demonstrated a 16% reduction in mortality and a 26% reduction in combined endpoint of death and hospitalization in heart failure [60]. An extension of the trial to evaluate the decade long benefits of enalapril in X-SOLVD, which included 6784 patients over 12 years, resulted in enalapril continuing to display a sustained, significant reduction in all-cause mortality compared to placebo [61].

Additional long-term clinical trials have demonstrated similar benefits of ACE inhibitors in systolic heart failure associated with acute coronary syndrome. The AIREX (Acute Infarction Ramipril Efficacy study eXtension) was notable for a 36% mortality reduction after three years in patients with clinical heart failure after an acute myocardial infarction [62]. The ACE-inhibitor Myocardial Infarction Collaborative Group prospectively evaluated the results of three post-infarction trials in patients with left ventricular dysfunction. The combined results of these trials after three years showed a significant reduction in mortality, readmission rates for heart failure, reinfarction, or the composite of these events [63].

As opposed to β-blockers, there is no data to suggest individual differences amongst specific types of ACE inhibitors [64]. ACE inhibitors should be started at low doses and titrated up as tolerated. A repeat serum chemistry panel within the 2 weeks of therapy initiation is indicated to monitor serum potassium and creatinine levels in particular. It is common to encounter patients who will not tolerate doses of ACE inhibitors at target doses identified in the clinical trials. This is often due to hypotension [65]. If hypotension is encountered, adjustment of concurrent medications, such as diuretics, should be made in an attempt to achieve target doses of beta blockers and ACE inhibitors given the established mortality benefits. Health care professionals frequently face the dilemma of which agents to start first, which should be increased first, or which should be decreased first if there is significant hypotension [66]. To date, there are no good guidelines or clinical trials that address these questions. However, combined administrations of multiple classes of systolic heart failure drugs are likely to improve survival. With regards to ACE inhibitors, every attempt should be made to titrate the ACE inhibitors to the target doses studied in the clinical trials [31] (Table **2**). It is important not to abruptly discontinue ACE inhibitors, as patients may encounter withdrawal effects, including hypertension [31].

Important side effects of ACE inhibitors include acute kidney injury, cough, angioedema, rash, and hyperkalemia. Renal disease as mentioned is a common comorbidity seen in patients with chronic systolic heart failure, especially in the elderly population. The role of ACE inhibitors or ARBs was studied in 1046 patients (age ≥65 years) with systolic heart failure (ejection fraction <45%) and chronic kidney disease (eGFR < 60 ml/min/1.73 m^2). After 8 years of follow-up, there was a modest reduction in all-cause mortality associated with ACE inhibitor or ARB use, including with those with advanced chronic kidney disease [67]. Careful monitoring of volume status may prevent the development of acute kidney injury. The pathogenesis of ACE inhibitor-related angioedema is partly due to low plasma amion-peptidase P. The pathogenesis of ACE inhibitor-related cough is possibly mediated *via* bradykinin and substance P stimulation, which increases vasopermeability. Furthermore, a systemic review and meta-analysis showed one gene region (XPNPEP2) was associated with ACE inhibitor-induced angioedema. There was no association found between ACE insertion/deletion polymorphism and ACE inhibitor-related cough [68]. A rare side effect of this class of drugs is the development of a rash. A case series published in 2013 described an eczematous reaction. The authors described a latent period of 4-30 months and these rashes were associated with moderate-severe itch, usually with no response to antihistamines [68].

Table 2. Major trials that studied ACE (angiotensin-converting enzyme) inhibitors for systolic heart failure patients.

Intervention	Clinical Trial	Patients	Follow-up	Results
Enalapril (uptitrated to 20mg bid if tolerated) *vs.* placebo	CONSENSUS [57]	N=253; NYHA IV; mean age 71y; clinical diagnosis of severe HF	(mean) 6 months	Significant reduction in mortality at 6 months in treatment group
Enalapril (uptitrated to 20mg daily if tolerated) *vs.* placebo	SOLVD prevention [59]	N=2111; mean age 59.1y; mean EF 28%; NYHA I-II; receiving diuretics, nitrates, and/or digoxin	(mean) 37.4 months	Significant reduction in HF and HF related hospitalizations; non-significant trend towards fewer deaths due to CV causes in treatment group
Enalapril (uptitrated to 40mg daily if tolerated) *vs.* placebo	SOLVD treatment [60]	N=253; mean age 70y; NYHA II-III; EF $\leq$ 35%; receiving vasodilators, digoxin, anti-arrhythmics, antiplatelets, and/or diuretics	(mean) 41.4 months	Significant reduction in mortality and HF hospitalizations in treatment group
Ramipril (uptitrated to 10mg daily if tolerated) *vs.* placebo	AIRE [62]	N=2006; mean age 65y; recent MI; NYHA IV	(mean) 15 months	Mortality from all causes was significantly lower for patients randomized to receive ramipril

EF = Ejection fraction; NYHA = New York Heart Association; HF = Heart Failure; CV = Cardiovascular; MI = Myocardial infarction.

If patients develop ACE inhibitor-related cough, ARBs can be considered as an alternative. There is concern those with a prior ACE-induced angioedema episode may develop angioedema with the use of ARBs. Although this is a possibility, caution should be taken with careful monitoring for signs of angioedema. There is a hypothetical cross-reactivity, but no substantial studies have demonstrated the degree to which this is true. It is also reasonable to consider ARBs as a first line therapy for patients with left ventricular systolic dysfunction, especially if patients are already taking ARBs for hypertension [31]. The development of ARBs occurred because it was thought angiotensin II continued to be produced through non-ACE pathways, even while patients are on ACE inhibitors. Research turned towards blocking the effects of angiotensin II. Later, it became clear the benefits ACE inhibitors provided were due to kinin level elevations rather than decreasing levels of angiotensin II.

Several trials have evaluated the benefit of ARBs, including reduced hospitalizations and mortality (Table **3**). Two meta-analysis have been performed which compared ACE inhibitors *versus* angiotensin receptor antagonists in heart failure patients with left ventricular systolic dysfunction [54]. The RESOLVD (Randomized Evaluation of Strategies of for Left Ventricular Dysfunction) was a prospective study that compared candesartan with enalapril in heart failure patients with NYHA class II-IV symptoms and left ventricular ejection fraction of <40%, and a six minute walk test (6MWD) < 500m. The trial demonstrated, after close to four years, that there was no difference in any of these cardiovascular outcomes. However, the trial was not powered to detect difference in survival [69]. The ELITE (Evaluation of Losartan in The Elderly) study was a 4 year study that investigated 722 HF patients over the age of 65 years with either losartan or captopril. There were similar outcomes in terms of renal failure, HF hospitalizations, NYHA functional class, but there was a 46% mortality rate reduction with losartan compared with captopril in the secondary outcomes [70]. ELITE II, which evaluated all-cause mortality in 3152 elderly HF patients with similar characteristics, demonstrated no difference in mortality between ACE inhibitors or ARBs, which attests to ARBs as a reasonable alternative to ACE inhibitors if limited by ACE inhibitor side effects [71].

Table 3. Major clinical trials comparing ACE (angiotensin converting enzyme) inhibitors and ARBs (angiotensin receptor blockers).

Intervention	Clinical Trial	Patients	Follow-up	Results
Candesartan (4,8, or 16mg) *vs.* Enalapril (20mg) *vs.* Combination (Enalapril 20mg/Candesartan 4 or 8mg)	RESOLVD [69]	N=768; mean age 63y; EF < 40%; NYHA II-IV	mean 43 weeks	No change in 6MWD, NYHA functional class, EF, or QOL with enalapril compared to candesartan alone
Losartan (uptitrated to 50mg daily as tolerated) *vs.* captopril (uptitrated to 50mg tid as tolerated)	ELITE [70]	N=722; mean age 73y; EF < 40%; NYHA II-IV; 6MWD < 500m	mean 48 weeks	A small reduction in mortality in losartan group *vs.* captopril; no difference in renal function and improvement in NYHA functional class is similar between groups
Losartan (uptitrated to 50mg daily as tolerated) *vs.* captopril (uptitrated to 50mg tid as tolerated)	ELITE II [71]	N=3152; mean age 71y; EF < 40%; NYHA II-IV	(median) 555 days	No significant differences in all-cause mortality or sudden death or resuscitated arrests between groups
Candesartan 32mg *vs.* placebo	CHARM-Added [72]	N=4576; mean age 64y; EF ≤40%; NYHA II-IV	mean 41 months	A small reduction in CV mortality and HF hospitalizations
Losartan 50mg daily *vs.* Captopril 50mg tid	OPTIMAAL [74]	N=5477; mean age 67y; early post-MI; signs/symptoms of HF and/or EF ≤35% or LVEDD > 65mm	mean 2.7 years	Non-significant difference in total mortality favoring captopril
Valsartan 320mg daily *vs.* Valsartan 160mg daily + Captopril 150mg daily *vs.* Captropril 150mg daily	VALIANT [75]	N= 14,703; mean age 64.8y; early post-MI; signs/symptoms of HF and/or EF ≤ 35%	(median) 24.7 months	No difference in all-cause mortality between the three groups

6MWD = 6 minute walk distance; NYHA = New York Heart Association; QOL = Quality of Life; EF = Ejection fraction; TID = Three times daily; CV = Cardiovascular.

It may be intuitive to combine ARBs and ACE inhibitors for the treatment of chronic systolic heart failure, as ARBs would target blockage of angiotensin II [54]. However, two clinical trials - Val-HeFT (VALsartan HEart Failure Trial) and CHARM (Candesartan in Heart Failure: Assessment of Reduction in Mortality and morbidity)-Added trial - showed the combination of an ACE inhibitor and an ARB was no more effective than an ACE inhibitor itself, especially on all-cause mortality. However, there was a significant reduction in the number of heart failure hospitalizations with the combination of an ACE inhibitor and ARB [72, 73]. Patients who are in the post-myocardial infarction setting usually receive an ACE inhibitor for mortality benefit. Studies, such as OPTI-MAAL (OPtimal Trial in Myocardial infarction with the Angiotensin II An-tagonist Losartan) and VALIANT (VALsartan in Acute myocardial iNfarction Trial), were designed as non-inferiority trials that evaluated the combination of an ARB and ACE inhibitor in systolic heart failure patients after myocardial infarction. The combination had more drug-related adverse effects, and no diff-erence in the primary outcome of all-cause mortality [74, 75].

The combination of neprilysin inhibitor with ARB was examined in the recent PARADIGM-HF (Prospective Comparison of ARNI [Angiotensin Receptor – Neprilysin Inhibitor] with ACEI to Determine Impact on Global Mortality and Morbidity in Heart Failure Trial). The investigators studied LCZ696, which is a fixed-dose combination of valsartan and AHU-377 (a neprilysin inhibitor pro-drug), to a target-dosed enalapril-based regimen. The study was remarkable for significant reduction in cardiovascular morbidity and mortality with use of LCZ696. The trial included NYHA class II-IV chronic systolic heart failure (ejection fraction < 40%) patients who were on optimal medical therapy. PARA-DIGM-HF offered a novel pharmacotherapy that has the potential to be an adjunct to the standard chronic systolic heart failure regimen. Furthermore, the trial may be applicable to a wide spectrum of patients [76]. If results hold true in sub-sequent studies, this novel approach may be the first new drug in over more than a decade to result in reduction in mortality in chronic heart failure population.

Diuretics

Several different diuretics are commonly used to treat patients with congestive heart failure as they rapidly decrease the congestive symptoms of heart failure and control fluid retention. Diuretics are the most commonly prescribed drugs for heart failure. When first introduced decades ago, diurctics allowed physicians to quickly treat fluid retention [77]. Diuretics have since become a standard part of the management of patients with congestive heart failure, despite the relative paucity of research studies and clinical trials on their effects and benefits. Although diuretics have not been shown to improve survival in patients with heart failure, smaller clinical trials have been performed on their risks and benefits [78]. Despite that, diuretics are a mainstay in the armamentarium of drugs for management of heart failure.

In the current era of heart failure therapy, diuretics are often used in combination with ACE inhibitors and B-blockers for symptom control. ACE inhibitors alone are unable to alter urinary sodium excretion because the shift in renal function is offset by the reduction in blood pressure. Odemuyiwa *et al.* demonstrated that diuretic requirements did not decline after the addition of ACE inhibitors in patients with stable heart failure symptoms [79]. Furthermore, diuretics have been shown to decrease the risk of heart failure in patients with hypertension [80, 81].

Diuretics improve the symptoms of congestive heart failure by producing hemodynamic changes and acting as vasodilators [82]. They reduce right atrial and pulmonary capillary wedge pressures quickly when administered intravenously. These initial improvements in hemodynamics may be secondary to the release of vasodilatory prostaglandins [83]. Studies have shown that loop diuretics, such as furosemide, directly dilate veins which can be inhibited by indomethacin, implying that local prostaglandins may contribute to its vasodilatory properties [84]. Diuretics stimulate renin secretion by inhibiting NaCl uptake into macula densa cells. Sodium chloride uptake *via* the Na^+-K^+-Cl^- cotransport system is a central component of the macula densa-mediated pathway for renin secretion. This leads to a volume independent increase in angiotensin II and aldosterone secretion. Further, diuretics also stimulate renal production of prostacyclin, which enhances renin secretion. Diuretics can also increase renin secretion by contracting the extra cellular fluid (ECF) volume [85]. Apart from furosemide acting at the loop of Henle, other diuretics inhibit the reabsorption of sodium or chloride at different sites along the nephron. Loop diuretics, such as furosemide, have been a preferred agent for diuresis in heart failure patients.

Torsemide has been shown to have less variation in bioavailability and a longer duration of action when compared to furosemide. A systematic review and meta-analysis of randomized controlled trials comparing torsemide *versus* furosemide in patients with systolic heart failure was performed. Two randomized trials in 471 patients with systolic heart failure were reviewed. Compared to furosemide, torsemide had a statistically significant reduction of total heart failure and cardiovascular readmissions. In addition, torsemide caused a 14% reduction in all-cause mortality [86]. Growing evidence demonstrates more favorable pharmacokinetic profiles of torsemide and bumetanide compared to furosemide. Not only has torsemide been shown to be more efficacious, but also safer. A prospective head-to-head trial comparing furosemide *versus* torsemide *versus* bumetanide has not been performed. Currently furosemide is recommended as first line loop diuretic for its easy accessibility and favorable cost profile compared to torsemide. Ethacrynic acid is another loop diuretic that is usually reserved for patients who experience a serious hypersensitivity reaction to the sulfa moiety as ethacrynic acid does not contain the sulfonamide component like the other loop diuretics. It is usually reserved after other loop diuretics have been used because of its high ototoxic potential [87].

Diuretic doses must be titrated based on the signs or symptoms of congestion. However, when patients become unresponsive to higher loop diuretic doses, it is important to identify factors attributable to the recurrence of fluid retention [31]. For example, a high salt diet or NSAID (nonsteroidal anti-inflammatory drugs) use can blunt the effects of loop diuretics, especially if poor renal perfusion exists [88]. Thus, limiting sodium intake or removing offending agents that inhibit the loop diuretic response will help while evaluating for alternative diagnoses as appropriate.

There is limited data suggesting low dose dopamine infusion in addition to loop diuretics may augment diuretic response; however, in most cases this is not effective [89]. If higher doses of loop diuretics are ineffective, a second diuretic, such as a thiazide, is added to improve the diuretic response [90]. For example, metolazone is commonly administered in conjunction with furosemide to augment the diuresis. Metolazone is characterized by a slow and erratic absorption, a large volume of distribution, and has a high renal clearance. These properties of metolazone in combination with a loop diuretic allow a strong diuretic effect, especially in those with chronic renal insufficiency [91]. Metolazone also has a long half-life. Therefore, it is imperative to closely monitor the net diuresis effect during its use to prevent adverse effects of overaggressive diuresis.

Thiazide diuretics are often prescribed for hypertensive patients with mild fluid retention. The ALLHAT (Anti-hypertensive and Lipid-Lowering Treatment to Prevent Heart Attack Trial) study showed lower rates of heart failure in the those treated with chlorthalidone compared to the three other antihypertensive medications (*e.g.* amlodipine, lisinopril, and doxazosin) [92]. Several arguments have been proposed to explain these findings. First, most of the patients were taking anti-hypertensive agents prior to the start of the trial, and the withdrawal of these agents may have been sufficient enough to unmask heart failure. Second, chlorthalidone was able to demonstrate a larger reduction of systolic blood pressure than the three other agents. It is known in high-risk hypertensive patients, higher systolic blood pressure is associated with higher rates of heart failure [93]. Hydro-chlorothiazide is another commonly prescribed anti-hypertensive drug that has a mild diuretic effect. Remote studies have tried to deteremine whether hydrochlorothiazide has a robust diuretic effect or an equivalent cardiac remodeling effect as spironolactone in patients who have myocardial infarction-induced congestive heart failure [94, 95]. However, these studies are too small to provide any meaningful contribution. Nevertheless, there are no prospective long term studies evaluating the mortality benefit of hydrochlorothiazide use in chronic systolic heart failure.

Table 4. Key side effects from diuretics.

Complications	Recommendations
Electrolyte abnormalities	Serial monitoring of chemistries when actively adjusting doses
Hyponatremia	Monitor volume status and daily weights
Azotemia	Monitor for medication cross-interaction
Ototoxicity	Limit rapid bolus of diuretics and limit rate of furosemide infusion to less than 240mg/day
Arrhythmias	Keep serum potassium close to 4 mmol/L and magnesium close to 2 mEq/L

The main adverse effects of diuretics are electrolyte disturbance and volume depletion that can lead to acute kidney injury and hypotension (Table **4**). Hypokalemia and hypomagnesemia are the major electrolyte disturbances. If the magnitude of electrolyte depletion is severe or rapid, cardiac arrhythmias may occur. The combination of multiple diuretics or other heart failure medications increases the risk of electrolyte disturbances and hypotension even further, though ACE inhibition may counteract the natural potassium depleting effects of loop diuretics. It is reasonable to add potassium and magnesium repletion strategies to reduce the risk of dangerous electrolyte abnormalities. Frequent serial assessments of serum chemistries are indicated in this situation.

A diuretic is the first recommended agent for patients with signs and symptoms of fluid retention as it provides the most rapid improvements in symptoms. When patients have mild to moderate severe heart failure or renal insufficiency, a loop diuretic is recommended. Addition of a thiazide diuretic may be necessary if high dose loop diuretics prove insufficient. However, there is limited data suggesting a true mortality benefit with diuretics. Diuretics should be utilized and adjusted for symptomatic relief, but should always be used in concert with mortality-reducing medications such as β-blockers, ACE inhibitors, and aldosterone antagonists.

Aldosterone Antagonists

The renin-angiotensin-aldosterone system (RAAS) is crucial in the pathogenesis of chronic heart failure. Neurohormonal activation of this system is thought to significantly contribute to left ventricular remodeling and eventual systolic dysfunction. ACE inhibitors carry a class I indication for chronic systolic heart failure, regardless of symptoms. Although ACE inhibitors help reduce the production of aldosterone, there are other non-RAAS dependent sources of aldosterone, such as the adrenal glands. Aldosterone antagonism blunts the detrimental effects of this neurohormonal activation. Aldosterone antagonists, such as spironolactone and eplerenone, have been studied extensively in several landmark trials - RALES, EPHESUS, and EMPHASIS-HF [25 - 27] (Table **5**). The two major benefits of aldosterone antagonism in chronic heart failure include reduced risk of arrhythmia attributable to higher potassium levels and reduction in LV remodeling and fibrosis [96].

These three trials demonstrated several morbidity and mortality benefits of aldosterone antagonists. The RALES trial examined the role of spironolactone in 1663 patients with systolic heart failure, NYHA class III-IV, with a mean left ventricular ejection fraction of 25%. Most of the patients were taking an ACE inhibitor; however, only 11% were on a β-blocker. RALES showed reductions in deaths due to heart failure, sudden cardiac death, and heart failure hospitalizations [25]. EPHESUS randomized 6642 systolic heart failure patients who are post-MI and with a mean ejection fraction ≤40% to eplerenone *versus* placebo. At 16 months, there was a modest reduction in cardiovascular deaths and heart failure hospitalizations [97]. The EMPHASIS-HF trial, though similar in design to RALES, focused on patients with NYHA II symptoms. In EMPHASIS-HF, 2737 patients with left ventricular ejection fraction ≤35%, elevated B-type natriuretic peptide (BNP) or recent heart failure hospitalization were followed for 1.8 years (median). As in EPHESUS, close to 90% of patients in EMPHASIS-HF were on an ACE inhibitor and β-blocker [27]. These three landmark trials demonstrated a clear indication for spironolactone and eplerenone in the setting of systolic heart failure. The ACCF/AHA 2013 heart failure guidelines have assigned a class I indication for the addition of spironolactone or eplerenone for all patients with NYHA II-IV systolic heart failure who are already on ACE inhibitor and β-blockers to reduce morbidity and mortality [31].

Table 5. Major clinical trials of aldosterone antagonists.

Intervention	Clinical Trial	Patients	Follow-up	Results
Spironolactone 25-50mg daily *vs.* placebo	RALES [25]	N=1663, NYHA class III-IV, EF ≤ 35%, on ACE inhibitor	mean 2 years	Significant reduction in all-cause mortality in spironolactone group
Eplerenone 25-50mg daily *vs.* placebo	EPHESUS [26]	N=6632, acute MI complicated by LVSD and HF	mean 1.3 years	Significant reduction of death from any cause or hospitalization from any cause in treatment group
Eplerenone up to 50mg daily *vs.* placebo	EMPHASIS [27]	N=2737, NYHA class II, EF ≤ 35%	mean 1.8 years	Significant reduction in composite endpoint of death from CV causes or HF hospitalizations in treatment group

EF = Ejection fraction; NYHA = New York Heart Association; MI = Myocardial infarction; LVSD = Left ventricular systolic dysfunction; ACE = Angiotensin converting enzyme; HF = Heart Failure; CV = Cardiovascular.

It is important to understand that all three trials excluded patients with a serum creatinine >2.5 mg/dL in men or >2 mg/dL in women or glomerular filtration rate <30 ml/min/1.73 m^2 and/or hyperkalemia (>5 mmol/L) [95]. The majority of patients (95% of patients) had a creatinine ≤1.7 mg/dL. Therefore, it is no surprise that hyperkalemia was a major side effect in these patients. Initiation of spironolactone or eplerenone should only be done in patients with an initial serum creatinine <2.5 mg/dL or glomerular filtration rate >30 ml/min/1.73 m^2. In addition, a patient with history of hyperkalemia (>5.0 mEq/L) should be monitored carefully. Furthermore, concomitant use of an ACE inhibitor with spironolactone increases the risk of hyperkalemia. The ACCF/AHA 2013 guidelines suggest starting with an initial dose of spironolactone 12.5mg daily or eplerenone 25mg daily with increases to targets of spironolactone 25mg or eplerenone 50mg daily as renal function and serum potassium levels allow. Alternatively, patients with concerns for hyperkalemia or borderline renal function, every-other-day dosing of spironolactone or eplerenone can be considered [31, 96]. There is no efficacy difference between spironolactone or eplerenone; however, the RALES trial showed a 10% incidence of gynecomastia due to spironolactone because of its nonselective antagonist properties [25]. In EPHESUS and EMPHASIS-HF, this effect was negligible (<1%) with the use of eplerenone because of its selective aldosterone antagonism properties [25, 27].

Digoxin

Digoxin has long been a mainstay of therapy in the setting of congestive heart failure. It was first introduced in the 19th century and had been used for symptomatic relief. Digitalis exerts its positive inotropic effect by increasing the availability of intracellular calcium by binding to the Na^+/K^+ ATPase and inhibiting its activity. Inhibition of the Na^+/K^+ ATPase leads to a reduced transmembrane sodium gradient, decreasing the activity of the Na^+/Ca^{++} exchanger. The resulting increased intracellular Na+ concentration in turn increases intracellular Ca^{2+} stores [196, 197].

However, it was not until relatively recently that its efficacy was evaluated in detail [1]. The Digitalis Investigation Group (DIG) studied ambulatory patients with chronic systolic heart failure and discovered digoxin reduces 30 day all-cause hospital admissions. This trial was conducted during a time when chronic systolic heart failure patients were being treated with ACE inhibitors and diuretics only [98]. The DIG trial was a randomized, double-blind, placebo-controlled trial designed to evaluate the effect of digoxin added to diuretics and ACE inhibitors on mortality from any cause and hospitalization for heart failure in patients with heart failure (EF less than 45%) and normal sinus rhythm over a three-to-five year follow up [198]. There had been additional prior studies that similarly examined the combined effects of digoxin, ACE inhibitors, and diuretics. Although the PROVED (Prospective Randomized Study of Ventricular Function and Efficacy of Digoxin) and RADIANCE (Randomized Assessment of Digoxin and Inhibitors of Angiotensin-Converting Enzyme) trials were not randomized trials, they shed light onto digoxin's efficacy in heart failure. These trials collected data on different therapeutic combinations and observed effects on exercise capacity, heart failure symptoms, and left ventricular function. Young *et al.* described the optimal overall combination as ACE inhibitors, diuretics, and digoxin. The group managed only with diuretics had the worst outcomes in terms of heart failure symptoms and exercise capacity [99].

The Digitalis Investigation Group (DIG) randomized trial showed that digoxin had no mortality benefit despite its reduction in hospitalizations for worsening heart failure compared to placebo, consistent with the findings in PROVED and RADIANCE trials. Digoxin use in elderly patients over the age of 65 with systolic heart failure also showed a significant reduction in all-cause hospital admissions. Digoxin should not be abruptly withdrawn from the medication regimen as its withdrawal from clinically stable chronic systolic heart failure patients taking ACE inhibitors and diuretics worsened functional capacity and quality of life outcomes [100].

Despite these studies, there are no randomized trials that clearly establish the role of digoxin in combination with ACE inhibitors, β-blockers, diuretics amongst chronic systolic heart failure patients, particularly if there is no concomitant atrial fibrillation. Regardless, several professional societies have issued clinical guidelines recommending the adjunctive use of digoxin in persistently symptomatic patients with an ejection fraction ≤40%, who are currently on optimal medical therapy [31].

A unique role of digoxin in chronic systolic heart failure concerns patients with atrial fibrillation, as it may be adjunctive therapy in controlling rapid ventricular response. In a small, randomized, double-blinded, placebo-controlled study that evaluated the combined effects of digoxin and carvedilol in symptomatic chronic systolic heart failure patients (mean left ventricular ejection fraction 24%) with atrial fibrillation, digoxin was associated with reduction in symptoms and controlling rapid ventricular rates. Improvement in left ventricular ejection fraction was also seen, which disappeared when digoxin was discontinued despite continuing carvedilol [101]. Therefore, it is reasonable to add digoxin in symptomatic chronic systolic heart failure patients, with or without atrial fibrillation, on current standard heart failure pharmacotherapy. This approach may help decrease heart failure symptoms and hospitalizations.

Heart failure, along with myocardial infarction and pneumonia, is one of the three conditions that has the highest 30 day readmission rate [102]. Since 2012, the Centers for Medicare and Medicaid Services has decreased reimbursements to hospitals for excessive readmissions for heart failure [103]. Ahmed and *et al.* reviewed 5153 Medicare patients hospitalized for acute heart failure who were not on digoxin prior to admission. Those patients who received digoxin upon discharge were found to have a lower 30-day all-cause readmission rate, and these effects were seen up to 1 year [104]. Future randomized trials are needed to examine the effects of digoxin with acute heart failure patients [105]. Its role and the evidence to date will be examined later in this chapter.

Digoxin therapy should be initiated at a low dose (0.125 to 0.25mcg daily or every other day) taking into account one's age, renal function, and other comorbidities. Lower doses or every other day dosing are advised if a patient's age >70 years old, has impaired renal function, low body mass index [106]. There are no prospective trials to help guide digoxin dosing according to serum digoxin levels. However, Rathore *et al.* performed a retrospective study that examined clinical outcomes associated with variable digoxin doses and at different serum concentrations. Higher serum digoxin concentrations were associated with a trend towards increasing mortality without any added clinical benefit [107]. A serum digoxin concentration in the range of 0.5 to 0.9 ng/mL has been recommended to avoid adverse effects of digoxin.

It is important to monitor for side effects of digoxin. Digoxin toxicities can occur at any dose or serum level. The major side effects include cardiac arrhythmias such as heart block, re-entrant arrhythmias, and ectopic atrial tachycardia. Gastrointestinal symptoms, such as anorexia, nausea, vomiting, can occur as well as neurological symptoms, such as visual changes and confusion. There is a high risk of developing these symptoms when the serum digoxin level is greater than 2 ng/mL. These adverse effects may be magnified with electrolyte disturbances such as hypokalemia or hypomagnesemia. Hypothyroidism can also precipitate digoxin toxicity possibly through lower glomerular filtration rates associated with hypothyroidism [31]. Drug-drug interactions are also common with digoxin. Medicines that are metabolized through the cytochrome p450 system, such as macrolides, amiodarone, calcium channel blockers, and antifungals can increase levels of digoxin. Therefore, a dose reduction in these cases may be indicated [108].

Hydralazine/Isosorbide Dinitrate

Endothelial dysfunction, impaired activation of nitric oxide, and increased oxidative stress have also been shown to play important roles in the pathogenesis of systolic heart failure [109 - 111]. Therefore, increases in nitric oxide levels and antioxidants to halt the progression of heart failure have been a therapeutic target.

The combination of isosorbide dinitrate and hydralazine was studied in 3 large randomized controlled trials: V-HeFT I (Vasodilator-Heart Failure Trial) [14], V-HeFT II [112], and A-HeFT (African-American Heart Failure Trial) [113] (Table **6**). In V-HeFT I, 642 patients with NYHA II-III symptoms and left ventricular dysfunction < 45% were included. Patients either received isosorbide dinitrate 40mg QID and hydralazine 75mg QID *versus* prazosin 20mg daily *versus* placebo in addition to baseline digoxin and diuretics. Half of these patients had ischemic heart disease. After 2 year follow up, there was a 34% reduction in mortality risk in the isosorbide dinitrate and hydralazine combination compared to placebo ($p < 0.038$) [14]. There was no significant effect on the rates of hospitalizations or exercise tolerance. The authors from VHeFT I also investigated isosorbide dinitrate and hydralazine combination against enalapril 20mg daily - a drug known to reduce the risk of death in patients with systolic dysfunction – in VHeFT II.

The intent of VHeFT II was to compare these two drugs that were known to have a mortality benefit [114]. Both VHeFT I and II were conducted before ACE inhibitors and β-blockers were part of the standard heart failure treatment. As with VHeFT I, most of the patients in VHeFT II had ischemic heart disease and the authors studied the same primary endpoints. Enalapril had a cumulative mortality rate of 18%, and isosorbide dinitrate and hydralazine combination had a mortality rate of 25% (p=0.016). As a result, ACE inhibitors became part of the standard heart failure treatment [112]. Sub-analyses based on ethnic backgrounds of the V-HeFT trials demonstrated there was a mortality benefit of 47% seen in VHeFT I when black patients were compared to non-black patients.

Table 6. Major clinical trials evaluating isosorbide and hydralazine combination in systolic heart failure patients.

Drug	Clincal Trial	Patients	Follow-up	Results
Isosorbide 40mg QID and hydralazine 75mg QID *vs.* prazosin 20mg daily *vs.* placebo	V-HeFT I [14]	N= 642 patients, NYHA II-III, EF < 45%, receiving digoxin and diuretics, ~ 50% ICM, 27% black patients	minimum 2 years	34% reduction in mortality risk in the isosorbide and hydralazine
Hydralazine 300 mg plus isosorbide dinitrate 160 mg daily *vs.* enalapril 20mg	V-HeFT II [113]	N=804 men, NYHA II-III, EF < 30%, receiving digoxin and diuretics, ~ 50% ICM, 27% black patients	60 months	Enalapril had a cumulative mortality rate of 18%, and isosorbide-hydralazine combination had a mortality rate of 25% (p=0.016)
Hydralazine 37.5 mg TID and isosorbide dinitrate 20 mg TID (uptitrated to 2 tabs TID as tolerated) *vs.* placebo	A-HeFT [114]	N=1050 men, NYHA III-IV, EF < 35%, 100% black patients, receiving ACE inhibitor,β-blocker, diuretics, and/or digoxin	18 months	study terminated early due to significant mortality benefit in the treatment group

EF = Ejection fraction; NYHA = New York Heart Association; ICM = Ischemic Cardiomyopathy; QID = Four times a day; TID = Three times a day; ACE = Angiotensin converting enzyme.

A-HeFT was subsequently designed to include only black patients. The major etiology of the symptomatic NYHA III-IV left ventricular dysfunction was due to hypertension rather than ischemic heart disease in this population. In addition, patients were receiving the current standard heart failure therapy at that time, which comprised of ACE inhibitors, β-blockers, and/or aldosterone blockers, in addition to diuretics and digoxin. The A-HeFT trial evaluated the primary outcome measures of mortality, heart failure hospitalizations, and quality of life. With an intention-to-treat analysis, the combination of isosorbide dinitrate and hydralazine had a significant better primary outcome compared to placebo (p=0.016) [113]. Therefore, the 2013 ACCF/AHA guidelines, addition of iso-sorbide dinitrate/hydralazine combination carries a class I indication when added to optimal medical therapy for black patients with NYHA III-IV systolic heart failure [31].

These results sprung the idea that the underlying pathophysiology of heart failure in African Americans may differ than non-African Americans. African Americans tended to be younger, often have more advanced left ventricular dysfunction, and have at times worse heart failure symptoms [115]. African Americans also have a reduced ability to produce endogenous nitric oxide, which may be associated with enhanced responsiveness to drugs that facilitate delivery of nitric oxide, such as isosorbide dinitrate. In addition, the combination with hydralazine provides additive benefit because of its antioxidant properties and prevents degradation of nitric oxide [116].

Despite these data, there are no studies to suggest that the benefit of the hydralazine and isosorbide dinitrate combination would be seen in those not already being treated with standard heart failure therapies. Therefore, if a patient is tolerating ACE inhibitors, β-blockers, and/or aldosterone blockers, the combination of hydralazine and isosorbide dinitrate should not be substituted for any of these agents. Aside from the lack of evidence for clear benefit, the fre-quency of dosing is a disadvantage when compared to ACE inhibitors, β-blockers, and aldosterone antagonists.

There has been debate in the differences of efficacy results in V-HeFT I [14], V-HeFT II [112], and A-HeFT [113] trials given the different doses of isosorbide dinitrate and hydralazine combination used. Furthermore, there has not been a study that compared the administration of isosorbide dinitrate and hydralazine as individual agents *versus* the fixed dose combination used in A-HeFT [116].

In the OPTIMIZE-HF registry, only 4.5% of the 5,108 African-American patients with ejection fraction < 40% received the combination of isosorbide dinitrate and hydralazine at hospital discharge despite the proven mortality benefit seen in V-HeFT I [14], V-HeFT II [112], and A-HeFT [114 - 117]. Unlike core performance measures in place for ACE inhibitors and beta blockers, there are no such measures for nitrates and hydralazine [118]. The most frequent adverse effects include hypotension, headache, dizziness, and gastrointestinal complaints; however, these are well-tolerated.

Ivabradine

Heart rate is an important factor in the pathophysiology of heart failure. An elevated heart rate can increase myocardial oxygen demand, deplete myocardial energy reserves, accelerate atherosclerosis and increase the risk of plaque rupture [119]. These effects potentiate the development and progression of heart failure and portends poor prognosis in patients with chronic heart failure. Therefore, an aim to reduce heart rate is an important target for heart failure therapies. β-blockers have already been established as an influential chronic systolic heart failure therapy that reduces mortality, delays progression of heart failure, and improves left ventricular dysfunction by decreasing chronotropy and controlling myocardial contractility. There are additional neurohormonal mechanisms that β blockers possess that likely delays heart failure progression independent of these hemodynamic effects. Still, the heart slowing effects of β-blockers likely play a role in their documented beneficial effects. Patients with continued symptomatic heart failure despite being on the conventional RAAS blockers and β-blockers retain high mortality risk. In real life clinical population, only a modest group of patients reach target β-blockers as studied in clinical trials. This is a result of hypotension, fatigue, dizziness and other side effects of β-blockers which limit up-titration of dose. Ivabradine is a new anti-anginal and anti-ischemic agent designed in Europe. It inhibits I_f current in the sino-atrial node and provides heart rate reduction without altering cardiac conduction and other hemodynamic properties, such as blood pressure [120].

Heart rate is determined by the rate of depolarization of the action potential in the sinoatrial node. Activation of the action potential is influenced by the I_f channel.

The selective binding of ivabradine ensures the drug has no other effects on myocardial contractility and systemic blood pressure [119, 120]. Computational models have shown that near-complete inhibition of the current can reduce heart rate without causing profound bradycardia [121]. This was evident in only 3-4% of the 6505 patients in SHIFT (Systolic Heart failure treatment with the I_f inhibitor ivabradine Trial) having had symptomatic bradycardia. In addition, there were extremely low rates of discontinuation of ivabradine due to bradycardia [122]. Ivabradine is well-tolerated and safe to administer as a monotherapy or in combination with atenolol, bisoprolol, or other therapies [123 - 127]. Furthermore, it is well tolerated in patients with other comorbidities, such as asthma, chronic obstructive pulmonary disease, and diabetes [128]. Visual changes are a common side effect with ivabradine, due to its effect on retinal ion channels (*Ih* current), which are in the same family as those responsible for the I_f current in the sino-atrial node [129]. In chronic heart failure, ivabradine can be started at 5mg twice daily, which can be increased to 7.5mg twice daily in 2 weeks if the heart rate is greater than 60 beats per minute. If the patient experiences symptomatic bradycardia or if the patient is older than 75 years, a dose of 2.5mg twice daily could be used with careful monitoring. Renal impairment does not require dose adjustment; however, caution is advised in moderate or severe hepatic impairment. Although ivabradine is metabolized by the cytochrome P450 enzyme, it is a weak inhibitor of this enzyme and does not seem to have clinically significant drug-drug interactions, such as with statins, digoxin, and calcium-channel blockers [119].

In 2012, ivabradine was approved by European Medicines Agency for the treatment of chronic heart failure. The European Society of Cardiology (ESC) guidelines for the treatment of chronic heart failure recommends ivabradine for patients with sinus rhythm, left ventricular systolic dysfunction ≤ 35% and a heart rate ≥ 70 bpm, who are persistently symptomatic while on a RAAS blocker and β-blocker [130]. The basis for this guideline is from SHIFT - a randomized, double-blind, multi-center, placebo-controlled study. The investigators initiated ivabradine at 5mg twice daily and titrated to a maximum of 7.5mg twice daily on patients on guideline-based heart failure therapy. The 6,658 patients were randomly assigned to ivabradine (n=3,268 patients) *versus* placebo (n=3,290 patients). The median follow-up was 22.9 months, and the primary endpoint was a composite of cardiovascular mortality or hospitalization for worsening heart failure. The study's primary endpoint was achieved with a significant reduction of cardiovascular death and hospitalizations due to worsening heart failure by 18%, in comparison to placebo ($p < 0.0001$). In addition, this important result was seen amongst all subgroups, such as the elderly, any cause of heart failure, diabetes mellitus, and hypertension [122]. A post-hoc analysis of SHIFT assessed the impact of a background β-blocker or mineralocorticoid receptor antagonist on the response to ivabradine. It was clear ivabradine improves outcomes in heart failure patients receiving multiple neurohormonal treatments - ACE inhibitors, β-blockers, and/or mineralocorticoid receptor antagonists - whose heart rate is ≥70 beats per minute. The authors concluded the magnitude of additional heart rate reduction achieved by ivabradine was responsible for the beneficial outcomes [131, 132]. In addition, subsequent studies on ivabradine suggest it can reverse cardiac remodeling which is a central feature of the progression of heart failure [133]. The CARVIVA HF (effect of CARVedilol, IVAbradine or their combination on exercise capacity in patients with Heart Failure) study suggested ivabradine with or without a β-blocker can improve exercise capacity, while the heart failure patients are receiving a maximal dose of an ACE inhibitor [134].

The evidence to date suggests ivabradine improves heart failure mortality, reduces heart failure hospitalizations, and improves quality of life. The European Society of Cardiology (ESC) has already recommended that ivabradine be used for patients with sinus rhythm, left ventricular systolic dysfunction ≤35% and a heart rate ≥70 bpm, who are persistently symptomatic while on a RAAS blocker and β-blocker. The ACCF/AHA has yet to include the drug into their guidelines and this drug has recently been approved by Food and Drug Administration for use in the United States.

Polyunsaturated Fatty Acids (PUFA)

Major risk factors for developing heart failure include coronary artery disease, hypertension, left ventricular hypertrophy, type II diabetes mellitus, and obesity [135]. There have been many animal and human studies that support the use of PUFA towards these risk factors because of its potential anti-inflammatory and cardioprotective effects. Therefore, n-3 polyunsaturated fatty acids (PUFA) have been studied as a potential ancillary heart failure therapy. The American Heart Association (AHA) supports the use of n-3 PUFA supplements with patients with coronary artery disease, which is the leading risk factor for heart failure [136]. Pro-inflammatory cytokines, such as TNF-α and IL-6, and its receptors are independent predictors of mortality in heart failure patients [137]. Furthermore, inflammatory mediators are associated with the pathophysiological mechanisms of heart failure. Specifically, they contribute to the reduced cardiac output, endothelial dysfunction, hypercoagulability, and resting heart variability, all of which are characteristic of heart failure. PUFA supplements may have a role in the management of heart failure to halt the progression and development of heart failure through its anti-inflammatory actions.

However, conflicting evidence exist from observational and randomized trials that have withheld full evidence-based support for the addition of n-3 PUFA supplementation in heart failure treatment. The major n-3 PUFA in the human diet are alpha-linolenic acid (ALA), eicosapentaenoic acid (EPA), and docosahexaenoic acid (DHA) [138]. Observational studies such as the Japan Collaborative Cohort Study and Cardiovascular Health Study (CHS) showed that higher intakes of fatty fish or fish oil supplements with high concentrates of DHA and EPA are associated with lower risk of heart failure and cardiovascular events [139, 140]. In the Japan Collaborative Cohort Study, 57,972 Japanese men and women followed an increased fish or EPA/DHA diet. Supplementation with EPA/DHA was associated with decreased risk of many cardiovascular events, including heart failure [139]. In a different population that examined 39,367 older and middle-aged Swedish men over a 7 year period, moderate intake of fatty fish and marine n-3 PUFA was associated with a reduced risk of heart failure [141]. A sub-analysis of Cardiovascular Health Study (CHS) involving 2,735 adults showed that plasma EPA was inversely associated with the incidence of chronic heart failure [139, 141]. In contrast, two other observational studies - Rotterdam Study and Women's Health Initiative Observational Study - demonstrated no or weak association between n-3 PUFA ingestion and the risk of heart failure [142, 143]. The Rotterdam Study followed 5,299 middle-aged men and women for four years to examine whether intake of EPA+DHA and fish was associated with the risk of heart failure. Although there was no clear relationship seen, borderline significance was found in a diabetic sub-population. In this group, an inverse association of EPA+DHA intake and the incidence of heart failure was found. The Women's Health Initiative Observational Study found no clear association when they involved 93,676 middle-aged women with an average follow-up of 10 years.

The results from randomized controlled trials demonstrate a dose-dependency of marine n-3 PUFA and its effects on risk factors in heart failure at high doses of 4g/d or even 8g/d [144]. In severe, non-ischemic chronic heart failure patients, 4g/d of n-3 PUFA decreased IL-6 concentration, increased left ventricular ejection fraction and oxygen consumption [145]. However, the GISSI-HF study, which is one of the largest randomized, double-blinded studies to investigate the effects of marine n-3 PUFA on mortality and morbidity in patients with symptomatic heart failure, did not demonstrate significant mortality benefit or reduction in hospital admissions with the use of 1g/d EPA+DHA [146]. Furthermore, several other studies show no benefit with increased doses of n-3 PUFA, including no effects on left ventricular ejection fraction and dimensions [147, 148]. The variability of responses, sometimes at the same dose, limits a clear understanding of n-3 PUFA's effects on chronic heart failure patients. In addition, most of the observational and randomized studies have used marine-derived n-3 PUFA and not plant-derived PUFA or alpha-linolenic acid (ALA). Use of n-3 PUFA therapy has been safe and generally well-tolerated with gastrointestinal effects being the most common adverse effect [149]. However, conclusive evidence of benefit has been elusive [32]. This uncertainty denotes further studies are needed to examine the optimal dose range and the efficacy of other derivatives of PUFA [148].

Statins

Numerous studies have demonstrated the benefits of statins in cardiovascular disease. Aside from lipid-lowering effects, their pleiotropic effects have also been extensively characterized [150]. This includes anti-inflammatory, anti-fibrotic, anti-oxidant effects, as well as improvement in endothelial dysfunction, inhibition of neurohormonal activity, and cardiac arrhythmia prevention [151, 152]. Heart failure is characterized by elevated levels of circulating inflammatory mediators (*e.g.* proinflammatory cytokines, complement levels, C-reactive protein), which in turn contribute to its pathogenesis.

In the management of heart failure, statin therapy has been implicated in the prevention of new-onset heart failure and reduction in heart failure admissions. Several observational studies and post-hoc analyses of randomized-controlled trials in patients with heart failure have indicated beneficial effects of statins with a variety of clinical endpoints, including mortality [153, 154]. Levy reviewed the results of observational statin use in clinical trials that studied systolic heart failure, post-myocardial infarction with left ventricular dysfunction, and in cardiac device trials. He showed that statin use had a wide range of reduction in clinical events from 20% to 60% [155]. Some data suggest statins might reduce heart failure hospitalization. For example, in the PROVE-IT trial that randomized 4162 patients with an acute myocardial infarction to pravastatin 40mg/day *versus* atorvastatin 80mg/day, patients receiving a high dose statin were associated with a 45% reduction in heart failure hospitalization ($p = 0.008$) [156]. Results, such as these, sprung additional studies to determine whether statins have any benefit in systolic heart failure patients.

Krum *et al.* performed a post-hoc analysis of 5010 patients enrolled in the Val-HeFT trial to determine whether meaningful outcome differences exist in congestive heart failure patients according to statin use. In this analysis, mortality was reduced by 19% in those receiving a statin. Furthermore, a retrospective trial performed by Hognestad *et al.* demonstrated that initiation of a β-blocker and statin treatment early after MI complicated by heart failure was associated with decreased morbidity and mortality. In fact, there was an additive benefit with combined use of a statin and a β-blocker [157].

Statin use in clinical device trials of patients with left ventricular systolic dysfunction showed a trend towards reduction in sudden death with statin therapy. The DEFINIT trial, a randomized trial of ICD *versus* no ICD in 458 nonischemic heart failure patients, showed a trend towards less sudden death (84%, $p = 0.08$). There was no added benefit of reduction of appropriate shocks in the patients with an ICD [158]. In a recent meta-analysis, including PRAISE, ELITE 2, CIBIS II, SCD-HeFT, and Val-HeFT trials, as well as observational databases and the randomized CORONA trial, the benefit of statins was similar in patients with either ischemic etiology (27%) or nonischemic etiologies (27%) [159]. Most of the data evaluating the clinical benefit of statins in patients with heart failure are derived from retrospective analyses. Although statin use consistently resulted in significant decreases in mortality rates, the majority of patients in these retrospective and observation trials had ischemic heart disease. Therefore, it is not surprising there was a mortality benefit with use of statins in heart failure. Moreover, retrospective studies of trials with coronary artery disease patients who did not have prior history of heart failure demonstrated a reduction in the risk of development of heart failure and heart failure hospitalizations in patients taking statins [155]. At this point, it had become clear prospective trials were needed to advance our understanding of the potential role of statins.

In the original statin trials, patients with systolic heart failure were generally excluded. However, two randomized trials - GISSI-HF [146] and CORONA [160] - examined the effects of statins in heart failure. These two trials were designed to include patients with systolic dysfunction. GISSI-HF is a randomized, double blind, placebo-controlled trial that enrolled symptomatic adult chronic heart failure patients, regardless of depressed LV systolic function. Approximately 40% of the patients in each arm had a history of ischemic heart disease. The patients were randomized to receive rosuvastatin 10mg daily or placebo. Primary endpoints were time to death and admission to the hospital for cardiovascular causes. Results showed statin use had no effect on mortality in patients with symptomatic chronic heart failure. Despite the known mortality benefit of statins in patients with a history of coronary artery disease, this trial showed no mortality benefit although close to half of the patients enrolled had ischemic cardiomyopathy. It did, however, reduce the number of heart failure related admissions. The authors argued the non-lipid, immu-nomodulatory effects of statins allowed stabilization of coronary artery disease, which had an impact in the progression of heart failure. Given there exists a range of potency in statins, the reduction in heart failure admissions may be dose dependent [155, 161].

Similar to the GISSI-HF trial, the CORONA trial examined the effect of rosuvastatin 10mg compared to placebo. However, CORONA enrolled patients with symptomatic NYHA II-IV ischemic, systolic heart failure. Furthermore, the patients in the CORONA trial were older and more symptomatic. In contrast to the GISSI-HF trial, the primary outcome was mortality from cardiovascular cause. Secondary outcomes included death from any cause and the number of hospitalizations. Despite these differences, the CORONA trial also showed reductions in the number of hospitalizations for heart failure, possibly *via* reductions in the number of acute coronary syndromes that could have led to heart failure admissions. Known pleiotropic effects may have also contributed to the findings [160]. Surprisingly, although there were more patients with ischemic heart disease, this did not change the outcome of mortality. These trials clearly showed no additional mortality benefit of statins with standard heart failure treatment. However, there was impact in reducing heart failure admissions. Although these trials showed no mortality benefit of statins with standard heart failure treatment, there were reduced heart failure admissions.

Statins are well established medications in the setting of coronary artery disease with proven mortality benefits. However, prospective trial data in the setting of heart failure to date has been disappointing. In general, statins should not be added as a primary treatment for heart failure without another clear indication for its use [31].

ACUTE DECOMPENSATED HEART FAILURE

Acute decompensated heart failure is a heterogeneous syndrome, encompassing a wide range of clinical presentations from *de novo* diagnosis of heart failure to an acute worsening of a chronic process. Hospitalization for acute decompensated heart failure represents a major public health issue with respect to its associated morbidity, mortality, and cost to the healthcare system [31, 162]. Heart failure is the primary diagnosis in greater than 1 million hospitalizations annually and cost billions of dollars each year [31, 163]. Patients hospitalized for heart failure who are subsequently discharged are at high risk for all-cause rehospitalization, with a 1-month readmission rate of 25% [31, 164].

Despite extensive clinical trials devoted to improving clinical outcomes in acute decompensated heart failure, results with meaningful improvements in morbidity and mortality have been elusive. Multiple pathophysiologic processes are potentially responsible for an acute decompensation leading to hospitalization.

These include, but are not limited to, acute coronary syndromes, malignant hypertension, right heart failure, medication nonadherence, arrhythmias, infections, excessive alcohol or illicit drug use. As a result, clinical trials have been limited in producing evidence-based data to guide patient management [162]. Furthermore, in the Acute Decompensated Heart Failure National Registry (ADHERE), one-half of the patients presenting with acute decompensated heart failure had preserved systolic function [165, 166]. Irrespective of the underlying cause, systemic and pulmonary congestion due to elevated left ventricular filling pressure, manifested by dyspnea, jugular venous distention, and edema is nearly universal. There may or may not be associated decreases in cardiac output. The therapeutic aims for management of acute decompensated heart failure must be targeted at identifying and controlling the precipitating factors. However, universal treatment objectives include: relieving systemic congestion and/or augmenting low cardiac output in those with evidence of end-organ damage, improvement of post-discharge mortality, and prevention of hospital readmission.

Evidence of congestion

Evidence of poor perfusion?		NO	YES
	NO	WARM and DRY	WARM and WET
	YES	COLD and DRY	COLD and WET

Fig. (1). Clincal status in acute decompensated heart failure.

Classification

Hospitalized patients with acute decompensated heart failure can be classified into subgroups based on their etiology of decompensation and their hemodynamic status. Therapies for those hospitalized for acute decompensated heart failure (*i.e.* secondary to myocardial ischemia *versus* an infection) should be tailored appropriately [31]. Assessment of the patient's hemodynamic status in terms of the degree of congestion as an approximation of left ventricular end disastolic pressure ("wet" *versus* "dry") and the adequacy of systemic perfusion displaying signs of decreased cardiac output ("cold" *versus* "warm") is also necessary to determine the appropriate targeted therapy [31] (Fig. **1**). This is a clinical designation that is made *via* thorough physical examination that will guide proper initiation of therapies to optimize symptom relief and reduce morbidity/mortality.

Management

Diuretics

Fluid removal with loop diuretics (*e.g.* furosemide, bumetanide, and torsemide) is the mainstay of therapy in acute decompensated heart failure. Patients admitted with signs and symptoms of congestion and fluid overload should be promptly treated with intravenous (IV) loop diuretics [31]. Intravenous therapy is initially preferred due to the potential lower absorption of the oral forms in the presence of bowel edema as well as reduced intestinal absorption in hypervolemic states [167, 168].

Early therapy, begun in the emergency department, has been associated with better outcomes [169]. Diuretics should be dosed sufficiently to relieve congestion without inducing intravascular volume depletion, which could lead to hypotension, kidney injury, or both. Patients already receiving loop diuretics prior to hospitalization should receive an initial intravenous dose that is equal to or exceeding their chronic oral dose [31].

When diuresis is inadequate with the initial dose of diuretics, a higher dose of IV loop diuretics or the addition of a second diuretic may be beneficial [31, 166, 170]. A thiazide-type diuretic (*e.g.* metolazone, hydrochlorothiazide, chlorthiazide, and bendro-flumethiazide) blocks the distal tubular sodium resorption by inhibiting the sodium-chloride co-transporter, resulting in significant augmentation of diuresis [170]. The benefits of augmented diuresis with this combination must be weighed against the risks of electrolyte and metabolic consequences, such as hypokalemia, hypomagnesemia, hypochloremic metabolic alkalosis, and hyponatremia [168, 170].

To guide the initial dosing of diuretics, the DOSE-AHF trial compared the effects of high *versus* low dose diuretic administration as a bolus or continuous infusion [172]. Patients' global assessment of symptoms assessed by the Visual Analog Scale as well as the change in serum creatinine was examined. High dose diuretics were defined as 2.5 times the patient's total oral dose in furosemide equivalents [171]. High dose loop diuretics provided better relief of congestion than low dose diuretics. However, there were no differences between bolus dosing or continuous infusion with regards to patients' assessment of symptoms, changes in serum creatinine, the clinical composite endpoint of death, or rehospitalization rates at 60 days [171].

Retrospective analysis of the ADHERE registry data evaluating the clinical outcomes associated with lower *versus* higher intravenous loop diuretic doses (less than 160mg *vs.* greater than 160mg per day) in patients with acute decompensated heart failure showed that in-hospital mortality risk was significantly lower in the lower dose group when compared to the high dose [171 - 173]. The lower daily dose was associated with less risk of significant kidney injury (defined as a rise in serum creatinine greater than 0.5 mg/dL), which is likely intimately linked to the decreased mortality risk.

Angiotensin-Converting Enzyme (ACE) Inhibitors/Angiotensin Receptor Blockers (ARBs)

The benefits of ACE inhibitors and ARBs in heart failure have been long established by landmark studies [174, 175]. Patients with chronic heart failure with reduced ejection fraction admitted with an acute decompensation should be continued on their guideline-directed medical therapy, including ACE inhibitors or ARBs [31]. However, for patients admitted with significant worsening of renal function (development of oliguric/anuric status, rise in serum creatinine), severe or symptomatic hypotension (*i.e.* systolic blood pressure less than 90mmHg), a temporary cessation or dose reduction of the ACE inhibitors or ARBs should be considered until the renal function or hypotension recovers [31, 176]. Once stabilized, the ACE inhibitor or ARB should be reinstituted and the dosage up-titrated as much as possible prior to discharge. Renal function and electrolyte levels should be closely monitored to prevent worsening renal dysfunction or development of hyperkalemia.

β-blockers

β-blockers are a cornerstone of therapy in the management of chronic heart failure. This class of medications has been shown to improve symptoms, reverse left ventricular remodeling, improve systolic function, reduce hospitalizations, and improve mortality [167, 177 - 180]. However, no strong data exist on the role of β-blockers in patients hospitalized with acute decompensated heart failure. Theoretical justification for discontinuation or dose adjustment of β-blockers during an acute decompensation exists given its negative inotropic effect, particularly in those with symptoms of worsening heart failure and low cardiac output. However, one must also consider the risk of abrupt β-blocker withdrawal leading to reflex tachycardia and worsening hemodynamics. The European Society of Cardiology guidelines for management of acute decompensated heart failure includes the recommendation to consider a temporary dose reduction or discontinuation particularly in those with hypotension and signs of hypoperfusion or need for positive inotropic drugs [168, 181]. However, data from randomized controlled trials specifically designed to address whether β-blockers should be continued or discontinued during hospitalization for acute decompensated heart failure are scarce.

Data on the role of β-blockers during hospitalization for acute decompensated heart failure are mostly from sub-studies of larger trials. For example, a sub-study of COMET, a randomized, double-blind, parallel-group trial comparing the effect on morbidity and mortality of carvedilol and metroprolol tartrate, divided the patients in three groups: those who received the same dose before and after hospitalization, those who had a dose reduction, and those whose β-blocker was discontinued. Out of 3029 patients, 25% (752: 361 in carvedilol group, 391 in metoprolol group) had a heart failure hospitalization. Of these, 61 patients (8%) had the beta-blocker discontinued, 162 (22%) had a dose reduction, and 529 (70%) had the dose continued. In this analysis, risk of death was higher in those whose beta-blocker therapy was discontinued or reduced. However, this may be reflective of a bias as those whose β-blockers had been completely withdrawn had a worse prognosis with more severe signs of decompensated heart failure. Given the paucity of data in this clinical study, the decision to alter β-blocker dosing in the setting of acute decompensated heart failure is left to clinical judgment.

However, given the effects of β-blockade withdrawal and the positive hemodynamic effects, continuation of β-blocker therapy is preferable in patients who do not display marked hemodynamic instability [182].

Table 7. Recommendations (expert opinion) of oral pharmacotherapy management in acute decompensated heart failure.

	Warm and Dry	Warm and Wet	Cold and Dry	Cold and Wet
Diuretics	↔ or ↓	↑ or add second diuretic	↓ or ↔	↔ or individualize management
ACE inhibitors/ARBs	↔ or ↑ (monitoring renal function)	↔ or careful up-titration	↓ or stop	stop
β-blockers	↔ or ↑	↔ or careful up-titration	↓ or stop may need inotropic therapy	stop may need inotropic therapy
MRA	↔ or ↑	↔ or careful up-titration	↓ or stop	stop
Digoxin	↔ or may not be used	↔	↔	↔

ACE= Angiotensin converting enzyme; ARB= Angiotensin receptor blocker; MRA = Mineralocorticoid receptor antagonist; ↓ = decrease dose of drug; ↑ = increase dose of drug; ↔ = maintain current dose of drug

Aldosterone Antagonists

Aldosterone receptor antagonists are recommended as part of guideline-directed medical therapy in patients with systolic dysfunction. During hospitalization for acute decompensated heart failure, patients not already receiving aldosterone antagonists should be started as soon as possible. Renal impairment, common in patients admitted with acute decompensated heart failure, must be monitored closely prior to initiating an aldosterone antagonist. Similar to ACE inhibitors, aldosterone antagonists are not recommended in setting of severe renal dysfunction or hyperkalemia. As aldosterone antagonists have minimal effect on blood pressure, the therapy may be started during hospitalization with plans for aggressive uptitration after discharge [168]. Patients who present with evidence of right heart failure will show signs of hepatic congestion, which is often associated with increased serum concentrations of aldosterone [184]. Therefore, use of aldosterone antagonists may prove beneficial in those admitted with acute decompensated heart failure secondary to right ventricular dysfunction (Table 7).

Vasopressin Antagonists

Tolvaptan, a vasopressin-2 antagonist, when added to standard therapy in patients with acute decompensated heart failure, has been shown to normalize serum sodium levels and modestly improve hemodynamics [183]. Patients hospitalized with volume overload who have persistent hyponatremia despite water restriction and maximized guideline-directed medical therapy may benefit from addition of a vasopressin antagonist to improve serum sodium levels and reduce the risk of active cognitive symptoms, including falls and attention deficits [31]. However, long-term therapy with a selective vasopressor antagonist did not improve mortality [184]. Though there may be a role for this therapy, it is not thoroughly understood at this time and should be deferred to clinical judgement.

Vasodilators

In the absence of symptomatic hypotension, intravenous vasodilators may be considered as adjunctive therapies for relief of symptoms in patients with acute decompensated heart failure [31].

Nitroglycerin is a nitric oxide prodrug that activates soluble guanylate cyclase leading to vasodilation [185, 186]. Adverse effects include hypotension, neurohormonal activation, and risk of tachyphylaxis. Nitroglycerin primarily lowers preload *via* venodilation, thereby reducing pulmonary congestion [185, 186]. In one randomized control trial, patients presenting with acute decompensated heart failure were randomized to high-dose isosorbide dinitrate (ISDN) with low dose furosemide *versus* low-dose ISDN with high dose furosemide. The primary composite outcome of in-hospital mortality, intubation within 12 hours, myocardial infarction at 24 hours was significantly lower in the high dose ISDN group [187]. However, this was a small study with a patient population that tended to be hypertensive. There is no large, randomized, double-blinded, placebo-controlled trial studying the effect of nitroglycerin on patients with acute decompensated heart failure. Therefore, use of intravenous nitroglycerin may be most appropriate for patients presenting with acute decompensated heart failure secondary to hypertensive crisis or acute coronary syndrome.

Nitroprusside lowers both preload *via* venodilation and afterload *via* arteriodilation [188]. Adverse effects include hypotension, possible coronary steal, and ventilation-perfusion mismatch through pulmonary arteriolar dilatation in nonventilated areas. Cyanide toxicity can occur with prolonged infusions or renal dysfunction. Clinical trial experience with nitroprusside has yielded mixed data with regards to its effect on mortality [188, 189]. Much like nitroglycerin, although nitroprusside use remains recommended in the recent guidelines for management of acute decompensated heart failure, no large, randomized, double-blinded, placebo-controlled study of nitroprusside is planned.

Natriuretic Peptides

Nesiritide, a recombinant human brain natriuretic peptide (BNP), acts at the natriuretic peptide A receptor to decrease preload, afterload, and pulmonary capillary wedge pressure (PCWP). Adverse effects include headache and hypotension [162]. It received FDA approval in 2001 for use in patients with acute heart failure based on studies that showed a reduction in PCWP and improvement in dyspnea at 3 hours [190]. The Vasodilator in the Management of Acute Heart Failure (VMAC) study showed that the combination of nesiritide with standard medical therapy led to significant decreases in subjective dyspnea as well as pulmonary capillary wedge pressure [191]. However, subsequent pooled analyses and multiple meta-analyses suggested that nesiritide was associated with worsening renal function as well as an increased mortality risk [192, 193]. Therefore, the Acute Study of Clinical Effectiveness of Nesiritide in De-compensated Heart Failure (ASCEND-HF) was designed to evaluate the effect of nesiritide in addition to standard medical therapy on rates of self-reported dyspnea, rehospitalization rates death from any cause, and renal dysfunction.

ASCEND-HF was a randomized, double-blind, placebo-controlled trial of nesiritide in addition to standard therapy for acute decompensated heart failure [194, 195]. There were two co-primary endpoints: the change in self-reported dyspnea using the Likert scale at 6 and 24 hours after nesiritide and the composite end-point of re-hospitalization for heart failure and death from any cause at 30 days. Enrolling 7141 patients who were hospitalized with acute decompensated heart failure, the use of nesiritide was shown to have no effect on the incidence of rehospitalization or death at 30 days. There was a suggestion for marginal improvement in self-reported dyspnea; however, the results did not meet the pre-specified criteria for statistical significance [196]. Therefore, given the lack of any effect on hospitalization with non-significant effect on dyspnea as well as increased rates of hypotension, nesiritide was no longer recommended as part of therapy for acute decompensated heart failure.

Inotropes

Patients presenting in acutely decompensated heart failure with evidence of end organ dysfunction due to decreased cardiac output may benefit from intravenous inotropic agents to improve hemodynamics and relieve symptoms. The ideal agent would be a short-acting agent that reliably improves cardiac function without the adverse effects of increasing myocardial oxygen demand or promoting arrhythmias. The most widely used inotropes in the United States include dobutamine, dopamine, milrinone, and norepinephrine [197].

Cardiac glycosides have been in use for management of heart failure for more than 200 years since its identification from the foxglove plant by William Withering in the late 18th century [198]. Digoxin was once a widely used agent for treatment of chronic systolic heart failure. The long-term effects of digoxin on mortality and hospitalization for heart failure were unknown until the DIG (Digitalis Investigation Group) trial in 1997 [199]. There were reductions in overall rates of hospitalization but no benefit of digoxin on mortality. It has not been evaluated in acutely decompensated heart failure. If being utilized, abrupt discontinuation is discouraged and currently occupies a limited role as an adjunctive option in acute decompensated heart failure for those with concomitant atrial fibrillation that require rate control.

Dobutamine is an intravenous beta-1 and beta-2 adrenergic agonist with no vasoconstrictor properties [197]. Dobutamine increases cardiac output, reduces left ventricular end diastolic pressure (LVEDP) with only a modest increase in heart rate [197]. Adverse effects include hypotension in some patients due to peripheral vasodilation. Prolonged infusions over 72 hours were associated with pharmacodynamic tolerance [197]. Moreover, infusions longer than 7 days was associated with a higher 6-month mortality [197]. However, these poorer outcomes with dobutamine are largely based on observational data. Clinical experience anecdotally has confirmed reduced survival in heart failure patients on long-term dobutamine therapy but this may be reflective of a sicker cohort of patients that require inotropic support. Long-term infusions with inotropes remain commonly in use as a bridge to either mechanical support or heart transplantation.

Milrinone is a bipyridine, non-catecholamine inotrope that exerts its actions *via* phosphodiesterase inhibition. It is both a positive inotrope and peripheral vasodilator. By inhibiting PDE-3, an enzyme that breaks down cyclic AMP (cAMP), it ultimately leads to increases in intracellular calcium entry as well as its removal, leading to increased myocardial contractility [197]. Through its modulation of cAMP, milrinone may also reduce pulmonary artery pressures *via* a vasodilator mechanism. Therefore, milrinone may be favored in patients with elevated pulmonary artery pressures and in need for inotropic support. It was found to be associated with increased adverse events compared with standard therapy in the Outcomes of a Prospective Trial of Intravenous Milrinone for Exacerbations of Chronic Heart Failure (OPTIME-HF) trial [200]. As milrinone can lead to hypotension, it should be avoided in patients with renal dysfunction, it also can be proarrhythmic. The OPTIME-CHF study showed that when compared to placebo, milrinone was associated with more sustained hypotension (10.7% *vs.* 3.2%), more atrial arrhythmias (4.6% *vs.* 1.5%), and there was no difference in in-hospital mortality (3.8% *vs.* 2.3%) [197, 200]. Therefore, milrinone may have a role in acute decompensated heart failure patients with preserved renal function, elevated pulmonary pressures, or on concomitant β-blocker therapy [200].

Levosimendan is a calcium-sensitizing agent that increases myocardial contractility by enhancing the sensitivity of myofilaments to calcium. It has been shown to have favorable hemodynamic effects in small studies on patients with acute decompensated heart failure. Levosimendan also has peripheral vasodilatory properties by opening smooth muscle ATP-dependent potassium channels. It may also have PDE-3 inhibitor activity similar to milrinone [201]. Increased myocardial calcium sensitivity appears to potentiate myofilament cross-bridge formation and relaxation [201, 202].

When compared to dobutamine, levosimedan infusion was superior to dobutamine in the Levosimedan Infusion *versus* Dobutamine (LIDO) study [201]. The LIDO trial showed that patients assigned to levosimendan had a lower risk of death than those assigned to dobutamine. However, the primary end point of the LIDO study was not the risk of death. Therefore, the SURVIVE study was designed as a prospective, randomized trial to evaluate the risk of all-cause mortality at 31 and 180 days for levosimendan compared to dobutamine in patients with acute decompensated heart failure [202]. The SURVIVE study demonstrated that although the levosimedan group had greater decreases in BNP level at 24 hours when compared to the dobutamine group, there were no statistical differences between treatment groups for all-cause mortality (26% *vs.* 28%, hazard ratio 0.91, confidence interval 0.74-1.13). Moreover, there were no differences in any secondary clinical outcomes, including all-cause mortality at 31 days, cardiovascular mortality at 180 days, number of days alive and out of the hospital, and patient assessment of dyspnea. There were higher incidences of atrial fibrillation, hypokalemia, and headache in the levosimendan group [202].

There is currently a lack of head-to-head trials to determine any preference for one inotrope over another. Milrinone may be preferred in patients that are on beta blockers as it acts independent of beta-adrenergic receptors unlike dobutamine. Given its effect on pulmonary vasodilation, milrinone may be preferred in those with pulmonary arterial hypertension. On the other hand, milrinone is renally cleared and is associated with hypotension and arrhythmias. Given its longer half-life, milrinone may not be ideal in those with underlying renal dysfunction. Dobutamine may be preferred in patients with significant hypotension. Clinical judgment must guide the choice of inotropic agent given the lack of evidence-based data.

Novel Agents for Acute Decompensated Heart Failure in Development

There remains much to be studied in the field of acutely decompensated heart failure. What follows are several novel agents currently under development. They remain at various stages of development and most have yet to be adopted into universal practice.

Istaroxime is a novel intravenous agent with both inotropic and lusitropic properties. It acts *via* two proposed mechanisms: inhibition of the Na^+/K^+ adenosine triphosphatase (ATPase) and stimulation of sarcoplasmic reticulum calcium ATPase [197, 203]. In HORIZON-HF, a phase II dose-finding trial, the addition of a six hour infusion of intravenous istaroxime to standard therapy in patients hospitalized with acute decompensated heart failure decreased the PCWP (pulmonary capillary wedge pressure) and RAP (right atrial pressure), increased the cardiac index and improved diastolic function [203]. There were no significant adverse effects with regards to hypotension or arrhythmias. However, this phase II trial did not assess any improvement in patients' subjective improvements in dyspnea. Furthermore, the effects of istaroxime on both in-hospital and long-term mortality remain unknown.

Omecamtiv mecarbil is a cardiac myosin activator, which is a new class of medications designed to increase myocardial contractility by increasing the duration of systole without changing the rate of left ventricular pressure development (dP/dt). As a selective activator of cardiac myosin, omecamtiv mecarbil increases the occupancy time of myosin on actin, leading to increased numbers of myosin molecules bound to actin. This causes prolongation of the contractile force without increasing dP/dt, thereby increasing the stroke volume and cardiac output [204]. In preclinical studies, cardiac myosin activators increased myocardial contraction and stroke volume without increasing myocardial oxygen consumption [204]. Instead of increasing the heart's demand for energy, it allows the myocardium to make more efficient use of energy [197]. Due to the lack of effect on beta-adrenergic receptors or calcium efflux, there appears to be no arrhythmogenic potential.

Cleland *et al.* performed a double-blind, placebo-controlled, crossover, dose-ranging phase II trial studying the effects of omecamtiv mecarbil on patients with left ventricular systolic dysfunction (ejection fraction of 40% or less). The primary aim of the study was to assess the safety and tolerability of the novel agent at a safely tolerated plasma concentration. The phase II trial had promising outcomes with dose-dependent increases in left ventricular ejection time, stroke volume, associated with a small reduction in heart rate when compared to placebo. There were no major safety issues aside from two cases of cardiac ischemia noted at very high plasma concentrations. Higher plasma concentrations were associated with reductions in end-systolic and end-diastolic volumes [204]. Based on this promising data, further randomized controlled trials evaluating the effects on dyspnea, patient global assessment, change in NT-proBNP, and incidence of worsening heart failure are underway (NCT01300013, ClinicalTrials.gov). Though additional data is pending, this remains an exciting agent that may well prove beneficial in the future.

Rolofylline is an adenosine A1 receptor antagonist. Initial trials using rolofylline indicated there was enhanced diuresis without worsening renal dysfunction in patients with acute decompensated heart failure. The PROTECT study was a multicenter, double-blind, placebo-controlled trial that evaluated the effect of rolofylline with respect to survival, heart-failure status, and changes in renal function. Secondary end points were post-treatment development of persistent renal impairment and 60 day rate of death or readmission from cardiovascular or renal causes [205]. Rolofylline did not provide any favorable effect with respect to diuresis, worsening renal function, or the incidence of death or readmission for cardiovascular or renal causes at 60 days. Its continued role as a potential therapy remains in question.

Cinaciguat is a novel soluble guanylate cyclase activator that acts on the oxidized, heme-free sGC independent of the nitric oxide-mediated pathway [206]. Soluble guanylate cyclase activation is an essential step in nitric oxide-mediated vasodilation. Animal studies showed the agent had potent vasodilation properties while preserving GFR (glomerular filtration rate) combined with initial clinical results demonstrating significant increased cardiac output and reductions in preload and afterload. Because of these results, cinaciguat was thought to be a promising agent [207]. However, Erdmann *et al.* showed in a placebo-controlled, phase IIb study that although cinaciguat significantly decreased the pulmonary capillary wedge pressure (-7.7mmHg *vs.* -3.7mmHg in placebo, $p<0.0001$), mean right atrial pressure (-2.7mmHg *vs.* -0.6mmHg in placebo, $p=0.0019$), peripheral vascular resistance, mean arterial pressure, and increased the cardiac index (all $p<0.0001$ *vs.* placebo); the trial had to be terminated prematurely due to high incidence of treatment-emergent hypotension [206]. Although the hypotension was initially attributed to high doses (>200 μg/h), other phase II dose-finding studies in patients with acute decompensated heart failure using doses <200μg/h were also terminated due to excessive hypotension [206, 208]. Therefore, cinaciguat is no longer being developed as an acute intravenous agent for use in acute decompensated heart failure.

Relaxin is a naturally occurring hormone related to pregnancy that increases renal perfusion and decreases systemic vascular resistance. Serelaxin, a recombinant human relaxin-2, is a peptide hormone that has several potentially beneficial effects in the treatment of acute decompensated heart failure [209]. Serelaxin binds to relaxin family peptide receptors (RXFP) located in the heart, blood vessels, and kidneys [209]. This, in turn, leads to nitric oxide activation, generation of cyclic AMP, which leads to vasodilation. In RELAX-AHF, a phase III, multi-center, randomized, double-blind, placebo-controlled trial of serelaxin in treatment of acute decompensated heart failure, infusion of serelaxin 30μg/kg/day for 48 hours in a selected population of patients with decompensated heart failure significantly improved signs and symptoms of congestion. There were shorter initial hospital stays, decreased progression of heart failure events, and fewer in-hospital complications [210]. However, there was no improvement in the rates of hospital readmission for heart failure or renal failure. Interestingly, an incidental observation from RELAX-AHF is that there was a 37% reduction in cardiovascular death and all-cause mortality in the treatment group at 180 days [210]. However, the study was inadequately powered for these endpoints and will need to be confirmed in an appropriately designed study. Moreover, such significant reductions in mortality occurred despite only a 48 hour IV infusion during an acute decompensation episode, raising hypothesis-generating questions regarding the mechanisms responsible for long-term effects of short-term treatments for acute decompensated heart failure.

Although new agents such as those reviewed here are on the horizon, investigating and demonstrating their safety and efficacy in a syndrome as heterogenous and complex as decompensated heart failure will undoubtedly prove challenging. Moreover, large enrollments in studies will be required to demonstrate meaningful benefit. This is particularly true to demonstrate any long-term survival benefit using short-acting or short-term infusion therapies during a hospitalization. The lack of clinically significant benefit from many of the agents reviewed in the acute decompensated heart failure cohort of patients is reflective of the heterogeneity underlying the etiologies for decompensation. Relieving congestion and providing inotropic support remain the mainstays of therapy in acutely decompensated heart failure.

HEART FAILURE WITH PRESERVED EJECTION FRACTION

Heart failure has traditionally been thought of as primarily a clinical syndrome due to left ventricular systolic dysfunction. The concept that heart failure only encompasses those with depressed left ventricular systolic function was challenged with the recognition that heart failure can occur with any ejection fraction, including in the near-normal range [211]. Heart failure with preserved ejection fraction (HF*p*EF) is associated with high morbidity and mortality, represents >50% of all heart failure, and is a growing entity that we do not understand as deeply as heart failure with reduced ejection fraction (HF*r*EF) [212].

Many of the clinical features of HF*r*EF are shared with HF*p*EF, such as elevated left atrial pressures, abnormal left ventricular filling pressures, dyspnea, impaired exercise tolerance, pedal edema, and frequent hospitalizations. Though they share clinical presentation features, there are important differences between the two syndromes. Patients with HF*p*EF are usually older, more likely to be women, less likely to have ischemia, and more likely to be associated with systemic hyper-tension [213]. HF*p*EF is a clinical syndrome and not a specific disease process. There are varying presentations of HF*p*EF and the associated comorbidities, such as hypertension and diabetes mellitus, influence outcomes in this cohort [214, 215]. Shah, in an editorial in JACC (Journal of the American College of Cardiology), characterized three different HF*p*EF patient types: exercise-induced diastolic dysfunction (*e.g.* exercise-induced rise in left ven-tricular filling pressure), chronic volume overload, and associated right heart failure or pulmonary hypertension. Each of these types may represent different stages of HF*p*EF [216]. Therapies proven to improve outcomes in HF*r*EF have not demonstrated similar results in patients with HF*p*EF (Table **8**). To date, the available data on treatments for patients suffering from heart failure with preserved ejection fraction is limited.

Table 8. Major clinical trials evaluating pharmacotherapy in patients with heart failure with preserved ejection fraction (HF*p*EF).

Intervention	Clinical Trial	Patients	Follow-up	Results
Perindopril titrated to 4mg/day if tolerated *vs.* placebo	PEP-CHF [220]	N=850; median age 75y; excluded patients with EF < 40%; hospitalized within last 6 months	mean 26.2 months	No difference in composite all cause mortality or HF hospitalization between perindopril *vs.* placebo; perindopril had a greater 6MWT at 52 weeks
Candesartan titrated to 32mg/day if tolerated *vs.* placebo	CHARM-Preserved [221]	N=3023; mean age 67y, NYHA class II-IV for at least 4wk, hospitalized, EF > 40%	median 36.6 months	No difference in cardiovascular death or HF admission
Irbesartan titrated to 300mg/day if tolerated *vs.* placebo	I-PRESERVE [222]	N=4128; mean age 72y, NYHA class II-IV, hospitalized, EF ≥ 45%	mean 49.5 months	No difference in all-cause death or hospitalization for cardiovascular cause
Verapamil titrated to 360mg/day if tolerated *vs.* placebo	Setaro (1990) [224]	N=20; males, mean age 68y, EF > 45%	2 weeks for each treatment, crossed over to the other arm with 4-day washout period	Significant improvement in exercise capacity from baseline in treatment group
Variable doses of digoxin *vs.* placebo	DIG ancillary [227]	N=988; mean age 67y, EF > 45%, normal sinus rhythm, NYHA class I-IV	Mean 37 months	No difference in composite of HF hospitalization or HF mortality
Carvedilol titrated to 20mg/day if tolerated *vs.* placebo	Takeda (2004) [219]	N=40; mean age 71.2y, NYHA class II or III and stage C HF, EF ≥ 45%	12 months	NYHA class and exercise capacity in METs improved significantly in the treatment arm
Nebivolol 10mg/day if tolerated *vs.* placebo	SENIORS [217]	N=752; mean age 76y; hospitalized for HF within last year or an EF ≤ 35% within previous 6 months (EF > 35% subgroup analysis performed as well)	mean 21 months	Lower rates of composite all-cause mortality or hospitalization for cardiovascular causes in the treatment arm - regardless of EF

(Table 8) contd.....

Intervention	Clinical Trial	Patients	Follow-up	Results
Propranolol titrated to 90mg/day if tolerated *vs.* placebo	Aronow (1997) [218]	N=158; mean age 81y, NYHA class II or III, prior Q-wave MI, EF ≥ 40%, on ACE inhibitors and diuretics for 2 months	32 months	Decreased all-cause mortality plus nonfatal MI in the treatment group

EF = Ejection fraction; MWT = Minute walk test; NYHA = New York Heart Association; HF = Heart Failure; METs = Metabolic equivalents; MI = Myocardial infarction; ACE = Angiotensin converting enzyme.

β-Blockers

The 2010 HFSA (Heart Failure Society of America) guidelines gave a grade "A" strength of evidence for the use of β-blockers in patients with prior myocardial infarction and grade "B" for those with hypertension in patients with HF*p*EF [217]. There are three randomized controlled trials that addressed the role of β-blockers in HF*p*EF. The largest trial was the SENIORS study, performed to assess the effects of nebivolol in elderly patients, regardless of the ejection fraction. Enrolling 2,218 patients, including those older than 70 years of age, with a history of either HF*p*EF or HF*r*EF (hospital admission for heart failure within the previous year or with an ejection fraction ≤35%) were randomized to nebivolol *versus* placebo. This cohort included 35% of whom had an ejection fraction > 35%. There was a modest improvement in all-cause mortality or cardiovascular hospital admissions in the nebivolol group. The interaction test showed that ejection fraction did not affect the outcome results, suggesting nebivolol has similar effects in patients with both HF*p*EF and HF*r*EF. However, it should be noted this sub-analysis was inadequately powered to fully evaluate the effect of nebivolol on different ranges of ejection fractions [218]. Regardless, nevibolol was shown to be a powerful, safe therapy in elderly patients with a history of coronary artery disease and with HF*p*EF or HF*r*EF.

Aronow *et al.* examined the addition of propanolol to conventional heart failure therapy *versus* no propanolol in elderly patients (mean age 81 years old) with heart failure with preserved ejection fraction (≥40%), prior myocardial infarction, who were on ACE inhibitors and diuretics. A significant benefit in all-cause mortality plus non-fatal myocardial infarction (59% *vs.* 82%; p=0.002) during a follow-up period of 32 months favoring propranolol was reported. However, there was no significant difference in cardiac deaths between the study and control groups [219]. These trials demonstrated a favorable effect of β-blockers in terms of mortality in post-myocardial infarction HF*p*EF patients.

Several studies have assessed β-blockers' impact towards morbidity and functional class. One small Japanese single-center trial enrolled 40 patients with mild or moderate heart failure and an ejection fraction ≥45%. The patients were randomized to receive carvedilol along with standard heart failure therapy *versus* conventional heart failure therapy, which included ACE inhibitors, diuretics, and/or digoxin. After 12 months of therapy, the study group improved all end points - plasma concentration of B-type natriuretic peptide (BNP), NYHA functional class, and exercise capacity. Although this study had a positive impact, it had several limitations (short follow up, small cohort) and only addressed subjective endpoints [220]. Future larger studies with objective endpoints should be conducted in an attempt to reproduce these results. These trials must be designed to elucidate the mechanisms underlying the benefit of β-blockers in HF*p*EF, such as improved myocardial relaxation.

Angiotensin-Converting Enzyme (ACE) Inhibitors/Angiotensin Receptor Blockers (ARBs)

The role of ACE inhibitors or ARBs in HF*p*EF patients is less significant when compared with their role in the management in chronic systolic heart failure. Angiotensin II is believed to contribute to left ventricular hypertrophy, fibrosis, and diastolic dysfunction that are paramount features in HF*p*EF. Inhibiting production or binding of angiotensin II by ACE inhibitors and/or ARBs may prevent or reverse the mechanisms underlying HF*p*EF.

PEP-CHF (Perindopril for Elderly People with Chronic Heart Failure) study is the largest trial examining the role of ACE inhibitors in HF*p*EF. PEP-CHF enrolled 850 elderly patients taking a diuretic due to diastolic dysfunction and were hospitalized within the last 6 months for a cardiovascular cause and randomized them to receive perindopril 2mg daily or placebo. After a mean follow-up of 26.2 months, there was no significant difference between the treatment group or placebo in the primary outcome of composite all-cause mortality or unplanned hospitalization for heart failure (p=0.545) [221]. Results were not significant between the groups for any secondary outcomes either, except decreased heart failure hospitalization and improved NYHA functional class in the perindopril group during the first year ($p \leq 0.033$) [221]. The primary endpoint was not met due to patients withdrawing from the study after the blinded treatment period of 18 months. This decreased the power to detect a difference in the primary or secondary outcomes to 35% [221]. Aronow *et al.* designed a similar, smaller study to assess the effect of enalapril on elderly patients with heart failure with preserved ejection. This cohort had NYHA class III symptoms and a history of myocardial infarction. Patients were on a consistent dose of furosemide for two weeks or greater before the initiation of the study, and were randomized to receive enalapril titrated up to 20mg daily *versus* placebo. The combination of enalapril with furosemide improved NYHA functional class and exercise time from baseline to 3 months ($p = 0.005$) [222]. Multiple smaller studies not reviewed here have shown conflicting results with regards to the role of ACE inhibitors in HFpEF. Therefore, larger randomized, double blinded studies are needed to define this issue.

As is in HF*r*EF, angiotensin II and the RAAS are believed to play a central pathophy-siological role in the development of HF*p*EF. Two major large, double-blinded, multicenter, randomized controlled trials (CHARM-Preserved [223] and I-PRESERVE [224]) assessed the effects of an ARB on patients >60 years of age and with moderate to severe heart failure symptoms. CHARM-Preserved enrolled 3023 patients, randomized them to candesartan *versus* placebo, and followed the patients for 36.6 months. There was no difference between the groups in terms of cardiovascular disease-related death. As a secondary endpoint, candesartan provided moderate benefit to patients with HF*p*EF by significantly reducing the number of heart failure hospital admissions [223]. The I-PRESERVE trial enrolled 4128 patients with HF*p*EF who were randomized to irbesartan *versus* placebo. After a mean follow-up 49.5 months, there was no significant difference in all-cause death, hospitalizations, composite heart failure outcomes, or cardiovascular death. The results of both trials were confounded with additional inhibitors of the RAAS - 39% of patients were taking ACE inhibitors and 28% of patients were receiving spironolactone. Furthermore, the benefit of ARBs was also reduced as 34% of patients in I-PRESERVE had discontinued the study drug before the end of the trial [224].

Reflective of this limited evidence on the use of ACE inhibitors or ARBs in HF*p*EF, the HFSA and AHA/ACC guidelines give a grade "C" strength of evidence for their use [31, 225]. Nevertheless, there is a stronger indication for the use of ACE inhibitors or ARBs if there exists a comorbidity along with HFpEF; such as diabetes, coronary artery disease, or hypertension.

Calcium Channel Blockers

Similar to β-blockers, non-dihydropyridine calcium-channel blockers (verapamil and diltiazem) may be beneficial with HF*p*EF patients for its potential to improve diastolic function through common negative chronotropic and inotropic mechanisms. Clinical data regarding the use of agents in this class, however, is limited.

Setaro and colleagues conducted a small prospective study with 20 patients with diastolic heart failure (EF >45% and abnormal diastolic filling patterns). They evaluated the efficacy of verapamil in this placebo-controlled, double-blinded 5-week crossover trial. Any evidence of valvular disease or ischemia was excluded by echocardiography and thallium-201 stress scintigraphy, respectively. Verapamil, compared to placebo, significantly improved patients' exercise capacity by 33% and peak ventricular filling rate by 30%. Mean ejection fraction rates were unchanged from baseline [226]. Although the trial showed verapamil had therapeutic efficacy, the small number of patients and the short duration follow-up limit the applicability of this result. Comparable improvements in symptoms and exercise tolerance were reported by Hung *et al.* in a study of similar design [227]. However, larger trials are needed to replicate the results.

The 2010 HFSA guidelines, as well as the 2013 ACC/AHA guidelines, give calcium channel blockers a grade "C" strength of evidence for patients with HF*p*EF and atrial fibrillation and hypertension, and a grade "A" for patients with symptom-limiting angina. Those with atrial fibrillation with a rapid ventricular response should be given verapamil or diltiazem if they are intolerant to β-blockers [31, 225]. Although there is limited evidence with the use of calcium channel blockers in HF*p*EF patients, calcium channel blockers are prescribed in approximately 50% of patients according to registry data [228]. Therefore, further trials are warranted to clarify the role of calcium channel blockers in HF*p*EF.

Digoxin

The role of digoxin was studied extensively amongst chronic systolic heart failure patients. Although the DIG study showed a reduced risk for hospitalization for worsening heart failure in those with systolic dysfunction, there was no benefit seen in those with preserved ejection fraction [199]. In an ancillary trial, 988 patients with LVEF >45% and normal sinus rhythm at baseline were enrolled, randomized to receive digoxin *versus* placebo and followed for approximately 3 years. No significant differences in the combined endpoint of heart failure hospitalization, heart failure mortality, all-cause mortality, or all-cause hospitalization were seen in the HF*p*EF cohort [229]. Despite the lack of strong evidence, digoxin is still used in approximately 30% of patients with preserved ejection fraction [228].

Aldosterone Antagonists

Aldosterone plays an important role in the development of left ventricular diastolic dysfunction and cardiac remodeling. Aldosterone's actions include sodium retention, endothelial dysfunction, vascular inflammation, fibrosis, and hypertrophy [230]. Spironolactone and eplerenone are two mineralocorticoid receptor antagonists that are well-studied in patients with chronic systolic heart failure and have been proven to reduce total and cardiovascular mortality [231, 232]. Preliminary small studies have suggested that these beneficial effects of aldosterone antagonists may translate to patients with HF*p*EF. The Aldosterone Receptor Blockade in Diastolic Heart Failure (Aldo-DHF) trial - a multi-center, randomized, placebo-controlled trial - enrolled 422 patients, aged ≥50 years, and followed the patients for over 1 year. Spironolactone improved diastolic function parameters, reduced blood pressure, and improved cardiac remodeling. However, there was no effect on exercise capacity, symptoms, or quality of life [233]. The lack of subjective improvement with spironolactone may be due to a short duration of follow up. Similarily, TOPCAT [234] investigators studied the effects of spironolactone in symptomatic heart failure patients (NYHA II-III) with preserved ejection fraction in a randomized, double-blind trial. The primary outcomes were composite death from cardiovascular causes, cardiac arrest, and hospitalization from heart failure. After a mean follow-up of 3.3 years, there was no significant difference in outcome between the spironolactone group and placebo [234]. These large studies illustrate the difficulty of one drug influencing outcomes in a heterogeneous patient population. More importantly, these neutral trials will help deepen our understanding of the complex pathophysiology of HF*p*EF. These results should also generate hypotheses that will lead to new therapies or direct our existing treatments towards a more well-defined patient population.

The challenge to discover an evidence-based therapy that improves mortality and/or morbidity stems chiefly from the heterogeneity of HF*p*EF. Though some recognized subtypes of HF*p*EF exist, no uniform definition of HF*p*EF exists that can be applied in clinical trials. Furthermore, in order to conduct a successful clinical trial, well-designed studies designed to understand the underlying pathophysiology of the syndrome are needed. The heterogenity of the syndrome is caused by the variety of underlying etiologies and associated comorbidities. Thus, the current management of HF*p*EF is focused on the treatment of comorbidities, modifying physiological factors that can affect ventricular relaxation, and symptom reduction.

MISCELLANEOUS DRUG THERAPIES

It is important to mention some pharmacological therapies that have had neutral or negative effects in heart failure patients (Table **9**). Direct renin inhibitors, such as alsikiren, have been studied extensively in the treatment of systemic hypertension. They are now being explored in heart failure. The ATMOSPHERE [235] and ASTRONAUT [236] trials were performed to study the effects of direct renin inhibitors in heart failure patients. The trials were designed based on the idea that chronic ACE-inhibitor therapy (or ARB therapy) results in a reflex renin increase and eventually overcome enzyme inhibition. However, the ASTRONAUT trial (ATMOSPHERE results have not been released) demonstrated no significant impact on outcomes in heart failure patients.

Ibopamine is a drug that has dopaminergic properties, and has been shown to improve heart failure symptoms. Its mechanism is not clearly understood but it has been suggested its active metabolite stimulates DA-1 and DA-2 receptors. Ibopamine was further investigated in the

PRIME II study to assess for its effects on survival in heart failure [237]. The trial was prematurely stopped due to a surprisingly increased risk of death in the ibopamine group. It is possible that the effects that were observed can be attributed to its use in severe heart failure patients. The effects are not well established in mild heart failure patients. Nevertheless, ibopamine has not been further studied since.

The role of antithrombotic and antiplatelet therapy in heart failure patients has been debated for many years. Original trials have clearly established the beneficial effects of anticoagulation in systolic heart failure patients with atrial fibrillation and valvular disease [238]. Investigators, such as Lip *et al.*, suggest heart failure is associated with a hypercoagulable state, and can explain unrecognized thrombotic events that lead to sudden deaths [239]. As a result, anticoagulation in chronic heart failure patients, even in sinus rhythm, may be beneficial. The WATCH [240] (Warfarin and Antiplatelet Therapy in Chronic Heart Failure) trial was designed to address this question. This prospective, randomized clinical trial demonstrated that there was no superiority of warfarin over aspirin, clopidogrel over aspirin, or warfarin over clopidogrel. Not surprisingly, warfarin was associated with fewer non-fatal strokes than aspirin or clopidogrel. Because enrollment was slow and there was no profound impact on outcomes at 1 year, the trial was stopped early.

Table 9. Miscellaneous drug therapies in heart failure.

Drug	Trial(s)	Mechanism of Action	Patients	Follow-up	Outcome	Comments
Alsikiren	ATMOSPHERE [233]	direct renin inhibitor	N=2347; EF ≤ 35%; NYHA II-IV; BNP ≥150 pg/mL or NT-proBNP > 600 pg/ml	12 months		trial on-going

(Table 9) contd.....

Drug	Trial(s)	Mechanism of Action	Patients	Follow-up	Outcome	Comments
	ASTRONAUT [234]	direct renin inhibitor	N=808; 65 y (mean); mean EF 28%; 41% DM; most patients were on diuretics, β-blockers, ACE-I, and MRA	6 and 12 months	12 months- 35.0% in aliskiren group (126 CV deaths, 212 HF rehospitalizations) and 37.3% in placebo group (137 CV deaths, 224 HF rehospitalizations; HR, 0.93; 95% CI, 0.79-1.09; P = 0.36)	
Ibopamine	PRIME II [235]	unclear; neurohoromonal effects	N=953; 64.6 y(mean); NYHA III/IV; EF < 35% or LVIDd > 6cm, FS < 20%, CTR > 50%	minimum 6 months	232 (25%) of 953 patients in the ibopamine group died;193 (20%) of 953 patients in the placebo group died (relative risk 1.26 [95% Cl 1.04–1.53], p=0.017)	trial stopped early due to increased risk of death in ibopamine group
Anti-coagulation	WATCH[238]	coagulation factor inhibition (II, VII, IX, X) and antiplatelet inhibition	N=1587; EF ≤ 35%; symptomatic HF in last 3 months	12 months	composite end points of 1st occurence to death, nonfatal MI, or nonfatal stroke: warfarin *versus* aspirin, 0.98 (95% CI, 0.86 to 1.12; *P*=0.77); for clopidogrel *versus* aspirin, 1.08 (95% CI, 0.83 to 1.40; *P*=0.57); and for warfarin *versus* clopidogrel, 0.89 (95% CI, 0.68 to 1.16; *P*=0.39)	trial stopped early due to slow enrollment

NYHA = New York Heart Association; EF= Ejection Fraction; DM= Diabetes mellitus; ACE-I= Angiotensin converting enzyme inhibitor, MRA= Mineralocorticoid receptor antagonists; CV = Cardiovascular; HF= Heart Failure; LVIDd = Left ventricular internal diastolic diameter; FS = Fractional shortening; CTR = Cardiothoracic ratio; NSAIDs = Non-steroidal anti-inflammatory drugs.

CONCLUSION

Heart failure is a global pandemic affecting millions of people worldwide. Ambulatory heart failure patients with reduced ejection fractions have benefited from advances in pharmacotherapy consisting of β-blockers, ACE inhibitors (or ARBs), hydralazine/isosorbide dinitrate, and aldosterone antagonists, all of which have become the standard of care for chronic systolic heart failure patients. These therapies have shown morbidity and mortality benefits. Diuretics continue to play a central role in relieving congestion and will remain a mainstay in the armamentarium.

The prevalence of heart failure patients with preserved ejection fraction (HF*p*EF) continues to grow. Attention should be directed to understand the pathophysiology underlying HF*p*EF to design trials to study potential therapies. The prognosis of HF*p*EF patients is similar to chronic systolic heart failure patients, and one current challenge remains to discover disease-modifying therapies for HF*p*EF patients.

Multiple factors contribute to an acute decompensation of chronic systolic or diastolic heart failure. This inherent heterogeneity makes development of novel pharmacological therapies challenging. Future clinical trials in this arena should be aimed at identifying a specific sub-cohort of patients within the hospitalized population based on their underlying etiology for decompensation to target the pharmacotherapy appropriately.

CONFLICT OF INTEREST

The authors confirm that they have no conflict of interest to declare for this publication.

ACKNOWLEDGEMENTS

Declared none.

REFERENCES

[1] Katz AM. The "modern" view of heart failure: how did we get here? Circ Heart Fail 2008; 1(1): 63-71. [http://dx.doi.org/10.1161/CIRCHEARTFAILURE.108.772756] [PMID: 19808272]

[2] Davis RC, Hobbs FD, Lip GY. ABC of heart failure. History and epidemiology. BMJ 2000; 320(7226): 39-42.
[http://dx.doi.org/10.1136/bmj.320.7226.39] [PMID: 10617530]

[3] Eknoyan G. A history of edema and its management. Kidney Int Suppl 1997; 59(S1): S118-26.
[PMID: 9185118]

[4] Pizza R. Developing diuretics: From mercurials to thiazides, these "urine promoters" have proved to be some of the most prescribed therapeutics. Modern Drug Discovery 2003; 19-20.

[5] Lesney M. Flowers for the heart. Modern Drug Discovery 2002; 5(3): 46-8.

[6] Coombs C. The aetiology of cardiac disease. Bristol Med Chir J 1926; 43: 1.

[7] Cohn A. Heart disease from the point of view of the public health. Am Heart J 1927; 2: 275-301.
[http://dx.doi.org/10.1016/S0002-8703(27)90293-2]

[8] Paul J. The Epidemiology of Rheumatic Fever. Metropolitan Life Insurance Company 1930.

[9] Wilson MG. Rheumatic Fever. New York: The Commonwealth Fund 1940.

[10] Cournand A. Cardiac catheterization; development of the technique, its contributions to experimental medicine, and its initial applications in man. Acta Med Scand Suppl 1975; 579: 3-32.
[PMID: 1101653]

[11] Mann D. Heart Failure: A Companion to Braunwald's Heart Disease: Expert Consult. St. Louis, Missouri: Saunders 2011.

[12] Gault JH, Ross J Jr, Braunwald E. Contractile state of the left ventricle in man: instantaneous tension-velocity-length relations in patients with and without disease of the left ventricular myocardium. Circ Res 1968; 22(4): 451-63.
[http://dx.doi.org/10.1161/01.RES.22.4.451] [PMID: 5652458]

[13] Katz AM. Regulation of cardiac muscle contractility. J Gen Physiol 1967; 50(6): 185-96.
[http://dx.doi.org/10.1085/jgp.50.6.185] [PMID: 4227923]

[14] Cohn JN, Archibald DG, Ziesche S, *et al.* Effect of vasodilator therapy on mortality in chronic congestive heart failure. Results of a Veterans Administration Cooperative Study. N Engl J Med 1986; 314(24): 1547-52.
[http://dx.doi.org/10.1056/NEJM198606123142404] [PMID: 3520315]

[15] Mann DL, Bristow MR. Mechanisms and models in heart failure: the biomechanical model and beyond. Circulation 2005; 111(21): 2837-49.
[http://dx.doi.org/10.1161/CIRCULATIONAHA.104.500546] [PMID: 15927992]

[16] Francis GS. Neurohormonal control of heart failure. Cleve Clin J Med 2011; 78(1) (Suppl. 1): S75-9.
[http://dx.doi.org/10.3949/ccjm.78.s1.13] [PMID: 21972336]

[17] Dzau VJ, Colucci WS, Hollenberg NK, Williams GH. Relation of the renin-angiotensin-aldosterone system to clinical state in congestive heart failure. Circulation 1981; 63(3): 645-51.
[http://dx.doi.org/10.1161/01.CIR.63.3.645] [PMID: 7006851]

[18] Swedberg K. History of Beta blockers in congestive heart failure. Heart 1998; 79 (Suppl. 2): S29-30.
[http://dx.doi.org/10.1136/hrt.79.2008.29S] [PMID: 18610472]

[19] The SOLVD Investigators. Effect of enalapril on survival in patients with reduced left ventricular ejection fractions and congestive heart failure. N Engl J Med 1991; 325(5): 293-302. [http://dx.doi.org/10.1056/NEJM199108013250501] [PMID: 2057034]

[20] Effects of enalapril on mortality in severe congestive heart failure. Results of the Cooperative North Scandinavian Enalapril Survival Study (CONSENSUS). N Engl J Med 1987; 316(23): 1429-35. [http://dx.doi.org/10.1056/NEJM198706043162301] [PMID: 2883575]

[21] Quirke V. Putting theory into practice: James Black, receptor theory and the development of the β-blockers at ICI, 1958-1978. Med Hist 2006; 50(1): 69-92. [http://dx.doi.org/10.1017/S0025727300009455] [PMID: 16502872]

[22] Waagstein F, Bristow MR, Swedberg K, *et al.* Beneficial effects of metoprolol in idiopathic dilated cardiomyopathy. Lancet 1993; 342(8885): 1441-6. [http://dx.doi.org/10.1016/0140-6736(93)92930-R] [PMID: 7902479]

[23] A randomized trial of beta-blockade in heart failure. Circulation 1994; 90(4): 1765-73. [http://dx.doi.org/10.1161/01.CIR.90.4.1765] [PMID: 7923660]

[24] Ménard J. The 45-year story of the development of an anti-aldosterone more specific than spironolactone. Mol Cell Endocrinol 2004; 217(1-2): 45-52. [http://dx.doi.org/10.1016/j.mce.2003.10.008] [PMID: 15134800]

[25] Pitt B, Zannad F, Remme WJ, *et al.* The effect of spironolactone on morbidity and mortality in patients with severe heart failure. N Engl J Med 1999; 341(10): 709-17. [http://dx.doi.org/10.1056/NEJM199909023411001] [PMID: 10471456]

[26] Pitt B, Remme W, Zannad F, *et al.* Eplerenone, a selective aldosterone blocker, in patients with left ventricular dysfunction after myocardial infarction. N Engl J Med 2003; 348(14): 1309-21. [http://dx.doi.org/10.1056/NEJMoa030207] [PMID: 12668699]

[27] Zannad F, McMurray JJ, Krum H, *et al.* Eplerenone in patients with systolic heart failure and mild symptoms. N Engl J Med 2011; 364(1): 11-21. [http://dx.doi.org/10.1056/NEJMoa1009492] [PMID: 21073363]

[28] Morrissey RP, Czer L, Shah PK. Chronic heart failure: current evidence, challenges to therapy, and future directions. Am J Cardiovasc Drugs 2011; 11(3): 153-71. [http://dx.doi.org/10.2165/11592090-000000000-00000] [PMID: 21619379]

[29] Go AS, Mozaffarian D, Roger VL, *et al.* American Heart Association Statistics Committee and Stroke Statistics Subcommittee. Heart disease and stroke statistics--2013 update: a report from the American Heart Association. Circulation 2013; 127(1): e6-e245. [http://dx.doi.org/10.1161/CIR.0b013e31828124ad] [PMID: 23239837]

[30] Nair AP, Timoh T, Fuster V. Contemporary medical management of systolic heart failure. Circ J 2012; 76(2): 268-77. [http://dx.doi.org/10.1253/circj.CJ-11-1424] [PMID: 22240600]

[31] Yancy CW, Jessup M, Bozkurt B, *et al.* American College of Cardiology Foundation; American Heart Association Task Force on Practice Guidelines. 2013 ACCF/AHA guideline for the management of heart failure: a report of the American College of Cardiology Foundation/American Heart Association Task Force on Practice Guidelines. J Am Coll Cardiol 2013; 62(16): e147-239.

[http://dx.doi.org/10.1016/j.jacc.2013.05.019] [PMID: 23747642]

[32] Ong HT, Kow FP. β-blockers for heart failure: why you should use them more. J Fam Pract 2011; 60(8): 472-7.
[PMID: 21814642]

[33] Di Lenarda A, Remme WJ, Charlesworth A, *et al.* Exchange of β-blockers in heart failure patients. Experiences from the poststudy phase of COMET (the Carvedilol or Metoprolol European Trial). Eur J Heart Fail 2005; 7(4): 640-9.
[http://dx.doi.org/10.1016/j.ejheart.2004.09.010] [PMID: 15921806]

[34] van Veldhuisen DJ, Cohen-Solal A, Böhm M, *et al.* Beta-blockade with nebivolol in elderly heart failure patients with impaired and preserved left ventricular ejection fraction: Data From SENIORS (Study of Effects of Nebivolol Intervention on Outcomes and Rehospitalization in Seniors With Heart Failure). J Am Coll Cardiol 2009; 53(23): 2150-8.
[http://dx.doi.org/10.1016/j.jacc.2009.02.046] [PMID: 19497441]

[35] Smart NA, Kwok N, Holland DJ, Jayasighe R, Giallauria F. Bucindolol: a pharmacogenomic perspective on its use in chronic heart failure. Clin Med Insights Cardiol 2011; 5: 55-66.
[http://dx.doi.org/10.4137/CMC.S4309] [PMID: 21792345]

[36] DiNicolantonio JJ, Lavie CJ, Fares H, Menezes AR, O'Keefe JH. Meta-analysis of carvedilol *versus* beta 1 selective β-blockers (atenolol, bisoprolol, metoprolol, and nebivolol). Am J Cardiol 2013; 111(5): 765-9.
[http://dx.doi.org/10.1016/j.amjcard.2012.11.031] [PMID: 23290925]

[37] Gattis WA, O'Connor CM, Gallup DS, Hasselblad V, Gheorghiade M. Predischarge initiation of carvedilol in patients hospitalized for decompensated heart failure: results of the Initiation Management Predischarge: Process for Assessment of Carvedilol Therapy in Heart Failure (IMPACT-HF) trial. J Am Coll Cardiol 2004; 43(9): 1534-41.
[http://dx.doi.org/10.1016/j.jacc.2003.12.040] [PMID: 15120808]

[38] Flannery G, Gehrig-Mills R, Billah B, Krum H. Analysis of randomized controlled trials on the effect of magnitude of heart rate reduction on clinical outcomes in patients with systolic chronic heart failure receiving β-blockers. Am J Cardiol 2008; 101(6): 865-9.
[http://dx.doi.org/10.1016/j.amjcard.2007.11.023] [PMID: 18328855]

[39] Waagstein F, Caidahl K, Wallentin I, Bergh CH, Hjalmarson A. Long-term beta-blockade in dilated cardiomyopathy. Effects of short- and long-term metoprolol treatment followed by withdrawal and readministration of metoprolol. Circulation 1989; 80(3): 551-63.
[http://dx.doi.org/10.1161/01.CIR.80.3.551] [PMID: 2548768]

[40] McAlister FA, Ezekowitz J, Tonelli M, Armstrong PW. Renal insufficiency and heart failure: prognostic and therapeutic implications from a prospective cohort study. Circulation 2004; 109(8): 1004-9.
[http://dx.doi.org/10.1161/01.CIR.0000116764.53225.A9] [PMID: 14769700]

[41] Ito H, Nagatomo Y, Kohno T, *et al.* Differential effects of carvedilol and metoprolol on renal function in patients with heart failure. Circ J 2010; 74(8): 1578-83.
[http://dx.doi.org/10.1253/circj.CJ-09-0865] [PMID: 20562496]

[42] Ghali JK, Wikstrand J, Van Veldhuisen DJ, *et al.* The influence of renal function on clinical outcome

and response to β-blockade in systolic heart failure: insights from Metoprolol CR/XL Randomized Intervention Trial in Chronic HF (MERIT-HF). J Card Fail 2009; 15(4): 310-8.
[http://dx.doi.org/10.1016/j.cardfail.2008.11.003] [PMID: 19398079]

[43] Castagno D, Jhund PS, McMurray JJ, *et al.* Improved survival with bisoprolol in patients with heart failure and renal impairment: an analysis of the cardiac insufficiency bisoprolol study II (CIBIS-II) trial. Eur J Heart Fail 2010; 12(6): 607-16.
[http://dx.doi.org/10.1093/eurjhf/hfq038] [PMID: 20354032]

[44] Ezekowitz J, McAlister FA, Humphries KH, *et al.* The association among renal insufficiency, pharmacotherapy, and outcomes in 6,427 patients with heart failure and coronary artery disease. J Am Coll Cardiol 2004; 44(8): 1587-92.
[http://dx.doi.org/10.1016/j.jacc.2004.06.072] [PMID: 15489090]

[45] Meyer P, Filippatos GS, Ahmed MI, *et al.* Effects of right ventricular ejection fraction on outcomes in chronic systolic heart failure. Circulation 2010; 121(2): 252-8.
[http://dx.doi.org/10.1161/CIRCULATIONAHA.109.887570] [PMID: 20048206]

[46] Desai RV, Guichard JL, Mujib M, *et al.* Reduced right ventricular ejection fraction and increased mortality in chronic systolic heart failure patients receiving β-blockers: insights from the BEST trial. Int J Cardiol 2013; 163(1): 61-7.
[http://dx.doi.org/10.1016/j.ijcard.2011.05.051] [PMID: 21704392]

[47] Tatli E, Kurum T, Aktoz M, Buyuklu M. Effects of carvedilol on right ventricular ejection fraction and cytokines levels in patients with systolic heart failure. Int J Cardiol 2008; 125(2): 273-6.
[http://dx.doi.org/10.1016/j.ijcard.2007.07.166] [PMID: 18053592]

[48] Arif SA, Mergenhagen KA, Del Carpio RO, Ho C. Treatment of systolic heart failure in the elderly: an evidence-based review. Ann Pharmacother 2010; 44(10): 1604-14.
[http://dx.doi.org/10.1345/aph.1P128] [PMID: 20841514]

[49] Dobre D, Haaijer-Ruskamp FM, Voors AA, van Veldhuisen DJ. beta-Adrenoceptor antagonists in elderly patients with heart failure: a critical review of their efficacy and tolerability. Drugs Aging 2007; 24(12): 1031-44.
[http://dx.doi.org/10.2165/00002512-200724120-00006] [PMID: 18020535]

[50] Haas SJ, Vos T, Gilbert RE, Krum H. Are β-blockers as efficacious in patients with diabetes mellitus as in patients without diabetes mellitus who have chronic heart failure? A meta-analysis of large-scale clinical trials. Am Heart J 2003; 146(5): 848-53.
[http://dx.doi.org/10.1016/S0002-8703(03)00403-4] [PMID: 14597934]

[51] Deedwania PC, Giles TD, Klibaner M, *et al.* Efficacy, safety and tolerability of metoprolol CR/XL in patients with diabetes and chronic heart failure: experiences from MERIT-HF. Am Heart J 2005; 149(1): 159-67.
[http://dx.doi.org/10.1016/j.ahj.2004.05.056] [PMID: 15660048]

[52] de Groote P, Lamblin N, Mouquet F, Bauters C. No gender survival difference in a population of patients with chronic heart failure related to left ventricular systolic dysfunction and receiving optimal medical therapy. Arch Cardiovasc Dis 2008; 101(4): 242-8.
[http://dx.doi.org/10.1016/S1875-2136(08)73699-4] [PMID: 18654099]

[53] Creagh-Brown B. Benefits of β blockers in chronic obstructive pulmonary disease and heart failure.

BMJ 2014; 348: g3316.
[http://dx.doi.org/10.1136/bmj.g3316] [PMID: 24840101]

[54] Demers C, Mody A, Teo KK, McKelvie RS. ACE inhibitors in heart failure: what more do we need to know? Am J Cardiovasc Drugs 2005; 5(6): 351-9.
[http://dx.doi.org/10.2165/00129784-200505060-00002] [PMID: 16259523]

[55] Sander GE, McKinnie JJ, Greenberg SS, Giles TD. Angiotensin-converting enzyme inhibitors and angiotensin II receptor antagonists in the treatment of heart failure caused by left ventricular systolic dysfunction. Prog Cardiovasc Dis 1999; 41(4): 265-300.
[http://dx.doi.org/10.1053/pcad.1999.0410265] [PMID: 10362349]

[56] Jorde UP, Ennezat PV, Lisker J, *et al.* Maximally recommended doses of angiotensin-converting enzyme (ACE) inhibitors do not completely prevent ACE-mediated formation of angiotensin II in chronic heart failure. Circulation 2000; 101(8): 844-6.
[http://dx.doi.org/10.1161/01.CIR.101.8.844] [PMID: 10694521]

[57] The CONSENSUS Trial Study Group. Effects of enalapril on mortality in severe congestive heart failure. Results of the Cooperative North Scandinavian Enalapril Survival Study (CONSENSUS). N Engl J Med 1987; 316(23): 1429-35.
[http://dx.doi.org/10.1056/NEJM198706043162301] [PMID: 2883575]

[58] Swedberg K, Kjekshus J, Snapinn S. Long-term survival in severe heart failure in patients treated with enalapril. Ten year follow-up of CONSENSUS I. Eur Heart J 1999; 20(2): 136-9.
[http://dx.doi.org/10.1053/euhj.1998.1098] [PMID: 10099910]

[59] The SOLVD Investigators. Effect of enalapril on mortality and the development of heart failure in asymptomatic patients with reduced left ventricular ejection fractions. The SOLVD Investigattors. N Engl J Med 1992; 327(10): 685-91.
[http://dx.doi.org/10.1056/NEJM199209033271003] [PMID: 1463530]

[60] The SOLVD Investigators. Effect of enalapril on survival in patients with reduced left ventricular ejection fractions and congestive heart failure. N Engl J Med 1991; 325(5): 293-302.
[http://dx.doi.org/10.1056/NEJM199108013250501] [PMID: 2057034]

[61] Jong P, Yusuf S, Rousseau MF, Ahn SA, Bangdiwala SI. Effect of enalapril on 12-year survival and life expectancy in patients with left ventricular systolic dysfunction: a follow-up study. Lancet 2003; 361(9372): 1843-8.
[http://dx.doi.org/10.1016/S0140-6736(03)13501-5] [PMID: 12788569]

[62] Hall AS, Murray GD, Ball SG. Follow-up study of patients randomly allocated ramipril or placebo for heart failure after acute myocardial infarction: AIRE Extension (AIREX) Study. Acute Infarction Ramipril Efficacy. Lancet 1997; 349(9064): 1493-7.
[http://dx.doi.org/10.1016/S0140-6736(97)04442-5] [PMID: 9167457]

[63] Flather MD, Yusuf S, Køber L, *et al.* ACE-Inhibitor Myocardial Infarction Collaborative Group. Long-term ACE-inhibitor therapy in patients with heart failure or left-ventricular dysfunction: a systematic overview of data from individual patients. Lancet 2000; 355(9215): 1575-81.
[http://dx.doi.org/10.1016/S0140-6736(00)02212-1] [PMID: 10821360]

[64] Garg R, Yusuf S. Overview of randomized trials of angiotensin-converting enzyme inhibitors on mortality and morbidity in patients with heart failure. JAMA 1995; 273(18): 1450-6.

[http://dx.doi.org/10.1001/jama.1995.03520420066040] [PMID: 7654275]

[65] Calvert MJ, Shankar A, McManus RJ, Ryan R, Freemantle N. Evaluation of the management of heart failure in primary care. Fam Pract 2009; 26(2): 145-53.
[http://dx.doi.org/10.1093/fampra/cmn105] [PMID: 19153098]

[66] Parwani P, Ryan J. Heart failure patients with low blood pressure: how should we manage neurohormonal blocking drugs? Circ Heart Fail 2012; 5(6): 819.
[http://dx.doi.org/10.1161/CIRCHEARTFAILURE.112.970889] [PMID: 23170021]

[67] Ahmed A, Fonarow GC, Zhang Y, *et al.* Renin-angiotensin inhibition in systolic heart failure and chronic kidney disease. Am J Med 2012; 125(4): 399-410.
[http://dx.doi.org/10.1016/j.amjmed.2011.10.013] [PMID: 22321760]

[68] Vena GA, Cassano N, Coco V, De Simone C. Eczematous reactions due to angiotensin-converting enzyme inhibitors or angiotensin II receptor blockers. Immunopharmacol Immunotoxicol 2013; 35(3): 447-50.
[http://dx.doi.org/10.3109/08923973.2013.797992] [PMID: 23672527]

[69] McKelvie RS, Yusuf S, Pericak D, *et al.* The RESOLVD Pilot Study Investigators. Comparison of candesartan, enalapril, and their combination in congestive heart failure: randomized evaluation of strategies for left ventricular dysfunction (RESOLVD) pilot study. Circulation 1999; 100(10): 1056-64.
[http://dx.doi.org/10.1161/01.CIR.100.10.1056] [PMID: 10477530]

[70] Pitt B, Segal R, Martinez F, *et al.* Randomised trial of losartan *versus* captopril in patients over 65 with heart failure: the ELITE Study investigators. Lancet 1997; 349: 747-52.
[http://dx.doi.org/10.1016/S0140-6736(97)01187-2] [PMID: 9074572]

[71] Pitt B, Poole-Wilson P, Segal R, *et al.* Effect of losartan compared with captopril on mortality in patients with symptomatic heart failure: randomized trial. Losartan Heart Failure Survival Study ELITE II: the ELITE II investigators. Lancet 2000; 355: 1582-7.
[http://dx.doi.org/10.1016/S0140-6736(00)02213-3] [PMID: 10821361]

[72] McMurray JJ, Ostergren J, Swedberg K, *et al.* CHARM Investigators and Committees. Effects of candesartan in patients with chronic heart failure and reduced left-ventricular systolic function taking angiotensin-converting-enzyme inhibitors: the CHARM-Added trial. Lancet 2003; 362(9386): 767-71.
[http://dx.doi.org/10.1016/S0140-6736(03)14283-3] [PMID: 13678869]

[73] Cohn JN, Tognoni G, Latini R, *et al.* Valsartan Heart Failure Trial Investigators. A randomized trial of the angiotensin-receptor blocker valsartan in chronic heart failure. N Engl J Med 2001; 345(23): 1667-75.
[http://dx.doi.org/10.1056/NEJMoa010713] [PMID: 11759645]

[74] Dickstein K, Kjekshus J. OPTIMAAL Steering Committee of the OPTIMAAL Study Group. Effects of losartan and captopril on mortality and morbidity in high-risk patients after acute myocardial infarction: the OPTIMAAL randomized trial. Lancet 2002; 360: 752-60.
[http://dx.doi.org/10.1016/S0140-6736(02)09895-1] [PMID: 12241832]

[75] Pfeffer MA, McMurray JJ, Velazquez EJ, *et al.* Valsartan in Acute Myocardial Infarction Trial Investigators. Valsartan, captopril, or both in myocardial infarction complicated by heart failure, left ventricular dysfunction, or both. N Engl J Med 2003; 349(20): 1893-906.

[http://dx.doi.org/10.1056/NEJMoa032292] [PMID: 14610160]

[76] McMurray JJ, Packer M, Desai AS, *et al.* PARADIGM-HF Investigators and Committees. Angiotensin-neprilysin inhibition *versus* enalapril in heart failure. N Engl J Med 2014; 371(11): 993-1004.
[http://dx.doi.org/10.1056/NEJMoa1409077] [PMID: 25176015]

[77] Patterson JH, Adams KF Jr, Applefeld MM, Corder CN, Masse BR. Torsemide Investigators Group. Oral torsemide in patients with chronic congestive heart failure: effects on body weight, edema, and electrolyte excretion. Pharmacotherapy 1994; 14(5): 514-21.
[PMID: 7997385]

[78] Domanski M, Norman J, Pitt B, Haigney M, Hanlon S, Peyster E. Studies of Left Ventricular Dysfunction. Diuretic use, progressive heart failure, and death in patients in the Studies Of Left Ventricular Dysfunction (SOLVD). J Am Coll Cardiol 2003; 42(4): 705-8.
[http://dx.doi.org/10.1016/S0735-1097(03)00765-4] [PMID: 12932605]

[79] Odemuyiwa O, Gilmartin J, Kenny D, Hall RJ. Captopril and the diuretic requirements in moderate and severe chronic heart failure. Eur Heart J 1989; 10(7): 586-90.
[PMID: 2670567]

[80] Moser M. Diuretics in the prevention and treatment of congestive heart failure. Cardiovasc Drugs Ther 1997; 11 (Suppl. 1): 273-7.
[http://dx.doi.org/10.1023/A:1007791814100] [PMID: 9211020]

[81] Multiple Risk Factor Intervention Trial Research Group. Multiple risk factor intervention trial. Risk factor changes and mortality results. JAMA 1982; 248(12): 1465-77.
[http://dx.doi.org/10.1001/jama.1982.03330120023025] [PMID: 7050440]

[82] Larsen FF. Haemodynamic effects of high or low doses of furosemide in acute myocardial infarction. Eur Heart J 1988; 9(2): 125-31.
[PMID: 3280315]

[83] Dikshit K, Vyden JK, Forrester JS, Chatterjee K, Prakash R, Swan HJ. Renal and extrarenal hemodynamic effects of furosemide in congestive heart failure after acute myocardial infarction. N Engl J Med 1973; 288(21): 1087-90.
[http://dx.doi.org/10.1056/NEJM197305242882102] [PMID: 4697939]

[84] Raftery EB. Haemodynamic effects of diuretics in heart failure. Br Heart J 1994; 72(2) (Suppl.): S44-7.
[http://dx.doi.org/10.1136/hrt.72.2_Suppl.S44] [PMID: 7946758]

[85] Skøtt O, Briggs JP. Direct demonstration of macula densa-mediated renin secretion. Science 1987; 237(4822): 1618-20.
[http://dx.doi.org/10.1126/science.3306925] [PMID: 3306925]

[86] DiNicolantonio JJ. Should torsemide be the loop diuretic of choice in systolic heart failure? Future Cardiol 2012; 8(5): 707-28.
[http://dx.doi.org/10.2217/fca.12.54] [PMID: 23013124]

[87] Wall GC, Bigner D, Craig S. Ethacrynic acid and the sulfa-sensitive patient. Arch Intern Med 2003; 163(1): 116-7.

[http://dx.doi.org/10.1001/archinte.163.1.116] [PMID: 12523926]

[88] Gottlieb SS, Robinson S, Krichten CM, Fisher ML. Renal response to indomethacin in congestive heart failure secondary to ischemic or idiopathic dilated cardiomyopathy. Am J Cardiol 1992; 70(9): 890-3.
[http://dx.doi.org/10.1016/0002-9149(92)90733-F] [PMID: 1529943]

[89] Giamouzis G, Butler J, Starling RC, *et al.* Impact of dopamine infusion on renal function in hospitalized heart failure patients: results of the Dopamine in Acute Decompensated Heart Failure (DAD-HF) Trial. J Card Fail 2010; 16(12): 922-30.
[http://dx.doi.org/10.1016/j.cardfail.2010.07.246] [PMID: 21111980]

[90] Sica DA, Gehr TW. Diuretic combinations in refractory oedema states: pharmacokinetic-pharmacodynamic relationships. Clin Pharmacokinet 1996; 30(3): 229-49.
[http://dx.doi.org/10.2165/00003088-199630030-00004] [PMID: 8882303]

[91] Sica DA. Metolazone and its role in edema management. Congest Heart Fail 2003; 9(2): 100-5.
[http://dx.doi.org/10.1111/j.1527-5299.2003.01907.x] [PMID: 12671341]

[92] Davis BR, Piller LB, Cutler JA, *et al.* Antihypertensive and Lipid-Lowering treatment to prevent heart attack trial collaborative research group. Role of diuretics in the prevention of heart failure: the Antihypertensive and Lipid-Lowering treatment to prevent heart attack trial. Circulation 2006; 113(18): 2201-10.
[http://dx.doi.org/10.1161/CIRCULATIONAHA.105.544031] [PMID: 16651474]

[93] Arnold JM, Yusuf S, Young J, *et al.* HOPE Investigators. Prevention of heart failure in patients in the heart outcomes prevention evaluation (HOPE) study. Circulation 2003; 107(9): 1284-90.
[http://dx.doi.org/10.1161/01.CIR.0000054165.93055.42] [PMID: 12628949]

[94] Dormans TP, Gerlag PG. Combination of high-dose furosemide and hydrochlorothiazide in the treatment of refractory congestive heart failure. Eur Heart J 1996; 17(12): 1867-74.
[http://dx.doi.org/10.1093/oxfordjournals.eurheartj.a014805] [PMID: 8960430]

[95] Luo J, Gao X, Peng L, Sun H, Dai G. Effects of hydrochlorothiazide on cardiac remodeling in a rat model of myocardial infarction-induced congestive heart failure. Eur J Pharmacol 2011; 667(1-3): 314-21.
[http://dx.doi.org/10.1016/j.ejphar.2011.06.012] [PMID: 21703256]

[96] Sayer G, Bhat G. The renin-angiotensin-aldosterone system and heart failure. Cardiol Clin 2014; 32(1): 21-32, vii.
[http://dx.doi.org/10.1016/j.ccl.2013.09.002] [PMID: 24286576]

[97] Butler J, Ezekowitz JA, Collins SP, *et al.* Heart Failure Society of America Guidelines Committee. Update on aldosterone antagonists use in heart failure with reduced left ventricular ejection fraction. J Card Fail 2012; 18(4): 265-81.
[http://dx.doi.org/10.1016/j.cardfail.2012.02.005] [PMID: 22464767]

[98] The Digitalis Investigation Group. Rationale, design, implementation, and baseline characteristics of patients in the DIG trial: a large, simple, long-term trial to evaluate the effect of digitalis on mortality in heart failure. Control Clin Trials 1996; 17(1): 77-97.
[http://dx.doi.org/10.1016/0197-2456(95)00065-8] [PMID: 8721804]

[99] Young JB, Gheorghiade M, Uretsky BF, Patterson JH, Adams KF Jr. Superiority of "triple" drug therapy in heart failure: insights from the PROVED and RADIANCE trials. Prospective randomized study of ventricular function and efficacy of Digoxin. Randomized assessment of Digoxin and inhibitors of Angiotensin-Converting enzyme. J Am Coll Cardiol 1998; 32(3): 686-92. [http://dx.doi.org/10.1016/S0735-1097(98)00302-7] [PMID: 9741512]

[100] Packer M, Gheorghiade M, Young JB, *et al.* Withdrawal of digoxin from patients with chronic heart failure treated with angiotensin-converting-enzyme inhibitors. RADIANCE Study. N Engl J Med 1993; 329(1): 1-7. [http://dx.doi.org/10.1056/NEJM199307013290101] [PMID: 8505940]

[101] Khand AU, Rankin AC, Martin W, Taylor J, Gemmell I, Cleland JG. Carvedilol alone or in combination with digoxin for the management of atrial fibrillation in patients with heart failure? J Am Coll Cardiol 2003; 42(11): 1944-51. [http://dx.doi.org/10.1016/j.jacc.2003.07.020] [PMID: 14662257]

[102] Jencks SF, Williams MV, Coleman EA. Rehospitalizations among patients in the Medicare fee-fo--service program. N Engl J Med 2009; 360(14): 1418-28. [http://dx.doi.org/10.1056/NEJMsa0803563] [PMID: 19339721]

[103] Stone J, Hoffman G. Medicare Hospital Readmissions: Issues, Policy Options and PPACA: Congressional Research Service Report for Congress. Members and Committees of Congress.

[104] Ahmed A, Bourge RC, Fonarow GC, *et al.* Digoxin use and lower 30-day all-cause readmission for Medicare beneficiaries hospitalized for heart failure. Am J Med 2014; 127(1): 61-70. [http://dx.doi.org/10.1016/j.amjmed.2013.08.027] [PMID: 24257326]

[105] Bourge RC, Fleg JL, Fonarow GC, *et al.* Digoxin reduces 30-day all-cause hospital admission in older patients with chronic systolic heart failure. Am J Med 2013; 126(8): 701-8. [http://dx.doi.org/10.1016/j.amjmed.2013.02.001] [PMID: 23490060]

[106] Jelliffe RW, Brooker G. A nomogram for digoxin therapy. Am J Med 1974; 57(1): 63-8. [http://dx.doi.org/10.1016/0002-9343(74)90769-4] [PMID: 4600984]

[107] Rathore SS, Curtis JP, Wang Y, Bristow MR, Krumholz HM. Association of serum digoxin concentration and outcomes in patients with heart failure. JAMA 2003; 289(7): 871-8. [http://dx.doi.org/10.1001/jama.289.7.871] [PMID: 12588271]

[108] Bizjak ED, Mauro VF. Digoxin-macrolide drug interaction. Ann Pharmacother 1997; 31(9): 1077-9. [PMID: 9296249]

[109] Cai H, Harrison DG. Endothelial dysfunction in cardiovascular diseases: the role of oxidant stress. Circ Res 2000; 87(10): 840-4. [http://dx.doi.org/10.1161/01.RES.87.10.840] [PMID: 11073878]

[110] Drexler H, Hayoz D, Münzel T, *et al.* Endothelial function in chronic congestive heart failure. Am J Cardiol 1992; 69(19): 1596-601. [http://dx.doi.org/10.1016/0002-9149(92)90710-G] [PMID: 1598876]

[111] Belch JJ, Bridges AB, Scott N, Chopra M. Oxygen free radicals and congestive heart failure. Br Heart J 1991; 65(5): 245-8. [http://dx.doi.org/10.1136/hrt.65.5.245] [PMID: 2039668]

[112] Cohn JN, Johnson G, Ziesche S, *et al.* A comparison of enalapril with hydralazine-isosorbide dinitrate in the treatment of chronic congestive heart failure. N Engl J Med 1991; 325(5): 303-10. [http://dx.doi.org/10.1056/NEJM199108013250502] [PMID: 2057035]

[113] Taylor AL, Ziesche S, Yancy C, *et al.* African-American Heart Failure Trial Investigators. Combination of isosorbide dinitrate and hydralazine in blacks with heart failure. N Engl J Med 2004; 351(20): 2049-57. [http://dx.doi.org/10.1056/NEJMoa042934] [PMID: 15533851]

[114] Swedberg K, Held P, Kjekshus J, Rasmussen K, Rydén L, Wedel H. Effects of the early administration of enalapril on mortality in patients with acute myocardial infarction. Results of the Cooperative New Scandinavian Enalapril Survival Study II (CONSENSUS II). N Engl J Med 1992; 327(10): 678-84. [http://dx.doi.org/10.1056/NEJM199209033271002] [PMID: 1495520]

[115] Vaccarino V, Gahbauer E, Kasl SV, Charpentier PA, Acampora D, Krumholz HM. Differences between African Americans and whites in the outcome of heart failure: Evidence for a greater functional decline in African Americans. Am Heart J 2002; 143(6): 1058-67. [http://dx.doi.org/10.1067/mhj.2002.122123] [PMID: 12075264]

[116] Cheng JW. A review of isosorbide dinitrate and hydralazine in the management of heart failure in black patients, with a focus on a new fixed-dose combination. Clin Ther 2006; 28(5): 666-78. [http://dx.doi.org/10.1016/j.clinthera.2006.05.007] [PMID: 16861089]

[117] Ferdinand KC, Elkayam U, Mancini D, *et al.* Use of isosorbide dinitrate and hydralazine in African-Americans with heart failure 9 years after the African-American Heart Failure Trial. Am J Cardiol 2014; 114(1): 151-9. [http://dx.doi.org/10.1016/j.amjcard.2014.04.018] [PMID: 24846808]

[118] Yancy CW, Abraham WT, Albert NM, *et al.* Quality of care of and outcomes for African Americans hospitalized with heart failure: findings from the OPTIMIZE-HF (Organized Program to Initiate Lifesaving Treatment in Hospitalized Patients With Heart Failure) registry. J Am Coll Cardiol 2008; 51(17): 1675-84. [http://dx.doi.org/10.1016/j.jacc.2008.01.028] [PMID: 18436120]

[119] Deedwania P. Selective and specific inhibition of If with ivabradine for the treatment of coronary artery disease or heart failure. Drugs 2013; 73(14): 1569-86. [http://dx.doi.org/10.1007/s40265-013-0117-0] [PMID: 24065301]

[120] Manz M, Reuter M, Lauck G, Omran H, Jung W. A single intravenous dose of ivabradine, a novel $I_{(f)}$ inhibitor, lowers heart rate but does not depress left ventricular function in patients with left ventricular dysfunction. Cardiology 2003; 100(3): 149-55. [http://dx.doi.org/10.1159/000073933] [PMID: 14631136]

[121] Mangoni E, Fontanaud P, Bouly M, *et al.* Relationship between I_f current inhibition by ivabradine and cardiac pacemaker activity. Eur Heart J 2006; 27 (Suppl. 1): 380.

[122] Swedberg K, Komajda M, Böhm M, *et al.* SHIFT Investigators. Ivabradine and outcomes in chronic heart failure (SHIFT): a randomised placebo-controlled study. Lancet 2010; 376(9744): 875-85. [http://dx.doi.org/10.1016/S0140-6736(10)61198-1] [PMID: 20801500]

[123] Tardif JC, Ford I, Tendera M, Bourassa MG, Fox K. INITIATIVE Investigators. Efficacy of

ivabradine, a new selective $I_{(f)}$ inhibitor, compared with atenolol in patients with chronic stable angina. Eur Heart J 2005; 26(23): 2529-36.
[http://dx.doi.org/10.1093/eurheartj/ehi586] [PMID: 16214830]

[124] Ruzyllo W, Tendera M, Ford I, Fox KM. Antianginal efficacy and safety of ivabradine compared with amlodipine in patients with stable effort angina pectoris: a 3-month randomised, double-blind, multicentre, noninferiority trial. Drugs 2007; 67(3): 393-405.
[http://dx.doi.org/10.2165/00003495-200767030-00005] [PMID: 17335297]

[125] Tardif JC, Ponikowski P, Kahan T. ASSOCIATE Study Investigators. Efficacy of the I(f) current inhibitor ivabradine in patients with chronic stable angina receiving beta-blocker therapy: a 4-month, randomized, placebo-controlled trial. Eur Heart J 2009; 30(5): 540-8.
[http://dx.doi.org/10.1093/eurheartj/ehn571] [PMID: 19136486]

[126] Amosova E, Andrejev E, Zaderey I, Rudenko U, Ceconi C, Ferrari R. Efficacy of ivabradine in combination with Beta-blocker *versus* uptitration of Beta-blocker in patients with stable angina. Cardiovasc Drugs Ther 2011; 25(6): 531-7.
[http://dx.doi.org/10.1007/s10557-011-6327-3] [PMID: 21830063]

[127] López-Bescós L, Filipova S, Martos R. Long-term safety and efficacy of ivabradine in patients with chronic stable angina. Cardiology 2007; 108(4): 387-96.
[http://dx.doi.org/10.1159/000108387] [PMID: 17890862]

[128] Tendera M, Borer JS, Tardif JC. Efficacy of I_f inhibition with ivabradine in different subpopulations with stable angina pectoris. Cardiology 2009; 114(2): 116-25.
[http://dx.doi.org/10.1159/000219938] [PMID: 19468225]

[129] Savelieva I, Camm AJ. I_f inhibition with ivabradine : electrophysiological effects and safety. Drug Saf 2008; 31(2): 95-107.
[http://dx.doi.org/10.2165/00002018-200831020-00001] [PMID: 18217787]

[130] McMurray JJ, Adamopoulos S, Anker SD, *et al.* ESC Committee for Practice Guidelines. ESC Guidelines for the diagnosis and treatment of acute and chronic heart failure 2012: The Task Force for the Diagnosis and Treatment of Acute and Chronic Heart Failure 2012 of the European Society of Cardiology. Developed in collaboration with the Heart Failure Association (HFA) of the ESC. Eur Heart J 2012; 33(14): 1787-847.
[http://dx.doi.org/10.1093/eurheartj/ehs104] [PMID: 22611136]

[131] Swedberg K, Komajda M, Böhm M, *et al.* SHIFT Investigators. Effects on outcomes of heart rate reduction by ivabradine in patients with congestive heart failure: is there an influence of beta-blocker dose?: findings from the SHIFT (Systolic Heart failure treatment with the $I_{(f)}$ inhibitor ivabradine Trial) study. J Am Coll Cardiol 2012; 59(22): 1938-45.
[http://dx.doi.org/10.1016/j.jacc.2012.01.020] [PMID: 22617188]

[132] Komajda M, Böhm M, Borer J, *et al.* Influence of background treatment with mineralocorticoid receptor antagonists on ivabradine's effects in patients with chronic heart failure. Eur J Heart Fail 2013; 15(1): 79-84.
[http://dx.doi.org/10.1093/eurjhf/hfs127] [PMID: 22892123]

[133] Tardif JC, O'Meara E, Komajda M, *et al.* SHIFT Investigators. Effects of selective heart rate reduction with ivabradine on left ventricular remodelling and function: results from the SHIFT echocardiography

substudy. Eur Heart J 2011; 32(20): 2507-15.
[http://dx.doi.org/10.1093/eurheartj/ehr311] [PMID: 21875858]

[134] Volterrani M, Cice G, Caminiti G, *et al.* Effect of Carvedilol, Ivabradine or their combination on exercise capacity in patients with Heart Failure (the CARVIVA HF trial). Int J Cardiol 2011; 151(2): 218-24.
[http://dx.doi.org/10.1016/j.ijcard.2011.06.098] [PMID: 21764469]

[135] Kenchaiah S, Narula J, Vasan RS. Risk factors for heart failure. Med Clin North Am 2004; 88(5): 1145-72.
[http://dx.doi.org/10.1016/j.mcna.2004.04.016] [PMID: 15331311]

[136] Kris-Etherton PM, Harris WS, Appel LJ. American Heart Association. Nutrition Committee. Fish consumption, fish oil, omega-3 fatty acids, and cardiovascular disease. Circulation 2002; 106(21): 2747-57.
[http://dx.doi.org/10.1161/01.CIR.0000038493.65177.94] [PMID: 12438303]

[137] Petersen JW, Felker GM. Inflammatory biomarkers in heart failure. Congest Heart Fail 2006; 12(6): 324-8.
[http://dx.doi.org/10.1111/j.1527-5299.2006.05595.x] [PMID: 17170586]

[138] Tur JA, Bibiloni MM, Sureda A, Pons A. Dietary sources of omega 3 fatty acids: public health risks and benefits. Br J Nutr 2012; 107(s2) (Suppl. 2): S23-52.
[http://dx.doi.org/10.1017/S0007114512001456] [PMID: 22591897]

[139] Yamagishi K, Iso H, Date C, *et al.* Japan Collaborative Cohort Study for Evaluation of Cancer Risk Study Group. Fish, omega-3 polyunsaturated fatty acids, and mortality from cardiovascular diseases in a nationwide community-based cohort of Japanese men and women the JACC (Japan Collaborative Cohort Study for Evaluation of Cancer Risk) Study. J Am Coll Cardiol 2008; 52(12): 988-96.
[http://dx.doi.org/10.1016/j.jacc.2008.06.018] [PMID: 18786479]

[140] Mozaffarian D, Psaty BM, Rimm EB, *et al.* Fish intake and risk of incident atrial fibrillation. Circulation 2004; 110(4): 368-73.
[http://dx.doi.org/10.1161/01.CIR.0000138154.00779.A5] [PMID: 15262826]

[141] Mozaffarian D, Lemaitre RN, King IB, *et al.* Circulating long-chain ω-3 fatty acids and incidence of congestive heart failure in older adults: the cardiovascular health study: a cohort study. Ann Intern Med 2011; 155(3): 160-70.
[http://dx.doi.org/10.7326/0003-4819-155-3-201108020-00006] [PMID: 21810709]

[142] Dijkstra SC, Brouwer IA, van Rooij FJ, Hofman A, Witteman JC, Geleijnse JM. Intake of very long chain n-3 fatty acids from fish and the incidence of heart failure: the Rotterdam Study. Eur J Heart Fail 2009; 11(10): 922-8.
[http://dx.doi.org/10.1093/eurjhf/hfp126] [PMID: 19789394]

[143] Belin RJ, Greenland P, Martin L, *et al.* Fish intake and the risk of incident heart failure: the Women's Health Initiative. Circ Heart Fail 2011; 4(4): 404-13.
[http://dx.doi.org/10.1161/CIRCHEARTFAILURE.110.960450] [PMID: 21610249]

[144] Mehra MR, Lavie CJ, Ventura HO, Milani RV. Fish oils produce anti-inflammatory effects and improve body weight in severe heart failure. J Heart Lung Transplant 2006; 25(7): 834-8.
[http://dx.doi.org/10.1016/j.healun.2006.03.005] [PMID: 16818127]

[145] Moertl D, Hammer A, Steiner S, Hutuleac R, Vonbank K, Berger R. Dose-dependent effects of omega-3-polyunsaturated fatty acids on systolic left ventricular function, endothelial function, and markers of inflammation in chronic heart failure of nonischemic origin: a double-blind, placebo-controlled, 3-arm study. Am Heart J 2011; 161(5): 915.e1-9. [http://dx.doi.org/10.1016/j.ahj.2011.02.011] [PMID: 21570522]

[146] Tavazzi L, Maggioni AP, Marchioli R, *et al.* Effect of n-3 polyunsaturated fatty acids in patients with chronic heart failure (the GISSI-HF trial): a randomised, double-blind, placebo-controlled trial. Lancet 2008; 372(9645): 1223-30. [http://dx.doi.org/10.1016/S0140-6736(08)61239-8] [PMID: 18757090]

[147] Zhao YT, Shao L, Teng LL, *et al.* Effects of n-3 polyunsaturated fatty acid therapy on plasma inflammatory markers and N-terminal pro-brain natriuretic peptide in elderly patients with chronic heart failure. J Int Med Res 2009; 37(6): 1831-41. [http://dx.doi.org/10.1177/147323000903700619] [PMID: 20146881]

[148] Poudyal H, Brown L. The role of n-3 polyunsaturated fatty acids in human heart failure. Endocr Metab Immune Disord Drug Targets 2013; 13(1): 105-17. [http://dx.doi.org/10.2174/1871530311313010013] [PMID: 23369143]

[149] Lavie CJ, Milani RV, Mehra MR, Ventura HO. Omega-3 polyunsaturated fatty acids and cardiovascular diseases. J Am Coll Cardiol 2009; 54(7): 585-94. [http://dx.doi.org/10.1016/j.jacc.2009.02.084] [PMID: 19660687]

[150] Mathur N, Ramasubbu K, Mann DL. Spectrum of pleiotropic effects of statins in heart failure. Heart Fail Clin 2008; 4(2): 153-61. [http://dx.doi.org/10.1016/j.hfc.2008.01.007] [PMID: 18433695]

[151] Jain MK, Ridker PM. Anti-inflammatory effects of statins: clinical evidence and basic mechanisms. Nat Rev Drug Discov 2005; 4(12): 977-87. [http://dx.doi.org/10.1038/nrd1901] [PMID: 16341063]

[152] Dilaveris P, Giannopoulos G, Riga M, Synetos A, Stefanadis C. Beneficial effects of statins on endothelial dysfunction and vascular stiffness. Curr Vasc Pharmacol 2007; 5(3): 227-37. [http://dx.doi.org/10.2174/157016107781024091] [PMID: 17627566]

[153] Levy WC. Observational studies of statins in systolic heart failure. Heart Fail Clin 2008; 4(2): 201-8. [http://dx.doi.org/10.1016/j.hfc.2008.01.006] [PMID: 18433700]

[154] Krum H, Latini R, Maggioni AP, *et al.* Statins and symptomatic chronic systolic heart failure: a post-hoc analysis of 5010 patients enrolled in Val-HeFT. Int J Cardiol 2007; 119(1): 48-53. [http://dx.doi.org/10.1016/j.ijcard.2006.07.106] [PMID: 17049646]

[155] Kjekshus J, Pedersen TR, Olsson AG, Faergeman O, Pyörälä K. The effects of simvastatin on the incidence of heart failure in patients with coronary heart disease. J Card Fail 1997; 3(4): 249-54. [http://dx.doi.org/10.1016/S1071-9164(97)90022-1] [PMID: 9547437]

[156] Scirica BM, Morrow DA, Cannon CP, *et al.* PROVE IT-TIMI 22 Investigators. Intensive statin therapy and the risk of hospitalization for heart failure after an acute coronary syndrome in the PROVE IT-TIMI 22 study. J Am Coll Cardiol 2006; 47(11): 2326-31. [http://dx.doi.org/10.1016/j.jacc.2006.03.034] [PMID: 16750703]

[157] Hognestad A, Dickstein K, Myhre E, Snapinn S, Kjekshus J. OPTIMAAL Investigators. Effect of combined statin and beta-blocker treatment on one-year morbidity and mortality after acute myocardial infarction associated with heart failure. Am J Cardiol 2004; 93(5): 603-6. [http://dx.doi.org/10.1016/j.amjcard.2003.11.027] [PMID: 14996587]

[158] Goldberger JJ, Subacius H, Schaechter A, *et al.* DEFINITE Investigators. Effects of statin therapy on arrhythmic events and survival in patients with nonischemic dilated cardiomyopathy. J Am Coll Cardiol 2006; 48(6): 1228-33. [http://dx.doi.org/10.1016/j.jacc.2006.05.053] [PMID: 16979011]

[159] Ramasubbu K, Estep J, White DL, Deswal A, Mann DL. Experimental and clinical basis for the use of statins in patients with ischemic and nonischemic cardiomyopathy. J Am Coll Cardiol 2008; 51(4): 415-26. [http://dx.doi.org/10.1016/j.jacc.2007.10.009] [PMID: 18222351]

[160] Kjekshus J, Apetrei E, Barrios V, *et al.* Rosuvastatin in older patients with systolic heart failure. N Engl J Med 2007; 357(22): 2248-61. [http://dx.doi.org/10.1056/NEJMoa0706201] [PMID: 17984166]

[161] Khush KK, Waters DD, Bittner V, *et al.* Effect of high-dose atorvastatin on hospitalizations for heart failure: subgroup analysis of the Treating to New Targets (TNT) study. Circulation 2007; 115(5): 576-83. [http://dx.doi.org/10.1161/CIRCULATIONAHA.106.625574] [PMID: 17261662]

[162] Givertz MM, Teerlink JR, Albert NM, *et al.* Acute decompensated heart failure: update on new and emerging evidence and directions for future research. J Card Fail 2013; 19(6): 371-89. [http://dx.doi.org/10.1016/j.cardfail.2013.04.002] [PMID: 23743486]

[163] Go AS, Mozaffarian D, Roger VL, *et al.* American Heart Association Statistics Committee and Stroke Statistics Subcommittee. Heart disease and stroke statistics--2013 update: a report from the American Heart Association. Circulation 2013; 127(1): e6-e245. [http://dx.doi.org/10.1161/CIR.0b013e31828124ad] [PMID: 23239837]

[164] Krumholz HM, Merrill AR, Schone EM, *et al.* Patterns of hospital performance in acute myocardial infarction and heart failure 30-day mortality and readmission. Circ Cardiovasc Qual Outcomes 2009; 2(5): 407-13. [http://dx.doi.org/10.1161/CIRCOUTCOMES.109.883256] [PMID: 20031870]

[165] Adams KF Jr, Fonarow GC, Emerman CL, *et al.* ADHERE Scientific Advisory Committee and Investigators. Characteristics and outcomes of patients hospitalized for heart failure in the United States: rationale, design, and preliminary observations from the first 100,000 cases in the Acute Decompensated Heart Failure National Registry (ADHERE). Am Heart J 2005; 149(2): 209-16. [http://dx.doi.org/10.1016/j.ahj.2004.08.005] [PMID: 15846257]

[166] Gheorghiade M, Pang PS. Acute heart failure syndromes. J Am Coll Cardiol 2009; 53(7): 557-73. [http://dx.doi.org/10.1016/j.jacc.2008.10.041] [PMID: 19215829]

[167] Vasko MR, Cartwright DB, Knochel JP, Nixon JV, Brater DC. Furosemide absorption altered in decompensated congestive heart failure. Ann Intern Med 1985; 102(3): 314-8. [http://dx.doi.org/10.7326/0003-4819-102-3-314] [PMID: 3970471]

[168] Piepoli M, Binno S, Villani GQ, Cabassi A. Management of oral chronic pharmacotherapy in patients hospitalized for acute decompensated heart failure. Int J Cardiol 2014; 176(2): 321-6. [http://dx.doi.org/10.1016/j.ijcard.2014.07.085] [PMID: 25129309]

[169] Peacock WF IV, Fonarow GC, Emerman CL, Mills RM, Wynne J. ADHERE Scientific Advisory Committee and Investigators; Adhere Study Group. Impact of early initiation of intravenous therapy for acute decompensated heart failure on outcomes in ADHERE. Cardiology 2007; 107(1): 44-51. [http://dx.doi.org/10.1159/000093612] [PMID: 16741357]

[170] Jentzer JC, DeWald TA, Hernandez AF. Combination of loop diuretics with thiazide-type diuretics in heart failure. J Am Coll Cardiol 2010; 56(19): 1527-34. [http://dx.doi.org/10.1016/j.jacc.2010.06.034] [PMID: 21029871]

[171] Felker GM, Lee KL, Bull DA, *et al.* NHLBI Heart Failure Clinical Research Network. Diuretic strategies in patients with acute decompensated heart failure. N Engl J Med 2011; 364(9): 797-805. [http://dx.doi.org/10.1056/NEJMoa1005419] [PMID: 21366472]

[172] Shakar SF, Lindenfeld J. Treatment approaches to congestion relief in acute decompensated HF: Insights after DOSE-AHF and CARRESS-HF. Curr Treat Options Cardiovasc Med 2014; 16(8): 330. [http://dx.doi.org/10.1007/s11936-014-0330-5] [PMID: 25063583]

[173] Peacock WF IV, De Marco T, Fonarow GC, *et al.* Cardiac troponin and outcome in acute heart failure. N Engl J Med 2008; 358(20): 2117-26. [http://dx.doi.org/10.1056/NEJMoa0706824] [PMID: 18480204]

[174] The CONSENSUS Trial Study Group. Effects of enalapril on mortality in severe congestive heart failure. Results of the Cooperative North Scandinavian Enalapril Survival Study (CONSENSUS). N Engl J Med 1987; 316(23): 1429-35. [http://dx.doi.org/10.1056/NEJM198706043162301] [PMID: 2883575]

[175] Cohn JN, Tognoni G. Valsartan heart failure trial investigators. A randomized trial of the angiotensin-receptor blocker valsartan in chronic heart failure. N Engl J Med 2001; 345(23): 1667-75. [http://dx.doi.org/10.1056/NEJMoa010713] [PMID: 11759645]

[176] Endre ZH. Acute kidney injury: definitions and new paradigms. Adv Chronic Kidney Dis 2008; 15(3): 213-21. [http://dx.doi.org/10.1053/j.ackd.2008.04.002] [PMID: 18565473]

[177] Packer M, Fowler MB, Roecker EB, *et al.* Carvedilol Prospective Randomized Cumulative Survival (COPERNICUS) Study Group. Effect of carvedilol on the morbidity of patients with severe chronic heart failure: results of the carvedilol prospective randomized cumulative survival (COPERNICUS) study. Circulation 2002; 106(17): 2194-9. [http://dx.doi.org/10.1161/01.CIR.0000035653.72855.BF] [PMID: 12390947]

[178] CIBIS-II Investigators and Committees. The Cardiac Insufficiency Bisoprolol Study II (CIBIS-II): a randomised trial. Lancet 1999; 353(9146): 9-13. [http://dx.doi.org/10.1016/S0140-6736(98)11181-9] [PMID: 10023943]

[179] Effect of metoprolol CR/XL in chronic heart failure: Metoprolol CR/XL Randomised Intervention Trial in Congestive Heart Failure (MERIT-HF). Lancet 1999; 353(9169): 2001-7. [http://dx.doi.org/10.1016/S0140-6736(99)04440-2] [PMID: 10376614]

[180] Flather MD, Shibata MC, Coats AJ, *et al.* SENIORS Investigators. Randomized trial to determine the effect of nebivolol on mortality and cardiovascular hospital admission in elderly patients with heart failure (SENIORS). Eur Heart J 2005; 26(3): 215-25.
[http://dx.doi.org/10.1093/eurheartj/ehi115] [PMID: 15642700]

[181] McMurray JJ, Adamopoulos S, Anker SD, *et al.* ESC Committee for Practice Guidelines. ESC Guidelines for the diagnosis and treatment of acute and chronic heart failure 2012: The Task Force for the Diagnosis and Treatment of Acute and Chronic Heart Failure 2012 of the European Society of Cardiology. Developed in collaboration with the Heart Failure Association (HFA) of the ESC. Eur Heart J 2012; 33(14): 1787-847.
[http://dx.doi.org/10.1093/eurheartj/ehs104] [PMID: 22611136]

[182] Metra M, Torp-Pedersen C, Cleland JG, *et al.* COMET investigators. Should beta-blocker therapy be reduced or withdrawn after an episode of decompensated heart failure? Results from COMET. Eur J Heart Fail 2007; 9(9): 901-9.
[http://dx.doi.org/10.1016/j.ejheart.2007.05.011] [PMID: 17581778]

[183] Udelson JE, Orlandi C, Ouyang J, *et al.* Acute hemodynamic effects of tolvaptan, a vasopressin V2 receptor blocker, in patients with symptomatic heart failure and systolic dysfunction: an international, multicenter, randomized, placebo-controlled trial. J Am Coll Cardiol 2008; 52(19): 1540-5.
[http://dx.doi.org/10.1016/j.jacc.2008.08.013] [PMID: 19007589]

[184] Konstam MA, Gheorghiade M, Burnett JC Jr, *et al.* Efficacy of Vasopressin Antagonism in Heart Failure Outcome Study With Tolvaptan (EVEREST) Investigators. Effects of oral tolvaptan in patients hospitalized for worsening heart failure: the EVEREST Outcome Trial. JAMA 2007; 297(12): 1319-31.
[http://dx.doi.org/10.1001/jama.297.12.1319] [PMID: 17384437]

[185] Carlson MD, Eckman PM. Review of vasodilators in acute decompensated heart failure: the old and the new. J Card Fail 2013; 19(7): 478-93.
[http://dx.doi.org/10.1016/j.cardfail.2013.05.007] [PMID: 23834924]

[186] Elkayam U, Janmohamed M, Habib M, Hatamizadeh P. Vasodilators in the management of acute heart failure. Crit Care Med 2008; 36 (1 Suppl): S95e105.
[http://dx.doi.org/10.1097/01.CCM.0000297161.41559.93]

[187] Cotter G, Metzkor E, Kaluski E, *et al.* Randomised trial of high-dose isosorbide dinitrate plus low-dose furosemide versus high-dose furosemide plus low-dose isosorbide dinitrate in severe pulmonary oedema. Lancet 1998; 351(9100): 389-93.
[http://dx.doi.org/10.1016/S0140-6736(97)08417-1] [PMID: 9482291]

[188] Mullens W, Abrahams Z, Francis GS, *et al.* Sodium nitroprusside for advanced low-output heart failure. J Am Coll Cardiol 2008; 52(3): 200-7.
[http://dx.doi.org/10.1016/j.jacc.2008.02.083] [PMID: 18617068]

[189] Cohn JN, Franciosa JA, Francis GS, *et al.* Effect of short-term infusion of sodium nitroprusside on mortality rate in acute myocardial infarction complicated by left ventricular failure: results of a Veterans Administration cooperative study. N Engl J Med 1982; 306(19): 1129-35.
[http://dx.doi.org/10.1056/NEJM198205133061902] [PMID: 7040956]

[190] Elkayam U, Akhter MW, Singh H, Khan S, Usman A. Comparison of effects on left ventricular filling

pressure of intravenous nesiritide and high-dose nitroglycerin in patients with decompensated heart failure. Am J Cardiol 2004; 93(2): 237-40.
[http://dx.doi.org/10.1016/j.amjcard.2003.09.051] [PMID: 14715359]

[191] Publication Committee for the VMAC Investigators (Vasodilatation in the Management of Acute CHF). Intravenous nesiritide *vs.* nitroglycerin for treatment of decompensated congestive heart failure: a randomized controlled trial. JAMA 2002; 287(12): 1531-40.
[PMID: 11911755]

[192] Sackner-Bernstein JD, Skopicki HA, Aaronson KD. Risk of worsening renal function with nesiritide in patients with acutely decompensated heart failure. Circulation 2005; 111(12): 1487-91.
[http://dx.doi.org/10.1161/01.CIR.0000159340.93220.E4] [PMID: 15781736]

[193] Sackner-Bernstein JD, Kowalski M, Fox M, Aaronson K. Short-term risk of death after treatment with nesiritide for decompensated heart failure: a pooled analysis of randomized controlled trials. JAMA 2005; 293(15): 1900-5.
[http://dx.doi.org/10.1001/jama.293.15.1900] [PMID: 15840865]

[194] Hernandez AF, O'Connor CM, Starling RC, *et al.* Rationale and design of the Acute Study of Clinical Effectiveness of Nesiritide in Decompensated Heart Failure Trial (ASCEND-HF). Am Heart J 2009; 157(2): 271-7.
[http://dx.doi.org/10.1016/j.ahj.2008.07.031] [PMID: 19185633]

[195] Ezekowitz JA. Novel pharmacologic therapies in development for acute decompensated heart failure. Curr Cardiol Rep 2013; 15(2): 329.
[http://dx.doi.org/10.1007/s11886-012-0329-z] [PMID: 23314727]

[196] O'Connor CM, Starling RC, Hernandez AF, *et al.* Effect of nesiritide in patients with acute decompensated heart failure. N Engl J Med 2011; 365(1): 32-43.
[http://dx.doi.org/10.1056/NEJMoa1100171] [PMID: 21732835]

[197] Francis GS, Bartos JA, Adatya S. Inotropes. J Am Coll Cardiol 2014; 63(20): 2069-78.
[http://dx.doi.org/10.1016/j.jacc.2014.01.016] [PMID: 24530672]

[198] Hauptman PJ, Kelly RA. Digitalis. Circulation 1999; 99(9): 1265-70.
[http://dx.doi.org/10.1161/01.CIR.99.9.1265] [PMID: 10069797]

[199] Digitalis Investigation Group. The effect of digoxin on mortality and morbidity in patients with heart failure. N Engl J Med 1997; 336(8): 525-33.
[http://dx.doi.org/10.1056/NEJM199702203360801] [PMID: 9036306]

[200] Felker GM, Benza RL, Chandler AB, *et al.* OPTIME-CHF Investigators. Heart failure etiology and response to milrinone in decompensated heart failure: results from the OPTIME-CHF study. J Am Coll Cardiol 2003; 41(6): 997-1003.
[http://dx.doi.org/10.1016/S0735-1097(02)02968-6] [PMID: 12651048]

[201] Follath F, Cleland J, Just H, *et al.* Efficacy and safety of the IV levosimendan compared to dobutamine in severe low output heart failure. Lancet 2002; 360: 196-202.
[http://dx.doi.org/10.1016/S0140-6736(02)09455-2] [PMID: 12133653]

[202] Mebazaa A, Nieminen MS, Packer M, *et al.* SURVIVE Investigators. Levosimendan *vs.* dobutamine for patients with acute decompensated heart failure: the SURVIVE Randomized Trial. JAMA 2007;

297(17): 1883-91.
[http://dx.doi.org/10.1001/jama.297.17.1883] [PMID: 17473298]

[203] Gheorghiade M, Blair JE, Filippatos GS, *et al.* HORIZON-HF Investigators. Hemodynamic, echocardiographic, and neurohormonal effects of istaroxime, a novel intravenous inotropic and lusitropic agent: a randomized controlled trial in patients hospitalized with heart failure. J Am Coll Cardiol 2008; 51(23): 2276-85.
[http://dx.doi.org/10.1016/j.jacc.2008.03.015] [PMID: 18534276]

[204] Cleland JG, Teerlink JR, Senior R, *et al.* The effects of the cardiac myosin activator, omecamtiv mecarbil, on cardiac function in systolic heart failure: a double-blind, placebo-controlled, crossover, dose-ranging phase 2 trial. Lancet 2011; 378(9792): 676-83.
[http://dx.doi.org/10.1016/S0140-6736(11)61126-4] [PMID: 21856481]

[205] Cotter G, Dittrich HC, Weatherley BD, *et al.* Protect Steering Committee, Investigators, and Coordinators. The PROTECT pilot study: a randomized, placebo-controlled, dose-finding study of the adenosine A1 receptor antagonist rolofylline in patients with acute heart failure and renal impairment. J Card Fail 2008; 14(8): 631-40.
[http://dx.doi.org/10.1016/j.cardfail.2008.08.010] [PMID: 18926433]

[206] Erdmann E, Semigran MJ, Nieminen MS, *et al.* Cinaciguat, a soluble guanylate cyclase activator, unloads the heart but also causes hypotension in acute decompensated heart failure. Eur Heart J 2013; 34(1): 57-67.
[http://dx.doi.org/10.1093/eurheartj/ehs196] [PMID: 22778174]

[207] Lapp H, Mitrovic V, Franz N, *et al.* Cinaciguat (BAY 58-2667) improves cardiopulmonary hemodynamics in patients with acute decompensated heart failure. Circulation 2009; 119(21): 2781-8.
[http://dx.doi.org/10.1161/CIRCULATIONAHA.108.800292] [PMID: 19451356]

[208] Gheorghiade M, Filippatos G, Erdmann E, *et al.* Treatment of acute decompensated heart failure with the soluble guanylate cyclase activator cinaciguat: The COMPOSE program: three randomized, controlled, phase IIb studies. J Card Fail 2011; 17: 971.
[http://dx.doi.org/10.1016/j.cardfail.2011.10.004]

[209] Díez J. Serelaxin: a novel therapy for acute heart failure with a range of hemodynamic and non-hemodynamic actions. Am J Cardiovasc Drugs 2014; 14(4): 275-85.
[http://dx.doi.org/10.1007/s40256-014-0069-0] [PMID: 24590581]

[210] Teerlink JR, Cotter G, Davison BA, *et al.* RELAXin in Acute Heart Failure (RELAX-AHF) Investigators. Serelaxin, recombinant human relaxin-2, for treatment of acute heart failure (RELAX-AHF): a randomised, placebo-controlled trial. Lancet 2013; 381(9860): 29-39.
[http://dx.doi.org/10.1016/S0140-6736(12)61855-8] [PMID: 23141816]

[211] Owan TE, Hodge DO, Herges RM, Jacobsen SJ, Roger VL, Redfield MM. Trends in prevalence and outcome of heart failure with preserved ejection fraction. N Engl J Med 2006; 355(3): 251-9.
[http://dx.doi.org/10.1056/NEJMoa052256] [PMID: 16855265]

[212] Steinberg BA, Zhao X, Heidenreich PA, *et al.* Get With the Guidelines Scientific Advisory Committee and Investigators. Trends in patients hospitalized with heart failure and preserved left ventricular ejection fraction: prevalence, therapies, and outcomes. Circulation 2012; 126(1): 65-75.
[http://dx.doi.org/10.1161/CIRCULATIONAHA.111.080770] [PMID: 22615345]

[213] Kitzman DW, Little WC, Brubaker PH, *et al.* Pathophysiological characterization of isolated diastolic heart failure in comparison to systolic heart failure. JAMA 2002; 288(17): 2144-50. [http://dx.doi.org/10.1001/jama.288.17.2144] [PMID: 12413374]

[214] Ather S, Chan W, Bozkurt B, *et al.* Impact of noncardiac comorbidities on morbidity and mortality in a predominantly male population with heart failure and preserved *versus* reduced ejection fraction. J Am Coll Cardiol 2012; 59(11): 998-1005. [http://dx.doi.org/10.1016/j.jacc.2011.11.040] [PMID: 22402071]

[215] Shah SJ, Gheorghiade M. Heart failure with preserved ejection fraction: treat now by treating comorbidities. JAMA 2008; 300(4): 431-3. [http://dx.doi.org/10.1001/jama.300.4.431] [PMID: 18647986]

[216] Shah SJ. Matchmaking for the optimization of clinical trials of heart failure with preserved ejection fraction: no laughing matter. J Am Coll Cardiol 2013; 62(15): 1339-42. [http://dx.doi.org/10.1016/j.jacc.2013.07.010] [PMID: 23916923]

[217] Heart Failure Society of America. 2010 HFSA heart failure practice guidelines. Section 11: evaluation and management of patients with heart failure and preserved left ventricular ejection fraction. J Card Fail 2010; 16: e126-33.

[218] Flather MD, Shibata MC, Coats AJ, *et al.* SENIORS Investigators. Randomized trial to determine the effect of nebivolol on mortality and cardiovascular hospital admission in elderly patients with heart failure (SENIORS). Eur Heart J 2005; 26(3): 215-25. [http://dx.doi.org/10.1093/eurheartj/ehi115] [PMID: 15642700]

[219] Aronow WS, Ahn C, Kronzon I. Effect of propranolol versus no propranolol on total mortality plus nonfatal myocardial infarction in older patients with prior myocardial infarction, congestive heart failure, and left ventricular ejection fraction > or = 40% treated with diuretics plus angiotensin-converting enzyme inhibitors. Am J Cardiol 1997; 80(2): 207-9. [http://dx.doi.org/10.1016/S0002-9149(97)00320-2] [PMID: 9230162]

[220] Takeda Y, Fukutomi T, Suzuki S, *et al.* Effects of carvedilol on plasma B-type natriuretic peptide concentration and symptoms in patients with heart failure and preserved ejection fraction. Am J Cardiol 2004; 94(4): 448-53. [http://dx.doi.org/10.1016/j.amjcard.2004.05.004] [PMID: 15325927]

[221] Cleland JG, Tendera M, Adamus J, Freemantle N, Polonski L, Taylor J. PEP-CHF Investigators. The perindopril in elderly people with chronic heart failure (PEP-CHF) study. Eur Heart J 2006; 27(19): 2338-45. [http://dx.doi.org/10.1093/eurheartj/ehl250] [PMID: 16963472]

[222] Aronow WS, Kronzon I. Effect of enalapril on congestive heart failure treated with diuretics in elderly patients with prior myocardial infarction and normal left ventricular ejection fraction. Am J Cardiol 1993; 71(7): 602-4. [http://dx.doi.org/10.1016/0002-9149(93)90520-M] [PMID: 8438750]

[223] Yusuf S, Pfeffer MA, Swedberg K, *et al.* CHARM Investigators and Committees. Effects of candesartan in patients with chronic heart failure and preserved left-ventricular ejection fraction: the CHARM-Preserved Trial. Lancet 2003; 362(9386): 777-81. [http://dx.doi.org/10.1016/S0140-6736(03)14285-7] [PMID: 13678871]

[224] Massie BM, Carson PE, McMurray JJ, *et al.* I-PRESERVE Investigators. Irbesartan in patients with heart failure and preserved ejection fraction. N Engl J Med 2008; 359(23): 2456-67. [http://dx.doi.org/10.1056/NEJMoa0805450] [PMID: 19001508]

[225] Heart Failure Society of America. 2010 HFSA heart failure practice guidelines. Section 11: evaluation and management of patients with heart failure and preserved left ventricular ejection fraction. J Card Fail 2010; 16: e126-33.

[226] Setaro JF, Zaret BL, Schulman DS, Black HR, Soufer R. Usefulness of verapamil for congestive heart failure associated with abnormal left ventricular diastolic filling and normal left ventricular systolic performance. Am J Cardiol 1990; 66(12): 981-6. [http://dx.doi.org/10.1016/0002-9149(90)90937-V] [PMID: 2220622]

[227] Hung MJ, Cherng WJ, Kuo LT, Wang CH. Effect of verapamil in elderly patients with left ventricular diastolic dysfunction as a cause of congestive heart failure. Int J Clin Pract 2002; 56(1): 57-62. [PMID: 11831838]

[228] Smith GL, Masoudi FA, Vaccarino V, Radford MJ, Krumholz HM. Outcomes in heart failure patients with preserved ejection fraction: mortality, readmission, and functional decline. J Am Coll Cardiol 2003; 41(9): 1510-8. [http://dx.doi.org/10.1016/S0735-1097(03)00185-2] [PMID: 12742291]

[229] Ahmed A, Rich MW, Fleg JL, *et al.* Effects of digoxin on morbidity and mortality in diastolic heart failure: the ancillary digitalis investigation group trial. Circulation 2006; 114(5): 397-403. [http://dx.doi.org/10.1161/CIRCULATIONAHA.106.628347] [PMID: 16864724]

[230] Edelmann F, Tomaschitz A, Wachter R, *et al.* Serum aldosterone and its relationship to left ventricular structure and geometry in patients with preserved left ventricular ejection fraction. Eur Heart J 2012; 33(2): 203-12. [http://dx.doi.org/10.1093/eurheartj/ehr292] [PMID: 21856682]

[231] Pitt B, Zannad F, Remme WJ, *et al.* Randomized Aldactone Evaluation Study Investigators. The effect of spironolactone on morbidity and mortality in patients with severe heart failure. N Engl J Med 1999; 341(10): 709-17. [http://dx.doi.org/10.1056/NEJM199909023411001] [PMID: 10471456]

[232] Zannad F, McMurray JJ, Krum H, *et al.* EMPHASIS-HF Study Group. Eplerenone in patients with systolic heart failure and mild symptoms. N Engl J Med 2011; 364(1): 11-21. [http://dx.doi.org/10.1056/NEJMoa1009492] [PMID: 21073363]

[233] Edelmann F, Wachter R, Schmidt AG, *et al.* Aldo-DHF Investigators. Effect of spironolactone on diastolic function and exercise capacity in patients with heart failure with preserved ejection fraction: the Aldo-DHF randomized controlled trial. JAMA 2013; 309(8): 781-91. [http://dx.doi.org/10.1001/jama.2013.905] [PMID: 23443441]

[234] Pitt B, Pfeffer MA, Assmann SF, *et al.* TOPCAT Investigators. Spironolactone for heart failure with preserved ejection fraction. N Engl J Med 2014; 370(15): 1383-92. [http://dx.doi.org/10.1056/NEJMoa1313731] [PMID: 24716680]

[235] Krum H, Massie B, Abraham WT, *et al.* ATMOSPHERE Investigators. Direct renin inhibition in addition to or as an alternative to angiotensin converting enzyme inhibition in patients with chronic

systolic heart failure: rationale and design of the Aliskiren Trial to Minimize OutcomeS in Patients with HEart failuRE (ATMOSPHERE) study. Eur J Heart Fail 2011; 13(1): 107-14. [http://dx.doi.org/10.1093/eurjhf/hfq212] [PMID: 21169387]

[236] Gheorghiade M, Böhm M, Greene SJ, *et al.* ASTRONAUT Investigators and Coordinators. Effect of aliskiren on postdischarge mortality and heart failure readmissions among patients hospitalized for heart failure: the ASTRONAUT randomized trial. JAMA 2013; 309(11): 1125-35. [http://dx.doi.org/10.1001/jama.2013.1954] [PMID: 23478743]

[237] Hampton JR, van Veldhuisen DJ, Kleber FX, *et al.* Second Prospective Randomised Study of Ibopamine on Mortality and Efficacy (PRIME II) Investigators. Randomised study of effect of ibopamine on survival in patients with advanced severe heart failure. Lancet 1997; 349(9057): 971-7. [http://dx.doi.org/10.1016/S0140-6736(96)10488-8] [PMID: 9100622]

[238] Al-Khadra AS, Salem DN, Rand WM, Udelson JE, Smith JJ, Konstam MA. Warfarin anticoagulation and survival: a cohort analysis from the Studies of Left Ventricular Dysfunction. J Am Coll Cardiol 1998; 31(4): 749-53. [http://dx.doi.org/10.1016/S0735-1097(98)00006-0] [PMID: 9525542]

[239] Lip GY, Gibbs CR. Does heart failure confer a hypercoagulable state? Virchow's triad revisited. J Am Coll Cardiol 1999; 33(5): 1424-6. [PMID: 10193748]

[240] Massie BM, Collins JF, Ammon SE, *et al.* WATCH Trial Investigators. Randomized trial of warfarin, aspirin, and clopidogrel in patients with chronic heart failure: the Warfarin and Antiplatelet Therapy in Chronic Heart Failure (WATCH) trial. Circulation 2009; 119(12): 1616-24. [http://dx.doi.org/10.1161/CIRCULATIONAHA.108.801753] [PMID: 19289640]

CHAPTER 3

Vasopressin and the Cardiovascular System: Receptor Physiology and Clinical Implications

Amit Agrawal*

Gandhi Medical College & Hamidia Hospital, Bhopal, MP, India

Abstract: Arginine vasopressin or antidiuretic hormone has got name "vasopressin" due to its vasoconstrictor properties. Vasopressin is a posterior pituitary hormone which is essential for the cardiovascular homeostasis. In normal physiological conditions, it helps in regulation of plasma osmolality and volume *via* its action on the kidney. Other important actions of vasopressin include regulation of vascular smooth muscle tone, control of circadian rhythm, thermoregulation, and adrenocorticotropic hormone release (ACTH).

In recent years, vasopressin has emerged as an important therapeutic option in the treatment of various shock states. Vasopressin has increasingly been used in both pediatric and adult critical care units for the management of central diabetes insipidus, bleeding abnormalities, oesophageal variceal haemorrhage, asystolic cardiac arrest, and various shock states *e.g.* shock due to ventricular fibrillation, hypovolaemia, sepsis and cardiopulmonary bypass.

Ongoing researches helped in increasing understanding of the endocrine response to shock and importance of vasopressin in their management. Prolonged vasodilatory shock is characterised by relative deficiency of endogenous vasopressin and marked vasopressor effects of the exogenously administered hormone. Sepsis and post cardiopulmonary bypass conditions are the most common causes of vasodilatory shock; however, vasodilation can be a common final pathway of any type of shock. Unlike other vasoconstrictors, vasopressin also exerts some vasodilatory properties which can be due to its action on various receptors, namely V1 vascular, V2 renal, V3 pituitary and oxytocin receptors, and the P2 purinergic receptors producing variable and seemingly contradictory responses.

* **Corresponding author Amit Agrawal:** Gandhi Medical College & Hamidia Hospital, Bhopal, MP, India; Tel: 0755-2680996; E-mail: agrawaldramit@yahoo.co.in

Atta-ur-Rahman and M. Iqbal Choudhary (Eds.)

To better understand the variable responses on the vascular system, which vasopressin exerts, it is prudent to acquire the knowledge of the physiology and action of the different vasopressin receptors. In this chapter, vascular actions of vasopressin along with distribution of the classic vasopressin receptors and signalling pathways will be explored.

Keywords: Arginine-vasopressin, Oxytocin receptors, Terlipressin, Vasopressin, Vasopressin receptors.

INTRODUCTION

Arginine vasopressin (AVP), also known as antidiuretic hormone (ADH), is one of the first described and structurally characterized neuropeptide hormones. Vasopressin plays an important role in many peripheral and central functions such as regulation of plasma osmolality and blood pressure through its peripheral actions, and central actions include memory, learning and stress-related disorders. Vasopressin is an important stress hormone that has both vasoactive as well as antidiuretic properties. Since its isolation and synthetic preparation vasopressin has been extensively studied, mainly to treat diabetes insipidus and variceal hemorrhage. The vasoactive properties of vasopressin have become an area of intense research when Landry and colleagues first reported a relative deficiency of vasopressin in septic shock and increase in blood pressure and urine output after infusion of low doses of vasopressin [1, 2]. Now, vasopressin has emerged as an important therapeutic option in the management of septic shock and vasodilatory shock from other causes [3 - 5].

Since its isolation, vasopressin has been extensively studied and found to be useful in the management of enuresis, variceal bleeding, septic shock, and cardiac arrest. Enormous work has been done to demonstrate the complex system of synthesis, storage, secretion and regulation of vasopressin, in addition to its many different functions on specific receptors distributed throughout the body in such a manner as to perform its main effects, the regulation of plasma osmolality and arterial blood pressure, in harmony with several other hormones. However in this chapter, only those clinical uses of vasopressin implicated in cardiovascular homeostasis will be discussed. The initial part will cover the physiology and pharmacology of the hormone including structure and distribution of vasopressin receptors and their signalling pathways as it is necessary to understand the seemingly paradoxical vasodilatory and vasoconstrictor actions of vasopressin. In the later part of the chapter, the mechanisms of action of vasopressin through different types of receptors leading to vasoconstriction or vasodilation of vascular smooth muscles will be discussed.

HISTORICAL ASPECTS

Vasopressin was first discovered by Oliver & Schafer in 1895 by observing the vasoconstrictor effect of an extract of the posterior pituitary [6]. Human vasopressin contains the amino acid arginine; therefore, it is also named as "Arginine Vasopressin". In 1906, Sir Henry Dale has discovered another pituitary hormone "oxytocin" by successfully demonstrating the contractions of the mammalian uterus by a component of the pituitary [7]. A few years later in 1913, Farini in Italy and von del Venden in Germany successfully treated the patients of diabetes insipidus by injection of neurohypophysis extract and independently demonstrated its antidiuretic effect [8, 9]. In 1951, Turner *et al.* succeeded in purification of vasopressin preparation and identified the nine amino acid sequences of vasopressin [10]. Two years later in 1953, Acher & Chauvet and du Vigneaud *et al.* proposed the structure of vasopressin [11, 12]. Very soon, the structure of related oxytocin was also identified by Tuppy and du Vigneaud *et al.* [13, 14]. In 1954, du Vigneaud *et al.* first synthesized the vasopressin in a laboratory and proved that both the vasopressor and antidiuretic effects were from the same hormone [15]. For this pioneering work, du Vigneaud also won the Nobel Prize in chemistry in 1955.

Following discovery of structure and amino acid sequences of vasopressin and oxytocin, attention of the researchers have turned to locate the site of synthesis of these hormones in human body. About a decade later, Sachs *et al.* in their studies demonstrated the hypothalamus as the site of synthesis of vasopressin and oxytocin and that from the hypothalamus these hormones are transported to the posterior pituitary [16 - 18]. Pioneering studies by Howard Sachs and his colleagues hypothesized that the vasopressin peptide was formed by the post-translational processing of a precursor protein [16 - 17]. Gainer and colleagues confirmed their hypothesis by reporting the first physical evidence for the existence of the oxytocin and vasopressin precursor proteins [19 - 21]. They identified a putative precursor protein in the hypothalamus that was subsequently processed to the peptides and neurophysins while travelling from the supraoptic nuclei to the posterior pituitary.

Very soon, Land and colleagues determined the definitive structures of their precursors by using recombinant DNA techniques which lead to the rapid progress in the identification of sequences of the vasopressin and oxytocin cDNAs, genes, and precursor proteins [22 - 24]. Subsequently, three vasopressin receptors were cloned which were responsible for vasopressin's pressor (V1), antidiuretic (V2) and adrenocorticotropin-releasing (V3) effects [25 - 27]. Following complete characterization of vasopressin genes, numerous studies were conducted to explore the regulation of these genes' expression. Subsequently, genes in mouse, rat, and human genomes were shown to be located on the same chromosome separated by a short (3.5 to 12 kb) intergenic region, and are in opposite transcriptional orientations [28].

PHYSIOLOGY OF VASOPRESSIN

Structure of Vasopressin and Related Peptides

Structure of Vasopressin

The vasopressin is a peptide consisting of nine amino acids (nonapeptides). Oxytocin and vasopressin (OT/AVP) like peptides are present in a wide range of species, both invertebrate and vertebrate. These have been isolated from seven vertebrate families and four invertebrate phyla and virtually all vertebrate species possess OT/AVP - like peptides [29]. These have been evolved from the ancestral vasotocin (VT) peptide *via* genc duplication with subsequent mutations some 600 million years ago which is supported by the presence of VT peptide ([Ile3]-vasopressin or [Arg8]-oxytocin) in the most primitive organism cyclostomata [30]. There is high sequence similarity between all the members of the OT/AVP and VT peptide family, namely an N-terminal six-residue ring, formed by a disulfide bond between two cysteine residues at positions 1 and 6, and a flexible C-terminal three residue tail with a highly conserved proline at 7 and a glycine amide at position 9 (CXXXXCPXG). Amino acid residue varies at positions 2 to 5 and at position 8 and these amino acid variations are presumably responsible for species selective recognition, binding and activation of the different receptors [31].

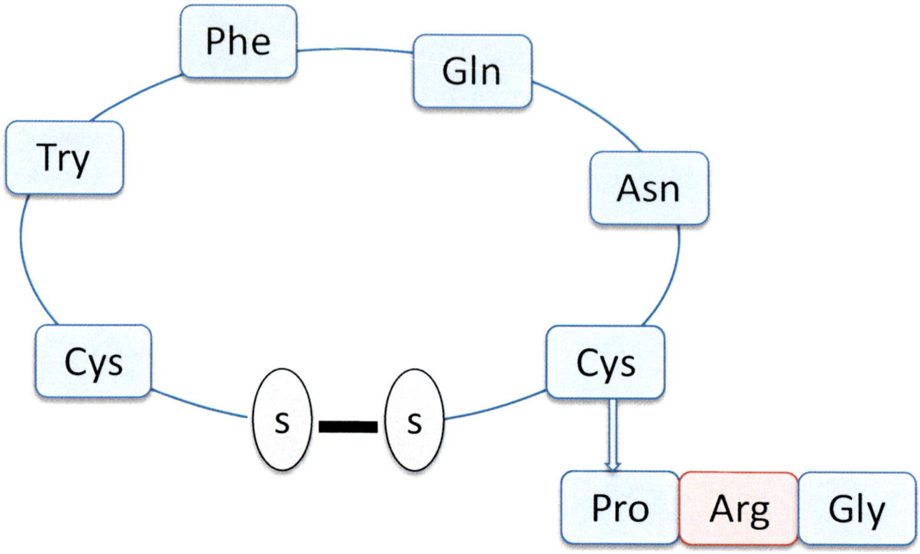

Fig. (1). Amino acid sequence of human vasopressin showing two cysteine residues at 1 and 6 positions forming a disulfide bond and arginine residue at the 8th position.

Human vasopressin contains the amino acid arginine at position 8, hence the name "Arginine Vasopressin". The amino acid sequence of human vasopressin is "Cys-Tyr-Phe-Gln-Asn-Cys-Pro-*Arg*-Gly-NH2", with two cysteine residues at 1 and 6 positions forming a disulfide bond between them. This results in formation of a peptide consisting of a cyclic part containing 6 amino acids and a C-terminal part containing 3 amino acids (Fig. **1**) [32]. The molecular formula of vasopressin is $C_{46}H_{65}N_{15}O_{12}S_2$ and it carries incomplete electron orbits due to which vasopressin molecule participates in H-bond reactions. After deprotonation, vasopressin contains a net charge of -1 and after protonation it has a net charge of +2. Vasopressin is a hydrophillic molecule so it can move freely in the blood without any carrier protein; however, it requires a carrier protein to travel along the axons. The molecular weight of vasopressin is 1084.2316 g/mol [33].

Structure of Related Peptides

Oxytocin

The oxytocin (a nonapeptide) is structurally similar to the vasopressin and its amino acid sequence differs at only two positions *i.e.* isoleucine at position 3rd and leucine at 8th position (Fig. **2**). The genes encoding these peptides are also located on the same chromosome at a relatively small distance in most species. The similarity of these two peptides can cause some cross-reactivity as evident by slight antidiuretic function of oxytocin and stimulation of uterine contractions by supraphysiological doses of vasopressin. However, in contrast to vasopressin, a bolus of oxytocin can produce hypotension, the cause of which is not well understood. Suggested underlying mechanisms include presence of chlorobutanol preservative, or due to the release of atrial natriuretic peptide. Its molecular formula is $C_{43}H_{66}N_{12}O_{12}S_2$ and the average molecular weight is 1007.18734 g/mol [34].

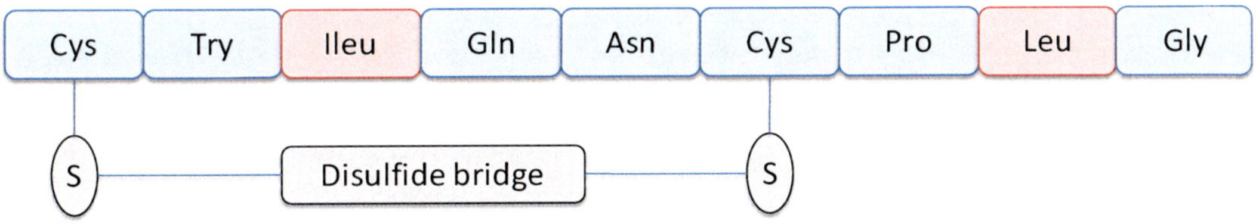

Fig. (2). Amino acid sequence of oxytocin showing isoleucine at 3rd position and leucine residue at the 8th position.

Terlipressin

Terlipressin (triglycyl lysine-vasopressin) is a longer acting synthetic analogue of the vasopressin which is slowly cleaved to lysine-vasopressin. As compared to vasopressin, it shows more affinity for V_1R than V_2R (2.2:1 compared to 1:1). Terlipressin is a longer molecule containing 12 amino acids with lysine at the 8th position in place of arginine and a disulphide bond between two cystiene residues (Fig. **3**). This lysine makes this molecule a triglycinc-lysine vasopressin, where glycines are cleaved by endothelial peptidases in liver and kidney over 4–6 hrs resulting in its breakdown into lysine-vasopressin. Molecular formula of

Terlipressin is $C_{52}H_{74}N_{16}O_{15}S_2$ and the average molecular weight is 1227.37216 g/mol [35].

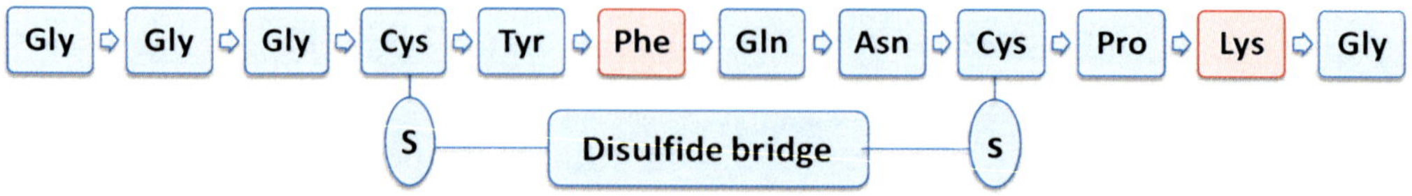

Fig. (3). Amino acid sequence of terlipressin containing 12 amino acids with lysine at 8th position and a disulphide bond between two cystiene residues.

Desmopressin

Desmopressin (*1-desamino-8-D-arginine vasopressin,* DDAVP) is a synthetic analogue of vasopressin. It is a selective V_2-agonist with an antidiuretic-t--vasopressor ratio 4000 times than that of vasopressin; therefore, it has prolonged antidiuretic properties with little vasopressor effects. As compared to vasopressin, first amino acid in desmopressin is deaminated, and the arginine at the eighth position is in the *dextro* rather than the *levo* form (Fig. **4**). It is thought that the substitution of a D-stereoisomer for arginine protects it from rapid metabolism by the various endothelial peptidases giving it a longer duration of action. Its molecular formula is $C_{48}H_{74}N_{14}O_{17}S_2$ and the average molecular weight is 1183.31476 g/mol [36].

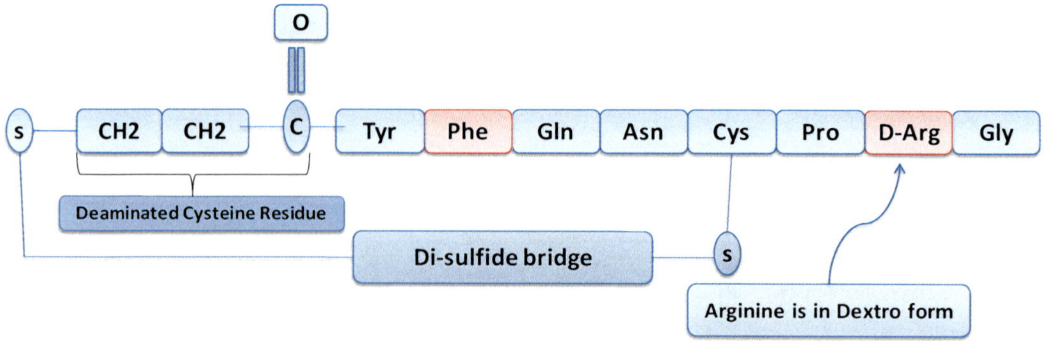

Fig. (4). Amino acid sequence of desmopressin showing deamination of first amino acid and *dextro* form of the arginine at 8th position.

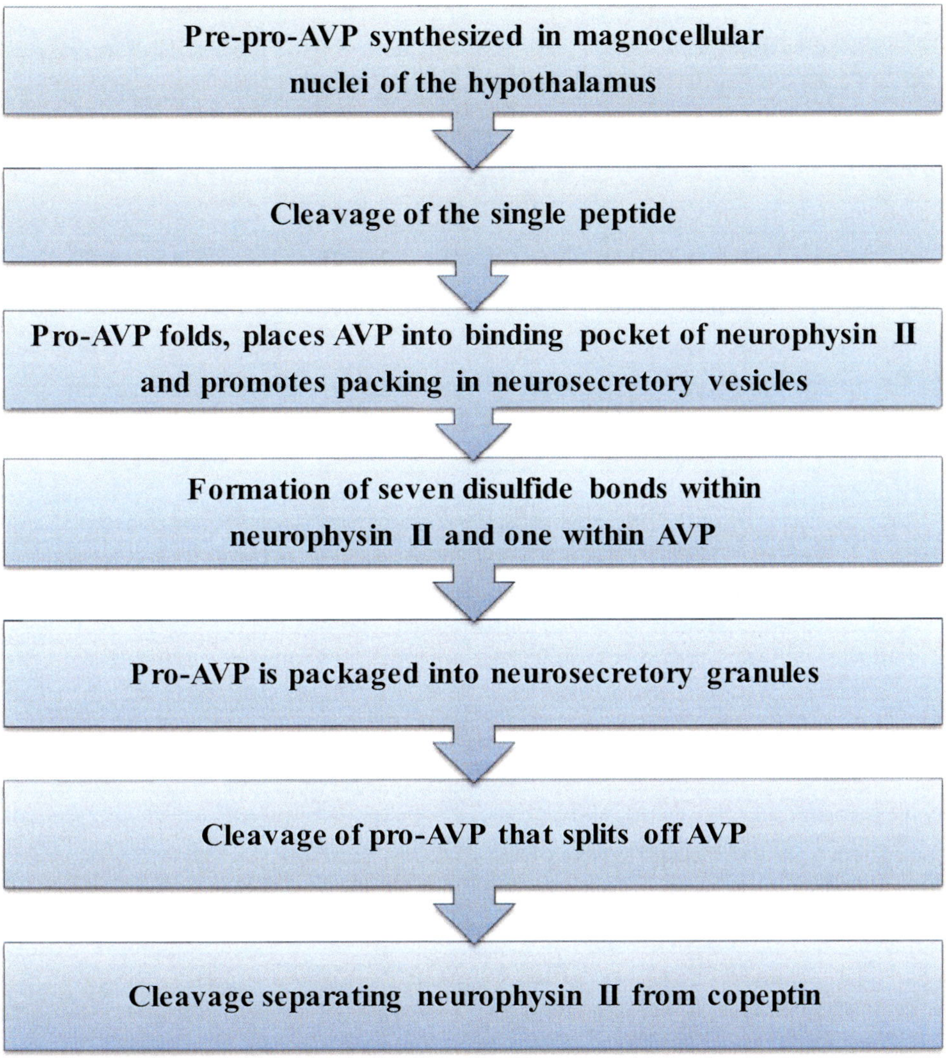

Fig. (5). Schematic presentation of the synthesis and release of the vasopressin. Last two processes occur during axonal transport from the hypothalamic nuclei to the neutrohypophysis.

Synthesis of Vasopressin

In humans, vasopressin is encoded by the mRNA to be synthesized as a prohormone "prepроneurophysin II" like many other hormones. This prohormone is synthesized in the parvocellular and magnocellular neurons of the supraoptic and paraventricular nuclei of the hypothalamus. Provasopressin is synthesized and packaged in neurosecretory granules along with an intragranular carrier protein, neurophysin, and transported along the supraoptic-hypophyseal tract to the axonal terminals of the magnocellualr neurons of the pars nervosa in the posterior pituitary [37, 38]. Subsequently, pre-provasopressin is converted to pro-vasopressin releasing two other substances namely, neurophysin II (95 amino acids) and a glycopeptide, copeptin (39 amino acids) followed by cleavage of provasopressin by subtilisin-like proprotein convertase (SPC3) releasing nine amino acids compound vasopressin (Fig. **5**). The final hormone is transported by the hypothalamo–neurohypophyseal neurons of the pituitary gland to its secretion site, *i.e.* the posterior hypophysis where it is stored in granule form. Only 10-20% of the intracellular vasopressin releases in response to appropriate stimuli; however, secretion diminishes with a sustained stimulus. The complete cycle of vasopressin synthesis, transport and storage takes about 1-2 hours.

Metabolism

Endogenous vasopressin is rapidly metabolised by renal and hepatic vasopressinase enzymes with a plasma half life of approximately 15-30 minutes. Its clearance is affected greatly by the renal and hepatic blood flows. The liver and the intestines share the splanchnic clearance of vasopressin equally. Approximately 5-15% of metabolic products are excreted through urine and vasopressin clearance can be affected by reduction in glomerular filtration rate as shown by animal studies. Exogenous vasopressin has a short half life (Nasal: 15 minutes; Parenteral: 5-15 minutes) but can go up to 35 min in certain situations [37]. Duration of action of nasal drug is 3-8 hours, intramuscular or subcutaneous is 2-8 hours while its pressor effect lasts for 30-60 minutes. In a physiological situation, adaptation of neurosecretion helps in alleviating the impact of variations in the metabolic clearance on circulating vasopressin levels [38].

Factors Affecting Vasopressin Release

The regulation of plasma vasopressin levels is an extremely complex phenomenon and factors stimulating its release differ in healthy and disease states. In healthy subjects, vasopressin release is primarily regulated by changes in serum osmolality (osmoregulation) while hypotension and hypovolemia are the other extremely potent stimuli which induce the release of vasopressin (baroregulation). Osmoregulation is a highly sensitive system, so that just 2% variations in the osmolality are enough to increase the secretion of vasopressin (upto 5pg/mL) and by virtue of its antidiuretic effect; vasopressin normalizes the osmolality [38 - 40]. On the contrary, more than 10% decrease in blood pressure is required for baroregulation to play a significant role in vasopressin secretion. As a result, vasopressin level can increase more than ten-fold to help restore the normal blood pressure, largely *via* its vasoconstriction action [39, 40]. Many other factors can stimulate or inhibit the release of vasopressin as shown in Table **1**.

Table 1. Factors affecting the vasopressin release.

Stimulate release	**Inhibit release**
Increasing plasma osmolality	Decreasing plasma osmolality
Reduced plasma volume	Increased plasma volume
Chemical mediators	Chemical mediators
Norepinephrine*, dopamine, acetylcholine, histamine, prostaglandins, angiotensin II, endotoxin, cytokines	Opioids, GABA, ANP, norepinephrine*
Pain, Stress, Exercise	
Hypoxia, hypercapnia, acidosis	

Note: * Norepinephrine can stimulate release through $\alpha 1$ receptors and inhibit release by $\alpha 2$ and β receptors stimulation

Osmoregulation

Plasma osmolality depends on the interaction between behavioral (hunger and thirst), and physiological responses (through the balance between vasopressin and atrial natriuretic peptide). The central osmoreceptors regulating vasopressin secretion are located near the supraoptic nucleus in the anterolateral hypothalamus near third ventricle in a region that is not protected by blood–brain barrier. The peripheral osmoreceptors are located in the hepatic portal venous system that can detect the osmotic impact of ingested foods and fluids. The afferent pathways reach the magnocellular neurons of the hypothalamus *via* vagus nerve. Furthermore, plasma hypertonicity directly depolarizes magnocellular neurons while hypotonic conditions hyperpolarize them [38, 41 - 43]. The circulating vasopressin levels are undetectable below the osmotic threshold of 280m Osmol/kg H_2O of mean extracellular osmolality and it increases in a linear fashion in relation to the osmolality beginning at approximately 290m Osmol/kg H_2O [41].

Baroregulation

Arterial hypotension and hypovolemia are the potent stimuli for vasopressin secretion which act *via* arterial baroreceptors located mainly in the left atrium, aortic arch and carotid sinus [44]. Afferent impulses originating from these receptors travel through the vagus and glossopharyngeal nerves toward the nucleus tractus solitarus, from there they reach to the supraoptic and paraventricular nuclei. Changes in the BP are sensed by the aortic arch and carotid sinus receptors while the change in plasma volume is sensed by the atrial and ventricular baroreceptors. Stimulation of these receptors tonically inhibits vasopressin secretion and in physiological situations, this inhibition is constant because of continuous discharge by these receptors. Vasopressin secretion increases only when stimulation diminishes *e.g.* due to hypovolemia [38]. In cases of hypotensive haemorrhages, a fall in blood volume is detected first by the cardiac baroreceptors resulting in secretion of atrial natriuretic peptide, norepinephrine and renin in an attempt to restore BP. If arterial pressure falls to the point that it can no longer be compensated by these mechanisms, then arterial baroreceptors finally register a fall in arterial BP resulting in release of vasopressin [38, 44 - 47]. In contrast to osmotic stimulation, hypotension and hypovolaemia stimulate vasopressin secretion exponentially without disturbing osmotic regulation as hypotension modifies the relationship between plasma osmolality and circulating vasopressin levels. It changes the sensitivity of osmoreceptors and lowers the osmotic threshold so elevated vasopressin levels are required to maintain the normal osmolality [38].

Neurohormonal Stimuli

Various hormonal stimuli play a role in the regulation of vasopressin secretion especially in septic shock and other critical illnesses which directly stimulate vasopressin release, *e.g.* dopamine and other catecholamines, histamine, acetylcholine, prostaglandins, nicotine, and angiotensin II [38, 48, 49]. The hypothalamic projections are predominantly noradrenergic; therefore, norepinephrine plays a critical role in vasopressin release but its effects are complex. At low concentrations, norepinephrine increases the secretion of vasopressin, an effect mediated by α_1- adrenergic receptors. On the other hand, high concentrations of norepinephrine inhibit the vasopressin release *via* its α_2-adrenoceptors or possibly β-adrenoreceptors mediated action [48, 49]. These opposing actions of noradrenergic inputs can be explained by differential distribution of α- and β-adrenergic receptors on the surface of magnocellular neurons [50]. Nitric oxide (NO) is also a powerful inhibitor of vasopressin release which acts *via* cyclic guanosine monophosphate (cGMP) pathway and is particularly important in the cases of septic shock [51].

There are several other stimuli such as hypoxia, hypercapnia, nausea, pain, hyperthermia, morphine and nicotine which can stimulate secretion of vasopressin and are relevant in critical illness and sepsis. [38]. High PaCO2 or low PaO2 elevate vasopressin levels by stimulating carotid chemoreceptors. Pain, nausea and pharyngeal stimuli are also capable of releasing vasopressin by acting through central afferent pathways. Furthermore, both endotoxin and cytokines enhance vasopressin production [48, 49]. Vasopressin stimulates the release of ACTH from the anterior pituitary resulting elevated glucocorticoid levels which in turn inhibits vasopressin release due to its negative feedback effect on the posterior pituitary [52]. Vasopressin inhibitors include opioids, alcohol, γ-aminobutyric acid (GABA), and atrial natriuretic peptide (ANP). Ethanol (alcohol) reduces vasopressin secretion by blocking voltage-gated calcium channels in neurohypophyseal nerve terminals. ANP inhibits its release by inhibiting angiotensin-II induced release of vasopressin. On the other hand, opioids and GABA exert their action through nitric oxide and cGMP pathway [48, 49].

Plasma Levels of Vasopressin

Vasopressin Levels in Health

Under normal conditions, mean serum vasopressin levels are approximately 2pg/mL and usually remain below 4pg/mL in overnight fasted, hydrated humans. Water deprivation increases plasma osmolality and as a result in raised vasopressin levels through osmoreceptors-renal mechanism upto 10pg/mL and can be increased maximally upto 20pg/mL to achieve maximal increase in urine osmolality. To produce vasoconstrictor effect, vasopressin levels can be increased upto 200 pg/mL [53, 54].

Vasopressin Levels During Illness

Vasopressin levels show a biphasic response in both septic and hemorrhagic shocks [1, 2, 55 - 61]. In the early phase, appropriately high levels of vasopressin (sometimes >500 pg/mL) are produced to help restoring the organ perfusion. However in later stage, paradoxical fall in vasopressin levels are seen due to still unclear reasons so that its plasma levels are close to the physiological concentrations. Several mechanisms have been proposed to explain this relative deficiency in established septic shock:-

- Depletion of neurohypophysial stores of vasopressin due to excessive stimulation of the baroreceptors [38, 62].
- Autonomic insufficiency as evidenced by lack of baroreflex - mediated bradycardia after vasopressin infusion [63, 64].
- Decreased vasopressin released to central inhibitory effect of increased norepinephrine levels (endogenous or exogenous) in patients with septic shock [48, 50].
- Inhibition of vasopressin production due to increased NO production by vascular endothelium of the posterior pituitary during sepsis [38, 65, 66].
- Tonic inhibition of vasopressin secretion by the atrial mechanoreceptors which are stimulated by cardiac volume variations caused by volume loading or mechanical ventilation [48, 67].
- Heme-oxygenase activation in sepsis may attenuate the elevation of vasopressin levels in patients with septic shock [68].
- Finally, decreased sensitivity of the vasopressin receptors, probably linked to the actions of proinflammatory cytokines, has also been demonstrated in rats with endotoxic shock [69].

Vasopressin levels increase early in septic shock because hypotension is the most potent stimulus for release and synthesis of vasopressin. Animal studies have shown that hypotensive hemorrhage in dogs and monkeys can rapidly increase vasopressin level (upto 100-1,000pg/mL) which is followed by decrease in its levels (upto 29 pg/mL) during prolonged (persisting for more than 5 hours) hemorrhagic shock [60, 61]. Similarly, acute endotoxin-induced shock and *Escherichia coli*-induced shock results in extremely high levels of vasopressin (>500 pg/mL in dogs and >300 pg/mL in baboons) within 15 minutes of initiation of sepsis [70]. Many human studies have also reported similar results and a large trial, Vasopressin and Septic Shock Trial (VASST), found that vasopressin levels remained very low for upto 7 days after the onset of septic shock [55]. Some evidences suggest that even very low plasma levels of vasopressin may not be associated with increased mortality in patients with septic shock and plasma vasopressin levels were significantly higher in non-survivors of septic shock [56]. Another study conducted in children with meningococcal septic shock showed that vasopressin level was higher in non-survivors than in survivors, and its level was not correlated with duration of shock, fluid expansion, or age-adjusted BP and sodium levels [71].

Measurement of Plasma Vasopressin Levels

Reliable measurement of circulating vasopressin levels is limited by several factors *e.g.* instability of the mature vasopressin hormone in isolated plasma, and it has a short half-life even at –20 °C. Secondly, more than 90% of the vasopressin is tightly attached to platelets, which are not measured in plasma. Therefore, the number of platelets can significantly influence the measured vasopressin levels and upto five to six times higher vasopressin concentration can be found in platelet-rich plasma than in platelet-depleted plasma [72 - 74]. Hence, interpretation of the static vasopressin levels may be misleading.

Co-peptin is C-terminal part of the precursor pre-provasopressin which contains 39-aminoacids. Co-peptin mirrors the vasopressin production as it is secreted into the circulation in an equimolar ratio to vasopressin. Therefore, it can be used as a surrogate biomarker of vasopressin secretion. Co-peptin remains stable in plasma as well as during storage and can be easily determined with several manual and automated assays. Many studies havc proposed co-peptin as a more sensitive and a potential prognostic marker of sepsis [72 - 74].

Vasopressin Receptors

Receptor Structure

Vasopressin receptors are the members of the G protein-coupled receptor superfamily as shown by molecular cloning of AVP/OT receptors. G-protein coupled receptors have seven hydrophobic transmembrane α-helices, with an extracellular amino-terminus, and a cytoplasmic carboxyl-terminus [75 - 78]. Guanine nucleotide-binding proteins (G-proteins) are the signal transducers which connect cell surface membrane receptors with ligands and stimulate intracellular signalling pathways. The human AVP/OT receptors show high sequence identity with approximately 102 invariant amino-acid residues among 370-420 amino-acids. These are members of the rhodopsin-like class A receptors and display all the structural hallmarks of these receptors. AVP/OT receptors contain palmitoylation motifs in C-terminal domain and glycosylation sites in the extracellular amino terminal domains, which participate in the binding of agonists [78, 79].

Due to structural similarity between vasopressin and oxytocin, and conservation of the binding sites of AVP/OT receptors throughout the family, there can be some cross-reactivity between them as evidenced by slight antidiuretic function of oxytocin and uterine contractions with high levels of AVP. The nature of some amino-acid residues and their location in the binding pockets can explain the differences in the selectivity of the different vasopressin receptors for their specific ligands. Stimulation of vasopressin receptors leads to interactions with G-protein-coupled receptor kinases and protein kinase C through specific motifs of the carboxyl terminals [78]. A single receptor can interact with one or more G-proteins leading to the activation of multiple second messenger pathways as evidenced by the functional characterization of the G-proteins, such as Gs, Gi/o, Gq/11, and G12/13. Vasopressin's signal is transmitted through both Gs and Gq/11 subtypes [75 - 79].

Receptor Subtypes

In 1979, Michell and colleagues proposed that there are two distinguished types of vasopressin receptors [80]. The first type was identified as the hepatic vasopressin receptor, which was termed as V_1 receptor and acts by increasing cytosolic free calcium through phosphatidylinositol - protein kinase C pathway. Second type *i.e.* renal vasopressin receptors were named as V_2 receptors which help in free water reabsorption by activation of adenylyl cyclase pathway. Later on, V_1 receptors were subdivided into V_{1A} (hepatic receptor) and V_{1B} (adenohypophysial receptor) subtypes by Jard *et al.* on the basis of their findings that vasopressin receptors of anterior pituitary which were involved in corticotropin release has different pharmacological profile than that of the hepatic/vascular receptor [81]. OT receptor displays unique pharmacological and tissue localization properties.

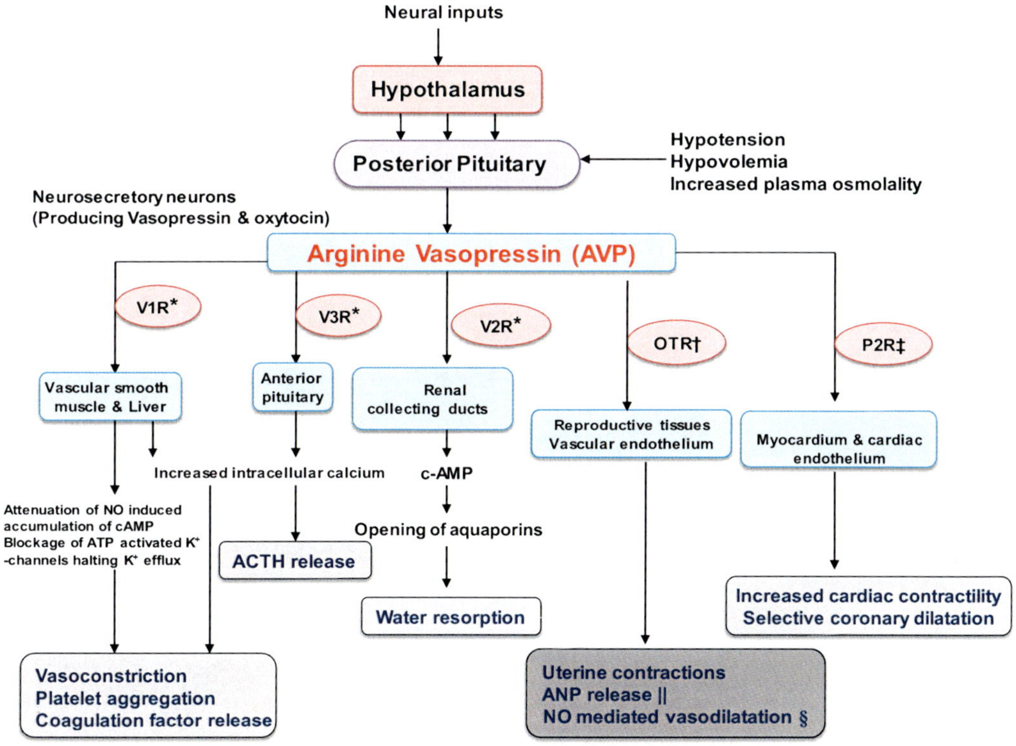

Fig. (6). Different types of receptors on which vasopressin may act and their corresponding actions. (*V1R – V1 receptor, V2R – V2 receptor, V3R – V3 receptor, † OTR – Oxytocin receptors, ‡ P2R – Purinergic 2 receptors, § NO – Nitirc oxide, cAMP – cyclic-Adenine Monophosphate, ATP – Adenine Triphosphate, ACTH – Adrenocartico tropic hormone, || ANP – Atrial Natriuretic Peptide).

Presently, vasopressin receptors are classified into $AVPR1_A$ or V1 (mainly vascular) receptor, AVPR2 or V2 (renal), and $AVPR1_B$ or V3 (mainly central or pituitary) on the basis of their location and second messenger pathways. Exogenous vasopressin also exerts some action *via* OTR (Oxytocin) and P2 (Purinergic) receptors at higher doses [38, 76, 77]. Physiology of vasopressin receptors has been presented in Table **2** and Fig. (**6**).

Table 2. Vasopressin receptors physiology.

Receptors	**Location**	**Effects**	**Intracellular Signalling/ transmitters**
V_1R (V_1 receptors, previously V_{1a} receptors)	Vascular smooth muscle	Vasoconstriction	Increased intracellular Ca $^{++}$ *via* Phosphoinositide pathway
	Myocardium	Inotropy	Increased intracellular Ca^{++}
	Platelets	Platelet Aggregation	
	Kidney (medullary interstitial cells, vasa recta, and epithelial cells of collecting ducts)	Diuresis	Selective renal efferent arteriolar constriction *via* local NO release
	Myometrium	Uterine contractions	
	Liver	Glycogenolysis	
	Bladder, spleen, adipocytes, testis	Vasodilation	
	Brain	Social memory, circadian rhythm, stress adaptation, emotional learning	
V_2R (V_2 receptors)	Renal collecting duct	Increased permeability to water	Increased cAMP *via* G protein
	Vascular smooth muscle	Vasodilation	
	Vascular endothelium	Release of von-Willebrand factor/VIII	NO mediated
V_3 R (V_1b Receptors)	Pituitary	Neurotransmitter (endorphins) release	Phosphokinase C pathway
		ACTH release	Increased cAMP *via* G protein

(Table 2) contd.....

Receptors	Location	Effects	Intracellular Signalling/ transmitters
Oxytocin(OTR) receptors	Uterus, mammary gland	Vasoconstriction	Phospholipase C mediated increased intracellular Ca^{++}
	Vascular endothelium	Vasodilation	NO mediated increase in cGMP level
	Heart	ANP release	
Purinergic (P_2R) receptors	Myocardium	Increased cardiac contractility	Increase in intracellular Ca^{++}
Purinergic (P_2R) receptors	Cardiac endothelium	Selective coronary vasodilation	NO mediated

Note – ACTH – Adrenocorticotropic hormone, ANP – atrial natriuretic peptide, NO – nitric oxide, cAMP – cyclic adenosine mono phosphate, cGMP - guanosine – cyclic monophosphate

V_{1A} Receptor

The V1A receptor (V1R) subtype was first isolated in 1992 from rat liver by cloning of its complementary DNA (cDNA). Two years later sequencing of the human V1R was done by cloning of the corresponding cDNA from a liver cDNA library [80, 81]. Human and rat receptors share 72% sequence identity. The V1R gene is located on chromosome 12q14-15. Functionally, the V1R activates the Gq/11 family of G proteins and the α-subunits of the receptors regulate the activity of β-isoforms of phospholipase C [82 - 84]. Mutations in V1R genes have been found to be linked with essential hypertension, generosity, and autism [85, 86]. V_{1A} receptor is expressed primarily on vascular smooth muscles, hepatocytes and platelets. These receptors are also expressed inother tissues such as heart, adrenal gland, testes, urinary bladder, brainstem, cerebral cortex, hippocampus, hypothalamus, olfactory bulb, and striatum [82]. Stimulation of V_{1A} receptor leads to cleavage of phosphatidylinositol bisphosphate into inositol triphosphate and diacylglycerol *via* activation of Gq protein and phospholipase C. These second messengers promote vasoconstriction by facilitating actin-myosin interactions by increasing intracellular calcium (Ca^{2+}) concentrations through various mechanisms (Fig. 7). Initial transient increase in cytoplasmic Ca^{2+} occurs by the emptying of Ca^{2+} stores within the sarcoplasmic reticulum whereas sustained increase is due to influx of extracellular Ca^{2+} through Ca^{2+} channels (receptor-operated and voltage-gated) activation *via* protein kinase C or indirectly by cell membrane depolarization [87, 88].

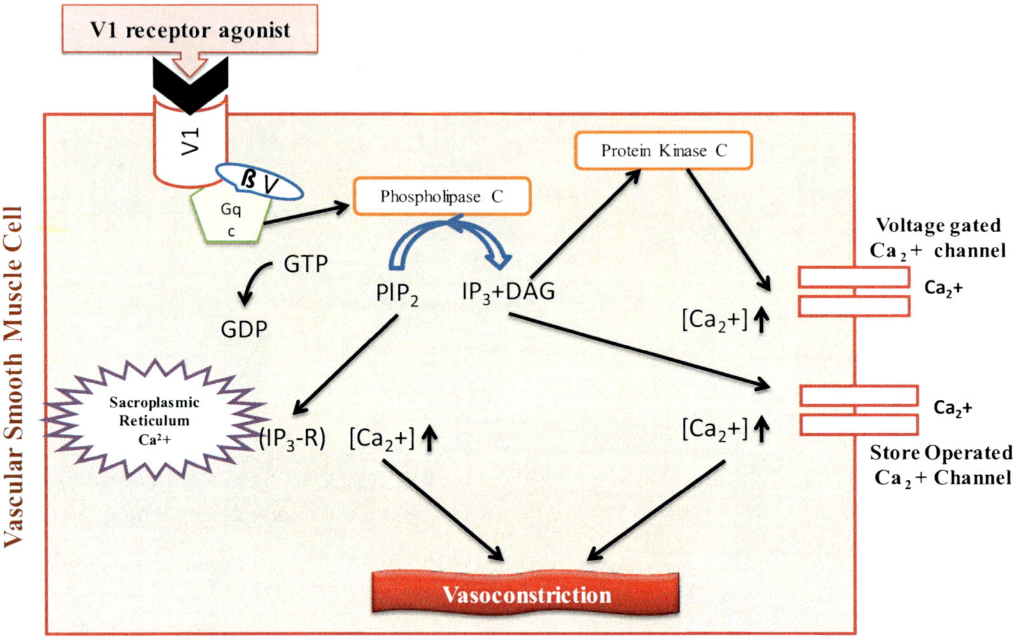

Fig. (7). Cellular mechanism of V1 receptor mediated vasoconstriction. Stimulation of V1R leads to hydrolysis of PIP2 to IP3 and DAG *via* activation of Gq protein and phospholipase C. These second messengers increase the concentrations of intracellular calcium (Ca^{2+}) which promote the vasoconstriction by facilitating actin-myosin interactions in smooth muscles. (DAG – diacylglycerol, IP3 - inositol triphosphate, PIP2 - phosphatidylinositol bisphosphate, GDP - guanosine diphosphate, GTP - guanosine triphosphate)

Stimulation of the V1R in coronary vessels and pulmonary vessels induces vasodilation of these vessels through nitric oxide release from endothelium [89 - 91]. V1R on platelets, upon stimulation, facilitates thrombosis by increasing intracellular calcium concentration; however, this aggregation response of normal human platelets to vasopressin varies tremendously [92, 93]. Stimulation of V1R in the brainstem modulates the autonomic nervous system and leads to baroreflex-mediated decrease in heart rate, which precludes a pressor effect of vasopressin on vascular smooth muscles in healthy people [94, 95]. Renal V1 receptors are present on medullary interstitial cells, vasa recta, and epithelial cells of the collecting duct and their stimulation reduces blood flow to the inner medulla without affecting blood flow to the outer medulla [96, 97]. V1R stimulation by vasopressin selectively contracts efferent arterioles only and not the afferent arteriole which increases glomerular filtration and probably accounts for the paradoxical increase in the urine output in patients with vasodilatory shock receiving vasopressin therapy [98, 99]. V1R knockout mice exhibit a decrease in BP and circulating blood volume, altered glucose homeostasis, and aldosterone secretion, and impaired spatial memory, and social recognition [100 - 103].

V_{1B} or V3 Receptor

The human V3 (previously known as V_{1B}) receptor was first cloned from a pituitary cDNA in 1994 followed by demonstration of extra-pituitary expression of V3 receptors (V3R) by cloning of corresponding rat V3 receptor [104, 105]. The 424-amino-acid sequence of V3R has 45%, 39%, and 45% identity with V1R, V2R, and OTR, respectively [104]. The V3R gene is located on chromosome region 1q32 [106]. These receptors are mostly present in the anterior pituitary gland (corticotroph cells), hippocampus and pancreatic beta cells. However, V3R is also found in other peripheral tissues such as kidney, thymus, heart, lung, spleen, uterus, adrenal gland and breast and multiple areas of the brain [76, 77]. Like V1R, V3R is primarily acts *via* activation of Gq protein and phospholipase C leading increased production of inositol triphosphate and diacylglycerol with resultant increase in cytosolic free calcium concentration and activation of protein kinase C. However, V3R have different pharmacologic profile than that of the human V1R. The human V3R activates several signalling pathways *via* different G proteins and more than one G-proteins may participate in signal transduction linked to V3R, depending on the level of receptor expression and the concentration of vasopressin. The V3R is also coupled to Gs and activation of adenylyl cyclase, although with a much lower potency [107 - 109]. Vasopressin releases ACTH by acting through V3R and interacts with the corticosteroid axis in response to stresses such as hypotension. Vasopressin and corticotrophin-releasing hormone (CRH) have synergistic effects on the release of ACTH which, although, act through different signalling systems. This is evidenced by demonstration of an impaired stress response of V3R knockout mice due to blunted ACTH response and overexpression of V3R in pituitary adenomas and ectopic ACTH syndrome [110, 111].

V2 Receptor

In 1992, human V2 receptors (V2R) were cloned using genomic expression cloning approach and rat V2Rs were cloned simultaneously from a rat kidney cDNA library [112, 113]. The human V2R gene is located on the long arm of the X chromosome (Xq28). More than150 mutations in the V2R gene have been reported to be associated with nephrogenic diabetes insipidus [113 - 115]. A high percentage identity is shown by V2R with all other AVP/OT receptors. The primary difference between V2R and V1R is the number of sites susceptible to N-linked glycosylation. The V1R has sites at both the amino-terminus and at the extracellular loop; whereas, the V2R has single site at extracellular amino terminus only [116]. The V2Rs are primarily expressed in the principal cells of renal collecting duct and are responsible for its antidiuretic effect. Vasopressin regulates water excretion from the kidney by increasing osmotic water permeability of the renal collecting duct. This effect is primarily mediated by coupling to Gs protein leading to activation of adenylyl cyclase followed by production of cyclic adenosine monophosphate (cAMP) and activation of protein kinase A. This increase in intracellular cAMP levels triggers the movement of aquaporin-2-bearing vesicles from cytoplasm and their fusion with apical membrane of the collecting duct cells. This process leads to increased water reabsorption (Fig. **8**) [117]. The V_2 receptor is secondarily coupled to Gq protein, although with a much lower potency, which leads to rise in cytosolic free calcium concentration. Vasopressin regulates water homeostasis by regulation of fast shuttling of aquaporin2 to the cell surface as well as by stimulating the synthesis of mRNA encoding the aquaporin2 proteins [118]. Vasopressin deficiency results in impaired water reabsorption due to internalization of aquaporin 2 channels from the apical membrane to subapical vesicles as well as due to decreased aquaporin 2 synthesis [119].

Although, V2Rs are primarily expressed in the renal collecting duct, existence of extra-renal V2Rs has also been proposed [120 - 123]. For example, V2R expressed in the internal ear may take part in regulating the hydraulic pressure of the endolymphatic system [123]. The V2R also mediates vasodilation by stimulating the nitric oxide pathway [124]. Expression of V2R in endothelium is supported by demonstration of release of von Willebrand factor and increased risk of clotting as well as vasodilation in response to high doses of potent V2R agonist desmopressin [125, 126].

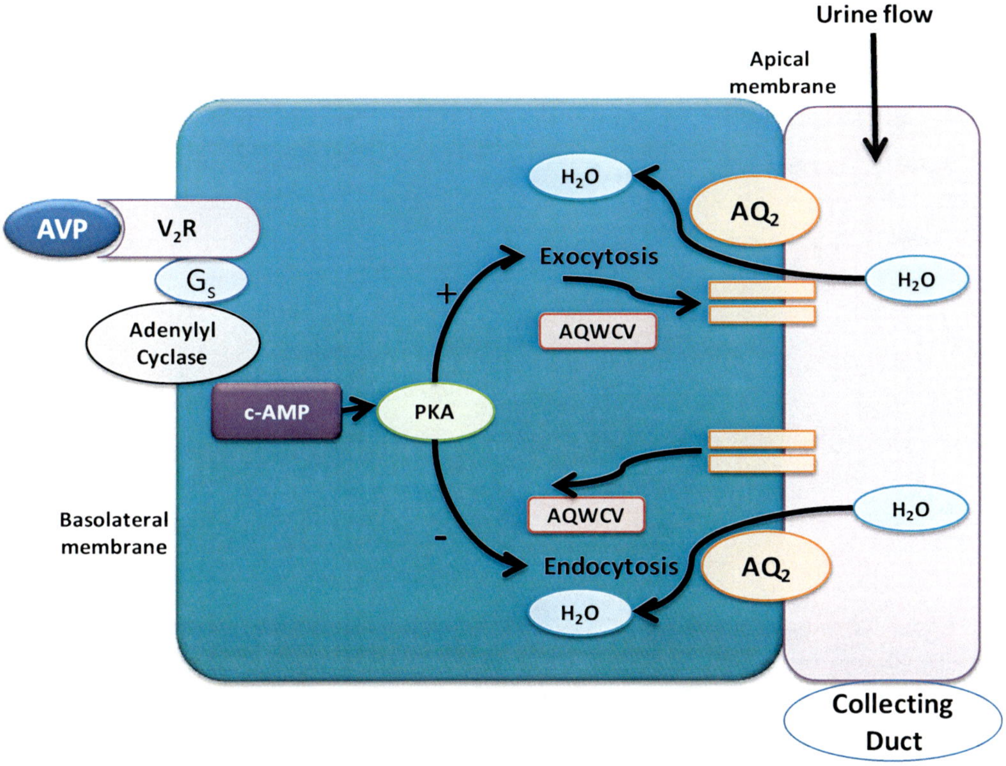

Fig. (8). V2 receptors mediated action of vasopressin leading to water reabsorption Schematic illustration of vasopressin mediated trafficking of aquaporin channels in the principal cells of the renal collecting duct. Binding of vasopressin to V2Rs present at basolateral membrane leads to activation of adenylate cyclase *via* Gs protein-mediated signalling. It results in increase in intracellular cAMP levels, and activation of protein kinase-A. This increases the exocytosis of aquaporin water channel–containing vesicles (AQMCV) and inhibits their endocytosis, resulting in increase in aquaporin 2 (AQ2) channel formation and apical membrane insertion. This event renders the cell permeable to water resulting in increased water reabsorption.

Oxytocin Receptor

The primary ligand for OT receptors (OTR) is oxytocin but it can also bind with vasopressin at higher concentrations. OTR has been identified in 1992 through human cDNA isolated by expression cloning [127]. The human OTR mRNA in mammary gland is 3.6 kb in size while it is 4.4 kb size in the ovary, uterine endometrium and myometrium [127, 128]. The OTRs are primarily expressed in the uterus and mammary gland, but these are also found in endothelial cells of umbilical vein, aorta, and pulmonary artery and in other peripheral organs such as skin, adipose tissue, ovaries, testes, and adrenal gland. These are also found to be present in brain areas like cerebral cortex, hippocampus, hypothalamus, olfactory bulb and striatum, suggesting a neurotransmitter-like activity for OT [129]. The OTRs are coupled to Gq/11 class binding proteins, and act through phosphatidyl-inositol pathway leading to rise in cytosolic calcium concentration. The OTR is also coupled to Gi leading to inhibition of adenylyl cyclase and decrease in cAMP levels [129]. This increased intracellular calcium leads to smooth muscle contraction through the calcium -calmodulin system [130].

The OTR present on endothelial cells mediates vasodilation *via* NO pathway, triggered by calcium-calmodulin complex activating neuronal and endothelial nitric oxide synthase to produce NO which in turn stimulates the soluble guanylate cyclase to produce cGMP and resulting in vasodilation [131]. In neurosecretory cells, increased intracellular calcium helps in neurotransmitter release by modulating cellular excitability and their firing patterns. Cardiac OT receptors are involved in natriuresis, regulation of blood pressure, and cell growth by atrial natriuretic peptide release [132]. Polymorphism in the OTR gene has been shown to be associated with autism [133]. OTR knockout female mice exhibit decreased lactation while male mice show deficits in social discrimination with elevated aggressive behaviour [134].

Purinergic Receptors

Vasopressin has been shown to act on the P2 class of purinergic receptors which belong to the seven-transmembrane-domain GPCR superfamily. At low doses, vasopressin acts on the purinergic receptors to mediate endothelial vasodilation while at higher doses; it mediates vasoconstriction through stimulation of the V1 receptors. Stimulation of endothelial P2 receptors by ATP released from platelets, endothelial cells and damaged myocardial cells activates phospholipase C leading to increased intracellular calcium levels. Intracellular calcium concentration results in vascular smooth muscle dilation through increased synthesis of prostacyclin and nitric oxide *via* stimulation of phospholipase A2 and NO synthase, respectively [135, 136]. Vasopressin stimulates the P2 receptors (P2X2, P2X3, P2X5 and P2Y1) present on cardiac endothelium to increase the cardiac contractility through ATP induced increase in intracellular calcium concentration [137 - 139]. ATP acts synergistically with norepinephrine through P2 receptors to stimulate the release of vasopressin, which may help in sustained release of vasopressin during hypotension [140, 141]. Purinergic receptors also modulate the antidiuretic effects of vasopressin through stimulation of P2Y1 and P2Y2 receptors expressed on convoluted tubule of the nephrons and P2Y2 knockout mice are shown to develop salt-resistant hypertension [142 - 144].

Down Regulation of Vasopressin Receptors

Binding of vasopressin receptors with the agonists lead to activation of these GPCRs followed by decrease in responsiveness (desensitization) of the receptors and this desensitization can reduce the signalling responsiveness by upto 70–80% [145]. Receptor desensitization occurs by two mechanisms which are coordinated by β-Arrestin proteins: 1) phosphorylation of activated receptors and binding to β-arrestin proteins thus inhibiting their interaction with G-proteins 2) degradation of cAMP by phosphodiesterases [146, 147]. Following exposure to vasopressin, V1Rs quickly desensitize, accompanied by sequestration of the receptors inside the cell. V1Rs recycle and resensitize rapidly as compared to V2Rs [148]. The interaction of β-arrestin with a specific motif in carboxyl terminal of the receptors determines the rate their recycling, and resensitization [148, 149].

Various studies of sepsis models demonstrated the downregulation of V1R expression. Continuous infusion of lipopolysaccharide decreased V1R expression by 43% [150, 151]. Downregulation of V1Rs in the lung, liver, kidney and heart is probably caused by increased TNFα, IL-1β, IL-6 and IFNγ [151, 152]. Sepsis also downregulates V2 and V3 receptors as evidenced downregulation of V2R expression in rat renal medulla and decrease in mRNA levels of V3R in the pituitary by lipopolysaccharide infusion [153, 154]. Ischemia–reperfusion injury down regulates the OTRs in the heart which gives the possible explanation for the potentially detrimental effects of vasopressin in conditions of myocardial ischemia–reperfusion [155].

Systemic Effects of Vasopressin

The distribution of AVP/OT receptors in the brain and in the periphery determines the physiological functions of vasopressin, the properties of which are summarized in Table **1**. Under normal physiological conditions, its main role is in osmoregulation and it has minimal effect on BP. The role of vasopressin has also been demonstrated in other physiological functions *e.g.* hemostasis, thermoregulation, memory, and sleep cycle, as well as in release of insulin and corticotropin. Vasopressin acts *via* V1Rs present on the systemic vascular smooth muscles and exerts a direct vasoconstrictor effect. However, vasopressin may lead to vasodilatation in some vascular regions at lower concentrations. Vasopressin also acts as a neurotransmitter [38 - 41].

Renal Effects

Antidiuresis is the most important physiological role of the vasopressin [156]. The renal effects of vasopressin are very complex and final effect depends on the interplay between osmoregulatory and renovascular effects. The antidiuretic effect is regulated by reabsorption of water in the kidney through V2R present at the basolateral membrane of renal tubules and collecting ducts. Vasopressin mediated V2R activation increases intracellular c-AMP levels through adenylate cyclase pathway. Intracellular c-AMP increases the intracellular water content by promoting fusion of aquaporin vesicles with luminal membrane. It further equilibrates osmotically with interstitial fluid resulting in concentrated urine [118,121]. Paradoxically, low dose vasopressin exerts diuretic effects in case of septic shock and congestive heart failure; the mechanism of which is not fully understood [98,157 - 159]. Proposed mechanisms include downregulation of the V2R; V1R mediated selective renal efferent arteriolar constriction, and NO mediated afferent arteriolar vasodilatation [97, 160, 161]. Animal studies have shown that in non-septic rats, elevated vasopressin concentrations provoked a dose-dependent fall in renal blood supply, glomerular filtration, and natriuresis [162, 163]. In clinical studies of vasopressin use in septic shock, beneficial renal effects were seen with minimal doses which allowed for the readjustment to achieve physiological concentrations [98, 157 - 158, 164, 165].

Vasoconstrictor Effects

In normal physiological conditions, vasopressin exerts minimal effect on the cardiovascular system. However, it affects the cardiovascular system in response to hemodynamic stress [3, 38 - 40]. Hypotension or hypovolemia sensed by baroreceptors stimulates vasopressin secretion from the posterior pituitary which in turn increases the arterial BP through V1Rs. Vasopressin binds to V1Rs in vascular smooth muscles and leads to vasoconstriction by increasing intracellular calcium levels through the Gq/11 pathway [166 - 168]. In vasodilatory shock states, vasopressin also restores vascular tone by following mechanisms 1) activation of V1 vascular receptors 2) dose dependent blockage of ATP-sensitive K^+ channels, 3) inhibition of cGMP mediated vasodilation by decreasing its levels through ameliorating inducible NO-synthase enzymes and 4) by potentiating effects of adrenergic and other vasoconstrictor agents [38 - 40, 169 - 172].

A variety of neurotransmitters and hormones regulate the contraction of vascular smooth muscle cells which use calcium as a signal for muscle contraction. Both the entry of extracellular calcium *via* voltage-gated calcium channels and release from intracellular stores lead to elevated cytosolic calcium concentrations. Intracellular calcium phosphorylates the light chain of myosin *via* calcium-calmodulin complex. Phosphorylated myosin leads to contraction of the muscles *via* cross-bridging of myosin with actin filaments. In contrast, vasodilators such as atrial natriuretic peptide (ANP) and NO produce vasodilation by activating a cGMP-dependent kinase which interacts with myosin phosphatase and dephosphorylates myosin to prevent the muscle contraction [173].

Tone of the vascular smooth muscles is primarily controlled through K+ channels and opening of K+ channels causes an efflux of potassium which hyperpolarizes the plasma membrane and prevents the entry of calcium into the cell by closing voltage gated calcium channels. Conversely, closure of K+ channels depolarizes the membrane and opens voltage-gated calcium channels increasing cytosolic Ca2+ concentration leading to constriction of vessels. Of the four types of K+ channels, the ATP gated K+ channel plays a critical role in vasodilatory shock states [171 - 175]. Vasopressin also potentiates the effects of other vasoconstrictors such as norepinephrine and angiotensin II by largely unknown mechanisms. Possible mechanisms are coupling between G-protein coupled receptors, interaction between G-proteins, and attenuation of downregulation of these receptors through arrestin trafficking [176 - 178]. Fig. (**9**) depicts the various mechanisms by which vasopressin acts to increase the blood pressure.

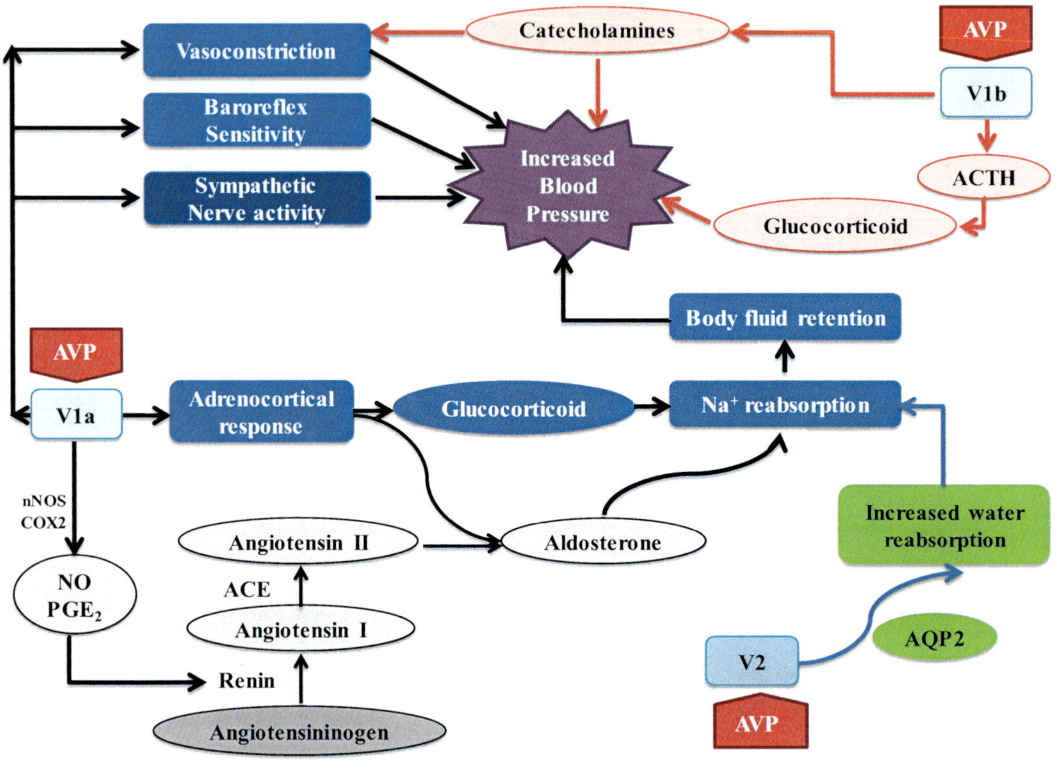

Fig. (9). Schematic illustration showing contributions of vasopressin and its receptors on regulation of blood pressure homeostasis. Hypotension and hypovolumemia stimulate secretion of vasopressin from the posterior pituitary which acts *via* V1, V1b (V3), and V2 receptors to maintain BP. Vasopressin increases blood pressure by stimulating vasoconstriction, aldosterone/ glucocorticoid release from the adrenal gland, renin production in the kidney, and elevated sympathetic nerve and baroreflex activity in the CNS, through the V1a receptors. Vasopressin mediated V3 receptor activation increases ACTH and catecholamine release from the anterior pituitary and adrenal gland, respectively. Vasopressin acts *via* the V2 receptor-AQP2 pathway to control BP by maintaining fluid retention. Vasopressin/ V1 receptor stimulates the expression of nNOS and COX-2, which leads to the production of NO and PGE2 to stimulate renin production. Renin stimulates subsequent increase in angiotensin II and aldosterone levels and promotes water reabsorption.

The vasoconstrictor effect of vasopressin is heterogeneous on a topographical level and at times it may produce vasodilation also. Vasopressin produces vasoconstriction mainly in skin, skeletal muscle, adipose tissue, pancreas and thyroid with less apparent effect on mesenteric, coronary and cerebral vessels. The ultimate vasoconstrictor or vasodilator effect depends on the vascular bed and receptor density on it (V1R *versus* OTR), as well as the dose and duration of vasopressin exposure [179 - 183]. Indeed, further research is needed to completely understand the opposing influences of various pathways that determine the final state of the vascular smooth muscle.

Vasodilator Effects

Unlike other vasoconstrictors, vasopressin induces vasodilation in many vascular beds especially pulmonary, renal and cerebral circulation. This vasodilatory effect is seen more at low doses unlike its dose dependent vasoconstrictor effect. Vasopressin acts through V2Rs or endothelial OTRs triggering activation of endothelial NOS resulting in NO release to induce vasodilation [89 - 91, 131, 180, 184 - 186]. Vasopressin induced cerebral vasodilatation has been shown to be more pronounced in the area of circle of Willis [91]. Vasopressin induces pulmonary artery vasodilatation through V1R mediated release of NO, both under physiological and hypoxic conditions [89 - 90, 186 - 188]. Vasopressin acts through ANP to decrease the pulmonary arterial pressure both in normal and hypoxic conditions [189]. These effects make vasopressin more useful in septic shock conditions due to presence of the increased pulmonary vascular tone and resistance in these situations.

Effects of Vasopressin on Heart

The actions of vasopressin on the heart are complex with contradictory results found in various studies. Vasopressin has been shown to induce coronary vasoconstriction or vasodilation and exert positive or negative inotropic effects, which probably depend on the experimental model, and dose and duration of vasopressin. Additionally, it has been also shown to exert mitogenic and metabolic effects on the heart [190 - 192].

Many studies using animal models [193] as well as with isolated human coronary arteries have demonstrated the V1R-mediated vasoconstriction of the coronary vascular bed [99, 194]. On the other hand, few studies have also demonstrated vasopressin-induced coronary vasodilation in isolated canine [195, 196] and primate [91] coronary arteries as well as in intact pigs [197]. Studies using pig model found the persistence of this coronary vasodilation during sinus rhythm, ventricular fibrillation, and after successful cardiopulmonary resuscitation (CPR). Coronary vasodilation is also results from V2Rs or endothelial OTRs mediated activation of endothelial NOS and NO release as seen in the pulmonary vasculature. A differential response to vasopressin has been reported depending upon coronary artery cell oxygen tensions, with vasoconstriction seen in normoxic state and vasodilation in hypoxic conditions [198]. Several studies on animal models of cardiac arrest have demonstrated superior resuscitation rates with vasopressin than with epinephrine [199 - 201]. Improved coronary blood flow due to vasopressin, mediated probably by improved coronary perfusion pressure rather than coronary vasodilation, was thought to be responsible for improvement in restoration of spontaneous circulation [202].

Studies have demonstrated both positive or negative inotropic effects of vasopressin on myocardium which probably depend on the dose used and the model studied. Studies conducted on isolated working heart models of rat [192], guinea pig [203] and dogs [204] showed that vasopressin infusion induced coronary vasoconstriction, negative inotropy with decrease in cardiac output and overall depression of cardiac performance. However, relevance of these observations in human vasodilatory shock is not very well understood. On the contrary, a direct positive inotropic effect of vasopressin has also been observed, which depends on its concentrations and the relative balance of its effect on the coronary circulation. Few clinical studies, conducted on patients with heart failure and vasodilatory shock due to milirinone therapy [205], post-cardiotomy refractory septic shock [206], and septic shock [99], demonstrated a positive inotropic effect of vasopressin. Regardless of the mechanism, low-dose vasopressin can improve cardiac performance.

To summarize, vasopressin induces coronary vasoconstriction in a dose-dependent manner through its V1Rs while at low doses, it may exerts coronary vasodilation and a positive inotropic effect *via* OTR or P2 receptors. However, further research is necessary to determine the significance of these observations in human heart, both healthy as well as diseased.

Endocrine Effects

In pharmacologic doses, vasopressin increases plasma cortisol levels by stimulating the ACTH release. This effect is most likely mediated *via* NO and c-GMP pathway *via* vasopressin mediated V3R stimulation, present at the surface of corticotroph cells [207, 208]. This effect can be beneficial in patients with septic shock, in whom adrenocortical dysfunction is common. Both vasopressin and CRH stimulate ACTH release by activating the hypothalamus-pituitar--adrenal (HPA) axis which then stimulates the glucocorticoid synthesis and secretion [209, 210]. Vasopressin itself is a weak upregulator of the ACTH secretion but it markedly potentiates the effects of CRH.

Vasopressin also mediates ANP and angiotensin-II secretion and stimulates prolactin and endothelin-I release [207]. Homeostatic control of the blood glucose levels is another important physiological process which is regulated by the vasopressin. Vasopressin can decrease blood glucose level through V3R mediated insulin release from the pancreatic beta cells or can increase it by promoting the glucagon release and by hepatic V1R mediated enhanced glycogenolysis [211, 212].

Effects on Coagulation System

Like other stress hormones, supraphysiological doses of vasopressin enhance the blood coagulation and acts as a platelet aggregating agent [213, 214]. This undesirable effect may further enhance the existing coagulation problems in septic shock. However, the doses used in clinical practice are less likely to provoke a significant aggregation effect. Vasopressin acts *via* V2R to stimulate the release of factor VIIIc, von Willebrand factor, and plasminogen activating factors from the vascular endothelial cells, and helps effective platelet adhesion. This effect of vasopressin has been utilized in clinical practice to treat bleeding due to functional platelet disorders; although, its use in these conditions has been limited by other physiological actions evoked by vasopressin. On the contrary, selective V2-agonist desmopressin (dDAVP) has fewer side effects than vasopressin and is widely used to treat bleeding disorders [215].

Other Effects

Apart from the hypothalamus, vasopressin is also produced in smaller amounts in many tissues locally. Therefore, vasopressin also exerts some autocrine and paracrine effects also apart from its endocrine effect. Vasopressin secreting neurohypophyseal tracts also innervates other areas of the brain and the spinal cord enabling vasopressin to exert some central actions apart from its well-known peripheral effects on blood glucose, lipid levels, and BP. Vasopressin may contribute in the regulation of physiologic changes relating to aging, abnormal social behaviour and cognitive function [216]. These effects may be mediated by V1R, V3R, and OT receptors found in the brain. The behavioural role of vasopressin such as in regulating pair bonding, mate guarding and paternal care in monogamous prairie voles has also been reported [217]. Many other human studies further suggested that vasopressin has a role in modulating social behaviour and cognition. It has been shown to enhance some aspects of social function in psychiatric disorders like autism [218]. Other actions include effects on pain perception and bone structure as well as on varied components of metabolic syndromes. Studies have also demonstrated the relationship of vasopressin with important cellular responses such as cell proliferation, inflammation, and control of infection. Vasopressin may also play a role in the progression of chronic kidney disease [219].

Table 3. Common indications and doses of vasopressin and analogs.

Indication	**Drug**	**Route**	**Dose (Children)**	**Dose (Adults)**
Nocturnal enuresis	DD-AVP	Intranasal	5-20 µg (in children > 6 yr)	-
		Oral	0.2-0.4 mg/d at bedtime	-
Central diabetes insipidus	DD- AVP	Intranasal	5-30 µg/d Q 8-12 hr	5-30 µg/d Q 8-12hr
		Oral	0.05-0.2 mg/d Q 8-12 hr	0.05-0.2 mg/d Q 8-12 hr
		IV/SC	2-4 µg/d Q 8-12 hr	2-4 µg/d Q 8-12 hr
	AVP	IM/SC	2.5-10U/dose 2-4 times/d	5-10U 2-4 times/d
		IV infusion	0.0005 U/kg/hr initially, double every 30 min up to 0.01 U/kg/hr	0.0005 U/kg/hr initially, double every 30 min up to 0.01 U/kg/hr

(Table 3) contd.....

Indication	Drug	Route	Dose (Children)	Dose (Adults)
Haemophilia-A, von Willebrand disease, platelet dysfunctions	DD- AVP	Intranasal	< 50 kg - 150 μg	> 50 kg - 300 μg
		IV	0.3 μg/kg (>3 months), repeat if needed, give 30 min before procedure	0.3 μg/kg over 15 - 30 min repeat if needed, give 30 min before procedure
Abdominal distension	AVP	IM	-	5 U stat then 10 U Q 3-4 hr
Bleeding esophageal varices	AVP	IV	Bolus 0.3 U/kg (max.- 20 U) then infusion: 0.002 - 0.01 U/kg/min	0.2 - 0.4 U, titrate upwards, continue for 12 hr then taper off in 48 hr
	TP	IV	10 - 20 μg/kg Q 4 - 6 hrs	1 - 2 mg Q 4-6 hr
Refractory vasodilatory shock	AVP	IV infusion	Variable (0.00005 to 0.008 U/kg/min)	0.01 - 0.1 Units/min
	TP	IV bolus	10 - 20 μg/kg Q 4 - 6 hrs	10 - 20 μg/kg Q 4 - 6 hrs
		IV infusion	10 μg/kg/hr	10 μg/kg/hr
Cardiac arrest	AVP	IV bolus	0.4 U/kg	40 U, Repeat after 3 min
	TP	IV bolus	10 - 20 μg/kg	
Pulseless VT/VF	AVP	IV bolus		40 U, single dose
		ET		40 U, single dose
	TP	IV bolus		

Note: DDAVP – Desmopressin, AVP – Arginine Vasopressin, TP – Terlipressin, VT – Ventricular Tachycardia, VF – Ventricular Firillation

Therapeutic Applications of Vasopressin

Approved uses for vasopressin and its analogues include management of diabetes insipidus (DI), nocturnal enuresis, variceal bleeding, and bleeding disorders such as haemophilia-A, von-Willebrand disease, and platelet function disorders. Although vasopressin is still not recognized as a standard of care, it has emerged as a potent vasopressor to treat vasodilatory shock states and cardiac arrest. Indications and doses of vasopressin/analogues are given in Table **3**.

Nocturnal Enuresis

Desmopressin and vasopressin are used to treat nocturnal enuresis, caused by maturational delay in normal nocturnal increase in vasopressin secretion [220].

Diabetes Insipidus

Diabetes insipidus can be of central or nephrogenic type and in both types; inability of the renal tubular collecting ducts to concentrate the urine is the characteristics finding. In cranial or central DI, there is congenital or acquired deficiency of vasopressin secondary to partial or complete destruction of the hypothalamus or pituitary gland. On the contrary, nephrogenic DI results from defective or absent vasopressin receptor sites or aquaporins leading to resistance of the kidney to vasopressin's action. Clinically, patient produces large quantities of dilute urine and urine osmolality is inappropriately low compared with the plasma osmolality [221].

In central DI, desmopressin forms the mainstay of treatment and reduces the polyuria, nocturia, and polydypsia. It enhances the renal reabsorption of water by increasing cellular permeability of collecting ducts. Vasopressin can safely be used to diagnose nephrogenic DI due to shorter half life and lesser risk of volume overload. Urine osmolality increase significantly in central DI; however, it remains low in nephorgeic DI. It is given by nasal, sublingual, intramuscular or intravenous routes. Serum/urinary sodium and osmolality, as well as urine output should be used as a guide to titrate the dose of vasopressin [222].

Bleeding Abnormalities

Vasopressin's action to increase factor VIII:c and VWF *via* extra-renal V2Rs has been utilized in treatment of certain types of von Willebrand disease and mild forms of haemophilia A. DDAVP can be used before minor surgical procedures in patients with impaired platelet function secondary to drugs such as aspirin or renal failure. These effects are probably mediated *via* increase in the factor VIII levels which allows activation of factor X and more efficient activation of platelets [223].

Oesophageal Varices Haemorrhage

In chronic liver disease, fibrosis of the liver results in increase in portal venous pressure resulting in opening of collateral circulation between portal and systemic circulation and formation of gastro-oesophageal varices. These varices might rupture and result in serious upper gastrointestinal bleeding [224]. Use of vasopressin is intended to decrease portal venous pressure, portal systemic collateral blood flow, and variceal pressure and to optimize clotting and hemostasis through its action of V1R. Vasopressin is considered as a second line of treatment in these situations as evidences do not show improved survival rate with its use [225]. Endoscopic sclerotherapy or band ligation is the first-line therapy followed by vasoactive drugs *i.e.* octreotide (somatostatin analogue), vasopressin and terlipressin [226]. The combined use of glyceryl trinitrate with vasopressin has been shown to reduce the side effects due to its vasoconstrictor actions. Terlipressin has been shown to more useful than vasopressin in treatment of variceal bleeding [227].

Abdominal Distension & Abdominal X-ray

Vasopressin may also be used to prevent and to treat post-operative as well as abdominal distension complicating pneumonia and other acute toxaemias. It has been used for dispelling gas interfering with the abdominal X-ray studies [228].

Vasodilatory Shock States

Vasodilatory shock forms a final common pathway following a variety of shock states such as septic shock, following cardiopulmonary bypass (CPB), cardiogenic shock prolonged hemorrhage, hypovolemia, anaphylaxis, and carbon monoxide poisoning. Vascular smooth muscle dysfunction and decreased responsiveness to catecholamines in these conditions are mediated by various common pathogenic mechanisms such as activation of ATP sensitive K^+-channels, NO-synthase stimulation and relative vasopressin deficiency [1, 169]. Vasopressin has been shown to reverse these mechanisms and therefore has emerged as a potential therapeutic option in vasodilatory shock states. Usual dose of vasopressin in adults with vasodilatory shock is 0.01 – 0.04 U/min. Doses of vasopressin or TP in pediatric vasodilatory shock are not very well documented and are primarily extrapolated from adult data. In various studies, vasopressin was used in a dose range of 0.0005-0.002 U/kg/min (from 0.00005 to as high as 0.008 U/kg/min) [229].

Septic Shock

Patients with septic shock develop hypotension due to multiple factors and inappropriate vasodilation compromises the organ perfusion. Fluid, vasoconstrictors (*e.g.* norepinephrine), and inotropes are the mainstay of therapy. Unfortunately, vasopressor action of catecholamines is often diminished in septic shock and advanced cardiovascular failure leads to death in more than half of the patients succumbing to sepsis. Increasing doses of norepinephrine produces adverse effects such as increased tissue oxygen demand, reduced renal and mesenteric blood flow, pulmonary hypertension, and arrhythmias. After demonstration of relative deficiency of vasopressin in septic shock and increase in BP and urine output with vasopressin infusion, it has emerged as a potential therapeutic option to improve BP in septic shock [1].

Vasopressin hypersensitivity has been demonstrated in patients with septic shock resulting in significant increase in BP which can be due to: 1) V_1R mediated vasoconstriction; 2) unlike catecholamine receptors, relative vasopressin deficiency in sepsis ensures the availability of V_1Rs as well as decrease their downregulation; 3) absent bradycardia reflex in critically ill patients with autonomic failure; 4) augmentation of vasopressor effects of catecholamines by decreasing the membrane hyperpolarization and vasodilation by blocking ATP sensitive K^+-channels; 5) Finally, vasopressin mediated increase in ACTH and cortisol release in these patients with septic shock having adrenocortical dysfunction [5, 38 - 40, 76, 207]. Vasopressin is found to be more beneficial in preserving vital organ functions in sepsis as compared to catecholamines due to its selective coronary, pulmonary, and cerebral vasodilator effects, along with its potential to improve urine output and creatinine clearance [89 - 91].

A large randomized controlled trial (RCT) showed a significant increase in mean arterial pressure (MAP), cardiac index, systemic vascular resistance index and left ventricular stroke work index as well as reduced norepinephrine requirement and heart rate in patients with catecholamine resistant vasodilatory shock who received combined vasopressin (4 IU/hour) and norepinephrine infusion than norepinephrine alone [230]. The vasopressin and septic shock trial (VASST), a multicenter, RCT which compared low-dose vasopressin with norepinephrine in

778 patients with septic shock showed no mortality benefit with the use of vasopressin but was shown to be as safe as norepinephrine. However in patients with less severe septic shock, vasopressin has lowered the mortality [231].

Vasopressin is acknowledged as an adjunct vasopressor in the *Surviving Sepsis Guidelines* 2012 according to which vasopressin (0.03 U/min) can be added to norepinephrine to either raise MAP to target or to decrease norepinephrine dose; however, it should not be used as the initial vasopressor therapy [232]. One fundamental concept of its use in sepsis is that the effects of vasopressin (both beneficial and adverse) depend on the volume status of the patients; therefore, adequate volume resuscitation of patients before starting vasopressin is of paramount importance [233]. Vasopressin can bridge the phase of advanced cardiovascular failure and can prevent the development of vicious cycle of high-dose catecholamine therapy in septic shock when it is used to supplement other vasopressor agents. Both the ideal dosage and timing of vasopressin use in septic patients are currently under investigation.

Usual timing of starting vasopressin therapy is the point when increasing norepinephrine doses are required to maintain MAP. This is supported by the one study which identified benefits of early goal-directed therapy when applied in the first 6 hours [234]. VASST also showed a trend to decreased mortality with vasopressin in patients treated within 12 hours suggesting that early treatment with vasopressin may optimize its benefits [231]. In advanced septic shock, institution of vasopressin therapy should not be guided by endocrinological but by hemodynamic indications [207]. Currently, there is inadequate evidence to recommend vasopressin as the first agent in septic shock due to scarcity of studies showing the safety and efficacy of vasopressin when used as the initial vasopressor agent in septic shock. Another retrospective cohort study of patients with septic shock found no difference in mortality between the groups receiving norepinephrine, vasopressin, or dopamine as the first vasopressor agent [235].

The ideal dosage of vasopressin in sepsis is currently under investigation and several investigators have explored the use of higher doses (0.06 U/min) of vasopressin [164 - 165, 206, 236, 237]. Vasopressin was found to decrease the use of norepinephrine and to increase the BP; however, it was also associated with increased adverse events such as decreased intestinal mucosal perfusion, digital ischemia, increased bilirubin, and serum transaminase levels, and decreased platelet counts [238]. Therefore, a large RCT is warranted to evaluate the safety and efficacy of higher doses of vasopressin in septic shock. Various studies have used vasopressin in the dose range of 0.01–0.04 IU/min to replace falling vasopressin levels. In most of the studies, vasopressin was slowly withdrawn once the cardiovascular function stabilized and norepinephrine could be decreased to dosages < 0.2-0.3 µg/kg/min.

Research using the synthetic vasopressin analog terlipressin for the treatment of septic shock has shown that outcome was better where terlipressin was used early as compared to when it was used as a last-resort treatment. A recent trial has compared continuous infusion of low-dose terlipressin with norepinephine or vasopressin as first-line therapy in septic shock patients and found it effective in increasing MAP and in reducing the requirement of norepinephrine [239]. Evidence from experimental and human studies suggests that continuous low-dose terlipressin therapy may help stabilize hemodynamics in patients with septic shock [240].

Vasopressin and terlipressin in pediatric patients with septic shock should be used judiciously as very limited data are available regarding their impact on outcome of these patients. The characteristic vasodilation of adult septic shock may not be recognised early in pediatric septic shock. Children with severe sepsis can present with low cardiac output and high systemic vascular resistance (SVR), high cardiac output and low SVR, or low cardiac output and low SVR shock [241]. Secondly, hemodynamic profile in children may change from one state to another with progression of the disease. According to recommendations from American College of Critical Care Medicine Clinical Guidelines 2007 for hemodynamic support of pediatric and neonatal septic shock, vasopressin/TP can be used in catecholamine-resistant shock with high cardiac index and low SVR. However, these agents should be used with cardiac output and mixed venous oxygen saturation ($ScvO_2$) monitoring as these agents can reduce cardiac output [242] *via* increased afterload.

Post-CPB/ Post - Cardiac Surgery Vasodilatory Shock

Vasodilatory shock following CPB or cardiac surgery not associated with primary cardiogenic or septic shock has been reported in approximately 10% of the cardiac surgeries [243]. These patients are more prone to postoperative blood loss due to CPB induced hemostatic derangements, relative depletion of coagulation factors and fibrinogen, and platelet dysfunction. The hemodynamic impact of postoperative blood loss is further exacerbated by CPB induced systemic inflammatory response secondary to endothelial injury, release of cytokines and other inflammatory mediators, and other nonspecific activators such as hypothermia, surgical trauma, and blood loss or transfusion [244]. Many other factors have been shown to contribute in the development of vasodilatory shock in these patients such as inappropriately low vasopressin secretion, prolonged duration of CPB, long-term ACE inhibitor or beta-blocker therapy, or post-bypass amiodarone and phosphodiestrase-III inhibitors [243, 244].

Various studies have found improved BP as well as restored catecholamines sensitivity with low dose vasopressin therapy by the mechanisms similar to that seen in septic shock [164,194, 243 - 246]. The unique benefits and risks of vasopressin therapy in these patients remain to be fully established. Vasopressin infusion has been found to have renal-protective effects and is associated with a reduction in markers of myocardial ischemia [245, 246]. Although not very common as suggested by available data, vasopressin may promote gastrointestinal ischemia, thrombogenesis and impaired microcirculation due to its vasoconstrictor and platelet aggregator effects. Many vasopressors such as norepinephrine, phenylephrine, vasopressin *etc.* have been shown to increase MAP in postcardiotomy hypotension, but none of them can bc suggested for use as an exclusive agent. However, existing data clearly place vasopressin among the therapeutic options [247].

Hemorrhagic Shock

Vasopressin and its analogs have been used in the management of trauma induced hemorrhagic shock utilizing its well known effect on controlling gastrointestinal hemorrhage. Patients with advanced hemorrhagic shock may develop resistant vasodilation secondary to metabolites produced during ischemic-reperfusion injury and the coexisting severe acidosis, which usually responds poorly to both volume administration and catecholamine therapy. By utilizing its potent vasopressor effect, vasopressin has been tried as a rescue therapy in such patients, which otherwise have an extremely poor prognosis. Vasopressin can be especially useful in patients with uncontrolled hemorrhage associated with subdiaphragmatic injury as it shifts the blood away from subdiaphragmatic areas to the vital organs [248].

Animal studies showed favourable results of vasopressin therapy for uncontrolled hemorrhagic shock such as enhanced renal perfusion and postresuscitation hemodynamic stability [249]. Results of a meta-analysis of randomized animal trials suggested that vasopressin and terlipressin improve survival in animal with early phases of hemorrhagic shock and vasopressin is more effective than all other treatments, including other vasopressor drugs [250]. These results are supported by the favourable impact of vasopressin when used during triage of human trauma victims as a temporary measure to support BP [251, 252]. However, its use may lead to adverse metabolic and hemodynamic consequences, including lactic acidemia and decreased cardiac index. Although no RCT is available currently, limited clinical and laboratory data support the use of vasopressin in selected patients with resistant hemorrhagic shock. A multicenter, RCT, the Vasopressin in Traumatic Hemorrhagic Shock (VITRIS) trial has been started to investigate the impact of vasopressin in the prehospital management of uncontrolled hemorrhagic shock. More definitive recommendations can be laid down on vasopressin use in hemorrhagic shock management once the results of this trial are available [253].

Anaphylactic Shock

Anaphylactic shock is characterized by systemic vasodilation and increased capillary permeability secondary to immune mediated release of inflammatory mediators [254]. Vasopressin has been found to be useful in epinephrine refractory anaphylactic shock due to its optimal vasoactive action *i.e.* vaso-constriction in skin and splanchnic circulation, along with the vasodilatation of coronary and cerebral vascular beds and renoprotective effects. No controlled trials or guidelines are currently available on vasopressin use in anaphylactic shock, and it is used only in case reports and laboratory studies in the dose range of 2-15 U (0.03-0.15 U/kg) [255 - 258].

Asystolic Cardiac Arrest

Epinephrine has been used as the first line drug in cardiopulmonary resuscitation (CPR) for more than 100 years due to its ability to improve blood flow to the heart by maintaining diastolic BP. However, clinical studies have failed to demonstrate any survival benefit of epinephrine use in these patients. On the contrary many studies have shown adverse effects with epinephrine such as increased myocardial oxygen consumption, myocardial dysfunction and ventricular arrhythmias, and ventilation–perfusion mismatch [259, 260]. A recent meta-analysis of RCTs showed no benefit of epinephrine in survival to discharge or neurological outcomes when used for out of hospital cardiac arrest. However, there were improved rates of survival to admission and return of spontaneous circulation (ROSC) with standard dose epinephrine over placebo and high dose epinephrine over standard dose epinephrine [261].

Vasopressin is proposed to be an alternative to epinephrine during CPR owing to its profound vasoconstriction effects which shunt the blood to the heart and the brain. Secondly, vasopressin may work better than epinephrine in the hypoxemic, acidotic conditions that accompanies cardiac arrest. Its use is further supported by the finding that vasopressin levels are higher in survivors of cardiac arrest than in non-survivors [262]. In contrast to epinephrine, vasopressin has been shown to enhance the myocardial oxygen delivery without marked increase in oxygen consumption and to improve cerebral perfusion with better neurologic outcomes and short term survival rates in animal studies [199 - 202].

A multicentre RCT compared the efficacy of vasopressin and epinephrine on 1186 out-of-hospital cardiac arrest patients. It showed better survival to hospital admission as well as discharge with vasopressin than epinephrine in asystole group of patients. There was no difference between these two in patients who suffered from pulseless electrical activity (PEA) or ventricular fibrillation (VF) cardiac arrests. They found that vasopressin followed by epinephrine was more effective than epinephrine alone in the treatment of refractory cardiac arrest [263].

Similarly, vasopressin has shown to have comparable efficacy to epinephrine in RCT of in-hospital arrests [264]. No consistent benefit was found in other studies using vasopressin in adult cardiac arrest; although, convincingly demonstrable harm was also not observed with vasopressin therapy. Poor initial CPR and differences in the time taken to provide advanced life support can explain the differences in outcome observed with different researchers. Available trend suggests a better outcome with vasopressin in patients receiving delayed or prolonged resuscitation. A recent meta-analysis showed a significantly better ROSC in "in-hospital" cardiac arrest patients with vasopressin use on comparing the efficacy of vasopressin containing regimen with epinephrine alone in a cohort of adult cardiac arrest patients. A subgroup analysis also showed a better ROSC, survival to hospital admission and discharge and favourable neurological outcome with repeated (up to 4-5 times) boluses of vasopressin; however, no overall survival benefit was seen in unselected cardiac arrest population [265].

The current American Heart Association guidelines 2010 have also recommended the use of 40 U of intravenous vasopressin as an alternative to either the first or second dose of epinephrine in treatment of all the cases of pulseless adult cardiac arrest (VF, pulseless VT, PEA and asystole) [266]. On the contrary, European Resuscitation Council guidelines 2010 did not support or refute the use of vasopressin or terlipressin as an alternative to or in combination with epinephrine in any cardiac arrest rhythm; however, these can be tried in cardiac arrest refractory to repeated doses of epinephrine [267].

Studies have been conducted to explore the potential benefit of combination of epinephrine and vasopressin to treat cardiac arrest which suggest a possible survival benefit with their combined use in comparison to using either drug alone [263]. A large RCT conducted on 3,000 patients with out-of-hospital cardiac arrest failed to show benefit of combined epinephrine and vasopressin than epinephrine alone in terms of ROSC, neurologic outcome at discharge, out-of-hospital and 1-year survival [268]. However, another RCT involving 100 patients with refractory in-hospital cardiac arrest demonstrated survival benefit on addition of intravenous corticosteroids to vasopressin and epinephrine [269]. Another RCT was conducted to determine the survival benefit, in terms of hospital discharge, with combined vasopressin-epinephrine use during CPR and corticosteroid supplementation during and after CPR in in-hospital cardiac arrest patients. This study found better survival to hospital discharge with favourable neurological status with combined vasopressin-epinephrine use along with methylprednisolone during CPR and stress-dose hydrocortisone in postresuscitation shock compared with epinephrine alone [270].

In comparison data available on vasopressin use in adult cardiac arrest, information regarding vasopressin use in pediatric cardiac arrest is limited. In adults, cardiac arrest is usually results from a sudden primary cardiac event where as in children; it is often the terminal result of progressive respiratory failure or shock. Prolonged CPR in children often has dismal prognosis with survivors having severe neurological impairment. Although, improved ROSC with vasopressin therapy was demonstrated in a few case reports [271 - 273], two larger studies failed to demonstrate any survival benefit of vasopressin in pediatric CPR [274, 275]. However, the results of these studies could have been biased due to the tendency for use of vasopressin as a "last resort" in children with prolonged CPR having more significant underlying pathology. Therefore, further research is necessary to evaluate the long term outcome and safety of vasopressin in pediatric CPR before recommending or refuting the use of vasopressin in this study population. Due to paucity of available data on vasopressin efficacy in pediatric cardiac arrest, American Heart Association guidelines have made no recommendations on its routine use in pediatric patients [276]. Similarly, European Resuscitation Council guidelines 2010 also did not support or refute the use of vasopressin or terlipressin as an alternative to or in combination with epinephrine in any cardiac arrest rhythm [277].

Other Uses

Anaesthesia Induced Hypotension

The sympathetic nervous system (SNS) response to hypotension can be altered by agents used for both general and neuraxial anaesthesia. Similarly, epidural anaesthesia also impairs the release of renin in response to hypotension by blocking the renal SNS discharge [278]. Animal studies showed that sympathetic blockade caused by epidural anaesthesia induces a compensatory rise in endogenous vasopressin secretion. On the basis of these findings, exogenous vasopressin infusion has been successfully used to treat catecholamine resistant hypotension in humans. It has been found to be more useful in treatment of hypotension in anesthetized patients who are receiving chronic angiotensin-converting enzyme (ACE) inhibitors or angiotensin receptor blockers therapy due to prevailing concomitant SNS and Renin – Angiotension - Aldosterone System (RAAS) dysfunction in them [279 - 282]. Supplementary opioids and α2-receptor agonists, frequently used during spinal/epidural anaesthesia, can inhibit endogenous vasopressin release. It was hypothesized that administration of vasopressin may mimic the physiological adaptation to the sympathetic block induced by epidural anaesthesia [283]

Prevention of Sedation Related Hypotension

Effect of vasopressin on redistribution of mesenteric blood was utilized in prevention of sedation/analgesia related hypotension in non-septic, hemo-dynamically stable but critically ill children in one study. However due to the side effects such as decreased urine output, hyponatremia, and rebound hypotension, the prophylactic use of vasopressin could not be recommended till further research show significant benefits [284].

Acute Brain Injury

Vasopressin has been used to ensure adequate cerebral perfusion pressure in perioperative setting due to its vasodilatory effects on arteries of the circle of Willis apart from systemic vasoconstriction. However, currently no large scale studies are available to support use of vasopressin in these patients and only few case reports available where vasopressin/TP has been used successfully in patients suffering from advanced vasodilatory shock after cerebeller and subarachnoid hemorrhage [285, 286].

Hormone Replacement in Brain-Dead Organ Donors

Vasopressin is used in brain-dead organ donors (dose - 1 IU bolus followed by 0.5-4 IU/hr) to treat DI and to achieve significant reduction in requirement of vasopressor and ionotropic drugs [287]. Low dose vasopressin infusion has also shown good pressure effects in critically ill children treated for DI during brain death and organ recovery without any adverse affect on transplant organ function [288].

Vasodilatory Shock After Pheochromocytoma Extirpation

Vasopressin has also been used in vasodilatory shock after resection of pheochromocytoma which is usually catecholamine resistant due to extensive downregulation of adrenergic receptors [289].

Hypotension Caused by Carcinoid Crisis

Vasopressin has been shown to be good alternative in patients with carcinoid tumours, where sympathomimetic vasoconstrictors are relatively contraindicated due to the risk of exaggeration of further peptide release via adrenergic receptor stimulation [290].

Pulmonary Hypertension

Vasopressin has been used successfully to improve BP and to decrease pulmonary artery pressure in children developing pulmonary hypertension secondary to congenital diaphragmatic hernia [291 - 293] and after correction of total anomalous pulmonary venous return which was refractory to other conventional therapies [294].

Adverse Effects/Precautions

Due to its potent vasoconstrictor action, vasopressin therapy may produce many side effects secondary to impaired capillary blood flow and tissue oxygenation. A number of adverse effects have been reported with vasopressin therapy depending upon the dose and duration, concurrent use of other vasopressor agents (more with moderate to high dose of norepinephrine), underlying disease process, and co-morbidities [38 - 40]. Severe skin necrosis after extravasation of vasopressin has been reported; therefore, peripheral administration of vasopressin should be discouraged [295]. Cardiovascular complications include venous thrombosis, severe hypertension, coronary ischemia, angina, and myocardial infarction, and ventricular arrhythmias (*e.g.* VT and asystole). Anaphylaxis, bronchospasm, urticaria angioedema, rashes, and severe GI ischemia leading to bowel necrosis have been reported with clinical use [296]. Other reported adverse effects include hyponatremia, irritation at the injection site, and cutaneous gangrene due to peripheral vasoconstriction [297]. Vasopressin therapy may also impair oxygenation in the gut mucosa and hepatic tissues with resultant increase in aminotransferase and bilirubin levels and a reduction in platelet count.

Teratogenic potential of vasopressin or terlipressin is currently unknown as no animal reproduction study has been conducted; however, few case reports are there on the use of vasopressin and desmopressin safely during pregnancy. It should be used with caution during lactation as it enters the breast milk. Similarly, safety data of vasopressin in children are also limited. Vasopressin is contra-indicated in patients with hypersensitivity to vasopressin or any component of the formulation. It should be used cautiously in patients with seizure disorders, migraine, asthma, cardiovascular disease, and chronic renal disease. Vasopressin infusion should be given through central venous catheters due to risk of tissue necrosis secondary to severe vasoconstriction if extravasated locally. In elderly patients, fluid intake should be restricted just to satisfy their thirst to avoid water intoxication and hyponatremia. In patients on vasopressin therapy, serum and urine sodium, urine specific gravity, urine and serum osmolality, fluid input and output, BP, heart rate should be closely monitored.

Future

Vasopressin is a potentially lifesaving drug to treat various vasodilatory shock states. Studies have shown the demonstrable efficacy of vasopressin therapy as a rescue agent to reverse the catecholamine refractory shock states due to sepsis or following cardiotomy/CPB. However, data is still limited to support its use in prolonged cardiac arrest and irreversible hypovolemic and anaphylactic shock. Before starting widespread use of vasopressin in critically ill patients, many questions have to be answered. First, whether the vasopressin should be used in all patients with septic shock? To answer this question in view of currently available evidences, is very difficult as none of the available clinical study including the VASST has demonstrated the overall mortality benefits in different sets of the patients treated with vasopressin. Secondly, should it be used as a vasopressor therapy, or endocrine support or both? As vasopressin binds to its own V1 vascular receptor, it can still act even if α1-receptors are downregulated in vasodilatory shock to improve BP and reduces catecholamine requirement. However, current evidence does not suggest its use as a first line vasopressor and to be titrated to increase BP; rather, it should be used at low fixed dosages. Thirdly, what should be the ideal time of initiation of vasopressin therapy? Present evidences support its use in early rather than in late stage of vasodilatory shock. Fourthly, what should be ideal dose of vasopressin infusion for the treatment of vasodilatory shock as few studies have shown better patient outcome with higher doses of vasopressin therapy. However, higher doses may further increase the chances of adverse affects of vasopressin.

Role of vasopressin in adult cardiac arrest has been accepted and supported by international guidelines. Still, more research is needed, particularly in humans, to establish full benefits of vasopressin use as an alternative to epinephrine in cardiac arrest victims. Another important area of research is to know the effects of vasopressin use in combination with other vasopressor such as epinephrine or corticosteroids. Few recent studies demonstrated the significantly increase hospital discharge rates when vasopressin was used in combination with epinephrine in cardiac arrest victims. Similarly, combined vasopressin and catecholamine therapy has been shown to improve hemodynamics in vasodilatory and hemorrhagic shock; however, survival benefits are yet to be established.

To conclude, vasopressin is still not a standard of care and it should only be used as a rescue therapy in patients with catecholamine-refractory shock and cardiac arrest under close monitoring. Further large scale controlled trials are necessary to define the efficacy, dosage, ideal initiation time, and safety profile in different disease states as well as different study population such as adults and pediatric population.

CONFLICT OF INTEREST

The author confirms that he has no conflict of interest to declare for this publication.

ACKNOWLEDGEMENTS

Declared none.

REFERENCES

[1] Landry DW, Levin HR, Gallant EM, *et al.* Vasopressin deficiency contributes to the vasodilation of septic shock. Circulation 1997; 95(5): 1122-5. [http://dx.doi.org/10.1161/01.CIR.95.5.1122] [PMID: 9054839]

[2] Landry DW, Levin HR, Gallant EM, *et al.* Vasopressin pressor hypersensitivity in vasodilatory septic shock. Crit Care Med 1997; 25(8): 1279-82. [http://dx.doi.org/10.1097/00003246-199708000-00012] [PMID: 9267938]

[3] Agrawal A, Singh VK, Varma A, Sharma R. Therapeutic applications of vasopressin in pediatric patients. Indian Pediatr 2012; 49(4): 297-305. [http://dx.doi.org/10.1007/s13312-012-0046-0] [PMID: 22565074]

[4] Treschan TA, Peters J. The vasopressin system: physiology and clinical strategies. Anesthesiology 2006; 105(3): 599-612. [http://dx.doi.org/10.1097/00000542-200609000-00026] [PMID: 16931995]

[5] Barrett LK, Singer M, Clapp LH. Vasopressin: mechanisms of action on the vasculature in health and in septic shock. Crit Care Med 2007; 35(1): 33-40. [http://dx.doi.org/10.1097/01.CCM.0000251127.45385.CD] [PMID: 17133186]

[6] Oliver G, Schäfer EA. On the physiological action of extracts of pituitary body and certain other glandular organs: preliminary communication. J Physiol 1895; 18(3): 277-9. [http://dx.doi.org/10.1113/jphysiol.1895.sp000565] [PMID: 16992253]

[7] Dale HH. On some physiological actions of ergot. J Physiol 1906; 34(3): 163-206. [http://dx.doi.org/10.1113/jphysiol.1906.sp001148] [PMID: 16992821]

[8] Farini F. Diabete insipido ed opoterapia. Gazz Osp Clin 1913; 34: 1135-9.

[9] Vongraven D. Die nierenwirkung von hypophysenextrakten meschen. Berl Klin Wochenscgr. 1913; 50: pp. 2083-6.

[10] Turner RA, Pierce JG, du VIGNEAUD V. The purification and the amino acid content of vasopressin preparations. J Biol Chem 1951; 191(1): 21-8. [PMID: 14850440]

[11] Acher R, Chauvet J. La structure de la vasopressine de boeuf. Biochim Biophys Acta 1953; 12(3): 487-8. [http://dx.doi.org/10.1016/0006-3002(53)90173-5] [PMID: 13115463]

[12] du Vigneaud V, Lawler HC, Popenoe EA. Enzymic cleavage of glycinamide from vasopressin and a proposed structure for this pressor antidiuretic hormone of the posterior pituitary. J Am Chem Soc 1953; 75(19): 4880-1. [http://dx.doi.org/10.1021/ja01115a554]

[13] Tuppy H. The amino-acid sequence in oxytocin. Biochim Biophys Acta 1953; 11(3): 449-50.

[http://dx.doi.org/10.1016/0006-3002(53)90071-7] [PMID: 13093758]

[14] Du Vigneaud V, Ressler C, Trippett S. The sequence of amino acids in oxytocin, with a proposal for the structure of oxytocin. J Biol Chem 1953; 205(2): 949-57.
[PMID: 13129273]

[15] du Vigneaud V, Gish DT, Katsoyannis PG. A synthetic preparation possessing biological properties associated with arginine-vasopressin. J Am Chem Soc 1954; 76: 4751-2.
[http://dx.doi.org/10.1021/ja01647a089]

[16] Sachs H, Takabatake Y. Evidence for a precursor in vasopressin biosynthesis. Endocrinology 1964; 75: 943-8.
[http://dx.doi.org/10.1210/endo-75-6-943] [PMID: 14236105]

[17] Takabatake Y, Sachs H. Vasopressin biosynthesis. 3. *in vitro* studies. Endocrinology 1964; 75: 934-42.
[http://dx.doi.org/10.1210/endo-75-6-934] [PMID: 14236104]

[18] Sachs H, Fawcett P, Takabatake Y, Portanova R. Biosynthesis and release of vasopressin and neurophysin. Recent Prog Horm Res 1969; 25: 447-91.
[PMID: 4902949]

[19] Gainer H, Sarne Y, Brownstein MJ. Biosynthesis and axonal transport of rat neurohypophysial proteins and peptides. J Cell Biol 1977; 73(2): 366-81.
[http://dx.doi.org/10.1083/jcb.73.2.366] [PMID: 858741]

[20] Gainer H, Sarne Y, Brownstein MJ. Neurophysin biosynthesis: conversion of a putative precursor during axonal transport. Science 1977; 195(4284): 1354-6.
[http://dx.doi.org/10.1126/science.65791] [PMID: 65791]

[21] Brownstein MJ, Russell JT, Gainer H. Synthesis, transport, and release of posterior pituitary hormones. Science 1980; 207(4429): 373-8.
[http://dx.doi.org/10.1126/science.6153132] [PMID: 6153132]

[22] Land H, Schütz G, Schmale H, Richter D. Nucleotide sequence of cloned cDNA encoding bovine arginine vasopressin-neurophysin II precursor. Nature 1982; 295(5847): 299-303.
[http://dx.doi.org/10.1038/295299a0] [PMID: 6276766]

[23] Land H, Grez M, Ruppert S, *et al.* Deduced amino acid sequence from the bovine oxytocin-neurophysin I precursor cDNA. Nature 1983; 302(5906): 342-4.
[http://dx.doi.org/10.1038/302342a0] [PMID: 6687626]

[24] Ivell R, Richter D. Structure and comparison of the oxytocin and vasopressin genes from rat. Proc Natl Acad Sci USA 1984; 81(7): 2006-10.
[http://dx.doi.org/10.1073/pnas.81.7.2006] [PMID: 6326097]

[25] Morel A, O'Carroll A-M, Brownstein MJ, Lolait SJ. Molecular cloning and expression of a rat V1a arginine vasopressin receptor. Nature 1992; 356(6369): 523-6.
[http://dx.doi.org/10.1038/356523a0] [PMID: 1560825]

[26] Lolait SJ, O'Carroll AM, McBride OW, Konig M, Morel A, Brownstein MJ. Cloning and characterization of a vasopressin V2 receptor and possible link to nephrogenic diabetes insipidus. Nature 1992; 357(6376): 336-9.
[http://dx.doi.org/10.1038/357336a0] [PMID: 1534150]

[27] Sugimoto T, Saito M, Mochizuki S, Watanabe Y, Hashimoto S, Kawashima H. Molecular cloning and functional expression of a cDNA encoding the human V1b vasopressin receptor. J Biol Chem 1994; 269(43): 27088-92.
[PMID: 7929452]

[28] Gainer H. Cell-type specific expression of oxytocin and vasopressin genes: an experimental odyssey. J Neuroendocrinol 2012; 24(4): 528-38.
[http://dx.doi.org/10.1111/j.1365-2826.2011.02236.x] [PMID: 21985498]

[29] Hoyle CH. Neuropeptide families and their receptors: evolutionary perspectives. Brain Res 1999; 848(1-2): 1-25.
[http://dx.doi.org/10.1016/S0006-8993(99)01975-7] [PMID: 10612694]

[30] Acher R, Chauvet J, Chauvet MT. Man and the chimaera. Selective *versus* neutral oxytocin evolution. Adv Exp Med Biol 1995; 395: 615-27.
[PMID: 8714026]

[31] Gruber CW, Koehbach J, Muttenthaler M. Exploring bioactive peptides from natural sources for oxytocin and vasopressin drug discovery. Future Med Chem 2012; 4(14): 1791-8.
[http://dx.doi.org/10.4155/fmc.12.108] [PMID: 23043476]

[32] Barberis C, Mouillac B, Durroux T. Structural bases of vasopressin/oxytocin receptor function. J Endocrinol 1998; 156(2): 223-9.
[http://dx.doi.org/10.1677/joe.0.1560223] [PMID: 9518866]

[33] Arginine Vasopressin. Available at: https://pubchem.ncbi.nlm.nih.gov/compound/644077 [Last accessed on 01/06/2015]

[34] Oxytocin. Available at: https://pubchem.ncbi.nlm.nih.gov/compound/439302#section=Top [Last accessed on 01/06/2015]

[35] Terlipressin. Available at: https://pubchem.ncbi.nlm.nih.gov/compound/Terlipressin#section=Top [Last accessed on 01/06/2015]

[36] Desmopressin. Available at: https://pubchem.ncbi.nlm.nih.gov/compound/46783812#section=Top [Last accessed on 01/06/2015]

[37] Share L, Kimura T, Matsui K, Shade RE, Crofton JT. Metabolism of vasopressin. Fed Proc 1985; 44(1 Pt 1): 59-61.
[PMID: 3967770]

[38] Holmes CL, Patel BM, Russell JA, Walley KR. Physiology of vasopressin relevant to management of septic shock. Chest 2001; 120(3): 989-1002.
[http://dx.doi.org/10.1378/chest.120.3.989] [PMID: 11555538]

[39] Russell JA. Bench-to-bedside review: Vasopressin in the management of septic shock. Crit Care 2011; 15(4): 226.
[http://dx.doi.org/10.1186/cc8224] [PMID: 21892977]

[40] Holmes CL, Landry DW, Granton JT. Science Review: Vasopressin and the cardiovascular system part 2 - clinical physiology. Crit Care 2004; 8(1): 15-23.
[http://dx.doi.org/10.1186/cc2338] [PMID: 14975041]

[41] Bourque CW, Oliet SH, Richard D. Osmoreceptors, osmoreception, and osmoregulation. Front Neuroendocrinol 1994; 15(3): 231-74.
[http://dx.doi.org/10.1006/frne.1994.1010] [PMID: 7859914]

[42] Schrier RW, Berl T, Anderson RJ. Osmotic and nonosmotic control of vasopressin release. Am J Physiol 1979; 236(4): F321-32.
[PMID: 373467]

[43] Robertson GL, Shelton RL, Athar S. The osmoregulation of vasopressin. Kidney Int 1976; 10(1): 25-37.
[http://dx.doi.org/10.1038/ki.1976.76] [PMID: 181630]

[44] Thrasher TN. Baroreceptor regulation of vasopressin and renin secretion: low-pressure versus high-pressure receptors. Front Neuroendocrinol 1994; 15(2): 157-96.
[http://dx.doi.org/10.1006/frne.1994.1007] [PMID: 7813742]

[45] Norsk P, Ellegaard P, Videbaek R, *et al.* Arterial pulse pressure and vasopressin release in humans during lower body negative pressure. Am J Physiol 1993; 264(5 Pt 2): R1024-30.
[PMID: 8498590]

[46] Goldsmith SR, Francis GS, Cowley AW, Cohn JN. Response of vasopressin and norepinephrine to lower body negative pressure in humans. Am J Physiol 1982; 243(6): H970-3.
[PMID: 7149050]

[47] O'Donnell CP, Thompson CJ, Keil LC, Thrasher TN. Renin and vasopressin responses to graded reductions in atrial pressure in conscious dogs. Am J Physiol 1994; 266(3 Pt 2): R714-21.
[PMID: 8160864]

[48] Leng G, Brown CH, Russell JA. Physiological pathways regulating the activity of magnocellular neurosecretory cells. Prog Neurobiol 1999; 57(6): 625-55.
[http://dx.doi.org/10.1016/S0301-0082(98)00072-0] [PMID: 10221785]

[49] Sklar AH, Schrier RW. Central nervous system mediators of vasopressin release. Physiol Rev 1983; 63(4): 1243-80.
[PMID: 6197715]

[50] Day TA, Randle JC, Renaud LP. Opposing α- and β-adrenergic mechanisms mediate dose-dependent actions of noradrenaline on supraoptic vasopressin neurones *in vivo*. Brain Res 1985; 358(1-2): 171-9.
[http://dx.doi.org/10.1016/0006-8993(85)90961-8] [PMID: 3000512]

[51] Reid IA. Role of nitric oxide in the regulation of renin and vasopressin secretion. Front Neuroendocrinol 1994; 15(4): 351-83.
[http://dx.doi.org/10.1006/frne.1994.1014] [PMID: 7534728]

[52] Wood CE, Chen HG. Acidemia stimulates ACTH, vasopressin, and heart rate responses in fetal sheep. Am J Physiol 1989; 257(2 Pt 2): R344-9.
[PMID: 2548408]

[53] Czaczkes JW, Kleeman CR, Koenig M. Physiologic studies of antidiuretic hormone by its direct measurement in human plasma. J Clin Invest 1964; 43: 1625-40.
[http://dx.doi.org/10.1172/JCI105038] [PMID: 14201546]

[54] Morton JJ, Padfield PL, Forsling ML. A radioimmunoassay for plasma arginine-vasopressin in man and dog: application to physiological and pathological states. J Endocrinol 1975; 65(3): 411-24. [http://dx.doi.org/10.1677/joe.0.0650411] [PMID: 168297]

[55] Russell JA, Walley KR, Singer J, *et al.* VASST Investigators. Vasopressin *versus* norepinephrine infusion in patients with septic shock. N Engl J Med 2008; 358(9): 877-87. [http://dx.doi.org/10.1056/NEJMoa067373] [PMID: 18305265]

[56] Jochberger S, Dörler J, Luckner G, *et al.* The vasopressin and copeptin response to infection, severe sepsis, and septic shock. Crit Care Med 2009; 37(2): 476-82. [http://dx.doi.org/10.1097/CCM.0b013e3181957532] [PMID: 19114902]

[57] Sharshar T, Blanchard A, Paillard M, Raphael JC, Gajdos P, Annane D. Circulating vasopressin levels in septic shock. Crit Care Med 2003; 31(6): 1752-8. [http://dx.doi.org/10.1097/01.CCM.0000063046.82359.4A] [PMID: 12794416]

[58] Argenziano M, Chen JM, Cullinane S, *et al.* Arginine vasopressin in the management of vasodilatory hypotension after cardiac transplantation. J Heart Lung Transplant 1999; 18(8): 814-7. [http://dx.doi.org/10.1016/S1053-2498(99)00038-8] [PMID: 10512533]

[59] Wang BC, Flora-Ginter G, Leadley RJ Jr, Goetz KL. Ventricular receptors stimulate vasopressin release during hemorrhage. Am J Physiol 1988; 254(2 Pt 2): R204-11. [PMID: 3278626]

[60] Morales D, Madigan J, Cullinane S, *et al.* Reversal by vasopressin of intractable hypotension in the late phase of hemorrhagic shock. Circulation 1999; 100(3): 226-9. [http://dx.doi.org/10.1161/01.CIR.100.3.226] [PMID: 10411844]

[61] Errington ML, Rocha e Silva M Jr. The secretion and clearance of vasopressin during the development of irreversible haemorrhagic shock. J Physiol 1971; 217(2): 43P-5P. [PMID: 5571938]

[62] Sharshar T, Carlier R, Blanchard A, *et al.* Depletion of neurohypophyseal content of vasopressin in septic shock. Crit Care Med 2002; 30(3): 497-500. [http://dx.doi.org/10.1097/00003246-200203000-00001] [PMID: 11990905]

[63] Zerbe RL, Henry DP, Robertson GL. Vasopressin response to orthostatic hypotension. Etiologic and clinical implications. Am J Med 1983; 74(2): 265-71. [http://dx.doi.org/10.1016/0002-9343(83)90625-3] [PMID: 6824005]

[64] Garrard CS, Kontoyannis DA, Piepoli M. Spectral analysis of heart rate variability in the sepsis syndrome. Clin Auton Res 1993; 3(1): 5-13. [http://dx.doi.org/10.1007/BF01819137] [PMID: 8386574]

[65] Corrêa PB, Pancoto JA, de Oliveira-Pelegrin GR, Cárnio EC, Rocha MJ. Participation of iNOS-derived NO in hypothalamic activation and vasopressin release during polymicrobial sepsis. J Neuroimmunol 2007; 183(1-2): 17-25. [http://dx.doi.org/10.1016/j.jneuroim.2006.10.021] [PMID: 17173980]

[66] Carnio EC, Moreto V, Giusti-Paiva A, Antunes-Rodrigues J. Neuro-immune-endocrine mechanisms during septic shock: role for nitric oxide in vasopressin and oxytocin release. Endocr Metab Immune Disord Drug Targets 2006; 6(2): 137-42.

[http://dx.doi.org/10.2174/187153006777442396] [PMID: 16787287]

[67] Cowley AW Jr, Switzer SJ, Guinn MM. Evidence and quantification of the vasopressin arterial pressure control system in the dog. Circ Res 1980; 46(1): 58-67. [http://dx.doi.org/10.1161/01.RES.46.1.58] [PMID: 7349918]

[68] Moreto V, Stabile AM, Antunes-Rodrigues J, Carnio EC. Role of heme-oxygenase pathway on vasopressin deficiency during endotoxemic shock-like conditions. Shock 2006; 26(5): 472-6. [http://dx.doi.org/10.1097/01.shk.0000230301.86139.6a] [PMID: 17047517]

[69] Bucher M, Hobbhahn J, Taeger K, Kurtz A. Cytokine-mediated downregulation of vasopressin V(1A) receptors during acute endotoxemia in rats. Am J Physiol Regul Integr Comp Physiol 2002; 282(4): R979-84. [http://dx.doi.org/10.1152/ajpregu.00520.2001] [PMID: 11893600]

[70] Wilson MF, Brackett DJ, Tompkins P, Benjamin B, Archer LT, Hinshaw LB. Elevated plasma vasopressin concentrations during endotoxin and E. coli shock. Adv Shock Res 1981; 6: 15-26. [PMID: 6760706]

[71] Leclerc F, Walter-Nicolet E, Leteurtre S, *et al.* Admission plasma vasopressin levels in children with meningococcal septic shock. Intensive Care Med 2003; 29(8): 1339-44. [http://dx.doi.org/10.1007/s00134-003-1868-y] [PMID: 12856123]

[72] Choong K, Kissoon N. Vasopressin in pediatric shock and cardiac arrest. Pediatr Crit Care Med 2008; 9(4): 372-9. [http://dx.doi.org/10.1097/PCC.0b013e318172d7c8] [PMID: 18496412]

[73] Morgenthaler NG, Müller B, Struck J, Bergmann A, Redl H, Christ-Crain M. Copeptin, a stable peptide of the arginine vasopressin precursor, is elevated in hemorrhagic and septic shock. Shock 2007; 28(2): 219-26. [http://dx.doi.org/10.1097/SHK.0b013e318033e5da] [PMID: 17515850]

[74] Bolignano D, Cabassi A, Fiaccadori E, *et al.* Copeptin (CTproAVP), a new tool for understanding the role of vasopressin in pathophysiology. Clin Chem Lab Med 2014; 52(10): 1447-56. [http://dx.doi.org/10.1515/cclm-2014-0379] [PMID: 24940718]

[75] Neves SR, Ram PT, Iyengar R. G protein pathways. Science 2002; 296(5573): 1636-9. [http://dx.doi.org/10.1126/science.1071550] [PMID: 12040175]

[76] Holmes CL, Landry DW, Granton JT. Science review: Vasopressin and the cardiovascular system part 1--receptor physiology. Crit Care 2003; 7(6): 427-34. [http://dx.doi.org/10.1186/cc2337] [PMID: 14624682]

[77] Mouillac B, Bichet D, Bouvier M, *et al.* Vasopressin and oxytocin receptors, introduction. IUPHAR/BPS Guide to PHARMACOLOGY. Available from: http://www.guidetopharmacology.org/GRAC/FamilyIntroductionForward?familyId=66 2015. [Accessed on 07/06/2015]

[78] Berrada K, Plesnicher CL, Luo X, Thibonnier M. Dynamic interaction of human vasopressin/oxytocin receptor subtypes with G protein-coupled receptor kinases and protein kinase C after agonist stimulation. J Biol Chem 2000; 275(35): 27229-37. [PMID: 10858434]

[79] Wheatley M, Simms J, Hawtin SR, *et al.* Extracellular loops and ligand binding to a subfamily of

Family A G-protein-coupled receptors. Biochem Soc Trans 2007; 35(Pt 4): 717-20. [http://dx.doi.org/10.1042/BST0350717] [PMID: 17635132]

[80] Michell RH, Kirk CJ, Billah MM. Hormonal stimulation of phosphatidylinositol breakdown with particular reference to the hepatic effects of vasopressin. Biochem Soc Trans 1979; 7(5): 861-5. [http://dx.doi.org/10.1042/bst0070861] [PMID: 510730]

[81] Jard S, Gaillard RC, Guillon G, *et al.* Vasopressin antagonists allow demonstration of a novel type of vasopressin receptor in the rat adenohypophysis. Mol Pharmacol 1986; 30(2): 171-7. [PMID: 3016500]

[82] Morel A, O'Carroll AM, Brownstein MJ, Lolait SJ. Molecular cloning and expression of a rat V1a arginine vasopressin receptor. Nature 1992; 356(6369): 523-6. [http://dx.doi.org/10.1038/356523a0] [PMID: 1560825]

[83] Thibonnier M, Auzan C, Madhun Z, Wilkins P, Berti-Mattera L, Clauser E. Molecular cloning, sequencing, and functional expression of a cDNA encoding the human V1a vasopressin receptor. J Biol Chem 1994; 269(5): 3304-10. [PMID: 8106369]

[84] Thibonnier M, Graves MK, Wagner MS, Auzan C, Clauser E, Willard HF. Structure, sequence, expression, and chromosomal localization of the human V1a vasopressin receptor gene. Genomics 1996; 31(3): 327-34. [http://dx.doi.org/10.1006/geno.1996.0055] [PMID: 8838314]

[85] Thibonnier M, Graves MK, Wagner MS, *et al.* Study of V(1)-vascular vasopressin receptor gene microsatellite polymorphisms in human essential hypertension. J Mol Cell Cardiol 2000; 32(4): 557-64. [http://dx.doi.org/10.1006/jmcc.2000.1108] [PMID: 10756113]

[86] Kim SJ, Young LJ, Gonen D, *et al.* Transmission disequilibrium testing of arginine vasopressin receptor 1A (AVPR1A) polymorphisms in autism. Mol Psychiatry 2002; 7(5): 503-7. [http://dx.doi.org/10.1038/sj.mp.4001125] [PMID: 12082568]

[87] Beech DJ. Actions of neurotransmitters and other messengers on Ca2+ channels and K+ channels in smooth muscle cells. Pharmacol Ther 1997; 73(2): 91-119. [http://dx.doi.org/10.1016/S0163-7258(97)87271-3] [PMID: 9131720]

[88] Koshimizu TA, Nakamura K, Egashira N, Hiroyama M, Nonoguchi H, Tanoue A. Vasopressin V1a and V1b receptors: from molecules to physiological systems. Physiol Rev 2012; 92(4): 1813-64. [http://dx.doi.org/10.1152/physrev.00035.2011] [PMID: 23073632]

[89] Russ RD, Walker BR. Role of nitric oxide in vasopressinergic pulmonary vasodilatation. Am J Physiol 1992; 262(3 Pt 2): H743-7. [PMID: 1558183]

[90] Evora PR, Pearson PJ, Schaff HV. Arginine vasopressin induces endothelium-dependent vasodilatation of the pulmonary artery. V1-receptor-mediated production of nitric oxide. Chest 1993; 103(4): 1241-5. [http://dx.doi.org/10.1378/chest.103.4.1241] [PMID: 8131474]

[91] Okamura T, Ayajiki K, Fujioka H, Toda N. Mechanisms underlying arginine vasopressin-induced

relaxation in monkey isolated coronary arteries. J Hypertens 1999; 17(5): 673-8.
[http://dx.doi.org/10.1097/00004872-199917050-00011] [PMID: 10403611]

[92] Filep J, Rosenkranz B. Mechanism of vasopressin-induced platelet aggregation. Thromb Res 1987; 45(1): 7-15.
[http://dx.doi.org/10.1016/0049-3848(87)90252-0] [PMID: 3105115]

[93] Lachant NA, Smith MR, Xie ZJ, Romani WR. Heterogeneity of the aggregation response of human platelets to arginine vasopressin. Am J Hematol 1995; 49(1): 56-66.
[http://dx.doi.org/10.1002/ajh.2830490110] [PMID: 7741139]

[94] Koshimizu TA, Nasa Y, Tanoue A, *et al.* V1a vasopressin receptors maintain normal blood pressure by regulating circulating blood volume and baroreflex sensitivity. Proc Natl Acad Sci USA 2006; 103(20): 7807-12.
[http://dx.doi.org/10.1073/pnas.0600875103] [PMID: 16682631]

[95] Peuler JD, Edwards GL, Schmid PG, Johnson AK. Area postrema and differential reflex effects of vasopressin and phenylephrine in rats. Am J Physiol 1990; 258(4 Pt 2): H1255-9.
[PMID: 2331015]

[96] Bankir L. Antidiuretic action of vasopressin: quantitative aspects and interaction between V1a and V2 receptor-mediated effects. Cardiovasc Res 2001; 51(3): 372-90.
[http://dx.doi.org/10.1016/S0008-6363(01)00328-5] [PMID: 11476728]

[97] Edwards RM, Trizna W, Kinter LB. Renal microvascular effects of vasopressin and vasopressin antagonists. Am J Physiol 1989; 256(2 Pt 2): F274-8.
[PMID: 2916660]

[98] Holmes CL, Walley KR, Chittock DR, Lehman T, Russell JA. The effects of vasopressin on hemodynamics and renal function in severe septic shock: a case series. J Intensive Care Med 2001; 27(8): 1416-21.
[http://dx.doi.org/10.1007/s001340101014] [PMID: 11511958]

[99] Patel B, Chittock D, Walley K. Vasopressin infusion in SIRS and septic shock: a randomized controlled trial. Am J Respir Crit Care Med 1999; 159: A608.

[100] Aoyagi T, Birumachi J, Hiroyama M, *et al.* Alteration of glucose homeostasis in V1a vasopressin receptor-deficient mice. Endocrinology 2007; 148(5): 2075-84.
[http://dx.doi.org/10.1210/en.2006-1315] [PMID: 17303660]

[101] Bielsky IF, Hu SB, Ren X, Terwilliger EF, Young LJ. The V1a vasopressin receptor is necessary and sufficient for normal social recognition: a gene replacement study. Neuron 2005; 47(4): 503-13.
[http://dx.doi.org/10.1016/j.neuron.2005.06.031] [PMID: 16102534]

[102] Birumachi J, Hiroyama M, Fujiwara Y, Aoyagi T, Sanbe A, Tanoue A. Impaired arginine-vasopressi--induced aldosterone release from adrenal gland cells in mice lacking the vasopressin V1A receptor. Eur J Pharmacol 2007; 566(1-3): 226-30.
[http://dx.doi.org/10.1016/j.ejphar.2007.03.022] [PMID: 17449028]

[103] Koshimizu TA, Nasa Y, Tanoue A, *et al.* V1a vasopressin receptors maintain normal blood pressure by regulating circulating blood volume and baroreflex sensitivity. Proc Natl Acad Sci USA 2006; 103(20): 7807-12.

[http://dx.doi.org/10.1073/pnas.0600875103] [PMID: 16682631]

[104] Sugimoto T, Saito M, Mochizuki S, Watanabe Y, Hashimoto S, Kawashima H. Molecular cloning and functional expression of a cDNA encoding the human V1b vasopressin receptor. J Biol Chem 1994; 269(43): 27088-92.
[PMID: 7929452]

[105] Saito M, Sugimoto T, Tahara A, Kawashima H. Molecular cloning and characterization of rat V1b vasopressin receptor: evidence for its expression in extra-pituitary tissues. Biochem Biophys Res Commun 1995; 212(3): 751-7.
[http://dx.doi.org/10.1006/bbrc.1995.2033] [PMID: 7626108]

[106] Rousseau-Merck MF, René P, Derré J, Bienvenu T, Berger R, de Keyzer Y. Chromosomal localization of the human V3 pituitary vasopressin receptor gene (AVPR3) to 1q32. Genomics 1995; 30(2): 405-6.
[PMID: 8586456]

[107] Thibonnier M, Preston JA, Dulin N, Wilkins PL, Berti-Mattera LN, Mattera R. The human V3 pituitary vasopressin receptor: ligand binding profile and density-dependent signaling pathways. Endocrinology 1997; 138(10): 4109-22.
[PMID: 9322919]

[108] Thibonnier M, Berti-Mattera LN, Dulin N, Conarty DM, Mattera R. Signal transduction pathways of the human V1-vascular, V2-renal, V3-pituitary vasopressin and oxytocin receptors. Prog Brain Res 1998; 119: 147-61.
[http://dx.doi.org/10.1016/S0079-6123(08)61568-X] [PMID: 10074787]

[109] Orcel H, Albizu L, Perkovska S, *et al.* Differential coupling of the vasopressin V1b receptor through compartmentalization within the plasma membrane. Mol Pharmacol 2009; 75(3): 637-47.
[http://dx.doi.org/10.1124/mol.108.049031] [PMID: 19047484]

[110] Lolait SJ, Stewart LQ, Jessop DS, Young WS III, O'Carroll AM. The hypothalamic-pituitary-adrenal axis response to stress in mice lacking functional vasopressin V1b receptors. Endocrinology 2007; 148(2): 849-56.
[http://dx.doi.org/10.1210/en.2006-1309] [PMID: 17122081]

[111] de Keyzer Y, Lenne F, Auzan C, *et al.* The pituitary V3 vasopressin receptor and the corticotroph phenotype in ectopic ACTH syndrome. J Clin Invest 1996; 97(5): 1311-8.
[http://dx.doi.org/10.1172/JCI118547] [PMID: 8636444]

[112] Birnbaumer M, Seibold A, Gilbert S, *et al.* Molecular cloning of the receptor for human antidiuretic hormone. Nature 1992; 357(6376): 333-5.
[http://dx.doi.org/10.1038/357333a0] [PMID: 1534149]

[113] Lolait SJ, O'Carroll AM, McBride OW, Konig M, Morel A, Brownstein MJ. Cloning and characterization of a vasopressin V2 receptor and possible link to nephrogenic diabetes insipidus. Nature 1992; 357(6376): 336-9.
[http://dx.doi.org/10.1038/357336a0] [PMID: 1534150]

[114] Seibold A, Brabet P, Rosenthal W, Birnbaumer M. Structure and chromosomal localization of the human antidiuretic hormone receptor gene. Am J Hum Genet 1992; 51(5): 1078-83.
[PMID: 1415251]

[115] Kambouris M, Dlouhy SR, Trofatter JA, Conneally PM, Hodes ME. Localization of the gene for X-linked nephrogenic diabetes insipidus to Xq28. Am J Med Genet 1988; 29(1): 239-46. [http://dx.doi.org/10.1002/ajmg.1320290138] [PMID: 2894172]

[116] Innamorati G, Sadeghi H, Birnbaumer M. A fully active nonglycosylated V2 vasopressin receptor. Mol Pharmacol 1996; 50(3): 467-73. [PMID: 8794883]

[117] Orloff J, Handler J. The role of adenosine 3′,5′-phosphate in the action of antidiuretic hormone. Am J Med 1967; 42(5): 757-68. [http://dx.doi.org/10.1016/0002-9343(67)90093-9] [PMID: 5337377]

[118] Knepper MA, Inoue T. Regulation of aquaporin-2 water channel trafficking by vasopressin. Curr Opin Cell Biol 1997; 9(4): 560-4. [http://dx.doi.org/10.1016/S0955-0674(97)80034-8] [PMID: 9261056]

[119] Rosenthal W, Antaramian A, Gilbert S, Birnbaumer M. Nephrogenic diabetes insipidus. A V2 vasopressin receptor unable to stimulate adenylyl cyclase. J Biol Chem 1993; 268(18): 13030-3. [PMID: 8514744]

[120] Hirasawa A, Nakayama Y, Ishiharada N, *et al.* Evidence for the existence of vasopressin V2 receptor mRNA in rat hippocampus. Biochem Biophys Res Commun 1994; 205(3): 1702-6. [http://dx.doi.org/10.1006/bbrc.1994.2864] [PMID: 7811254]

[121] Juul KV, Bichet DG, Nielsen S, Nørgaard JP. The physiological and pathophysiological functions of renal and extrarenal vasopressin V2 receptors. Am J Physiol Renal Physiol 2014; 306(9): F931-40. [http://dx.doi.org/10.1152/ajprenal.00604.2013] [PMID: 24598801]

[122] Nonoguchi H, Owada A, Kobayashi N, *et al.* Immunohistochemical localization of V2 vasopressin receptor along the nephron and functional role of luminal V2 receptor in terminal inner medullary collecting ducts. J Clin Invest 1995; 96(4): 1768-78. [http://dx.doi.org/10.1172/JCI118222] [PMID: 7560068]

[123] Kumagami H, Loewenheim H, Beitz E, *et al.* The effect of anti-diuretic hormone on the endolymphatic sac of the inner ear. Pflugers Arch 1998; 436(6): 970-5. [http://dx.doi.org/10.1007/s004240050731] [PMID: 9799415]

[124] Aki Y, Tamaki T, Kiyomoto H, *et al.* Nitric oxide may participate in V2 vasopressin-recepto--mediated renal vasodilation. J Cardiovasc Pharmacol 1994; 23(2): 331-6. [http://dx.doi.org/10.1097/00005344-199402000-00023] [PMID: 7511766]

[125] Kaufmann JE, Iezzi M, Vischer UM. Desmopressin (DDAVP) induces NO production in human endothelial cells via V2 receptor- and cAMP-mediated signaling. J Thromb Haemost 2003; 1(4): 821-8. [http://dx.doi.org/10.1046/j.1538-7836.2003.00197.x] [PMID: 12871421]

[126] Kaufmann JE, Oksche A, Wollheim CB, Günther G, Rosenthal W, Vischer UM. Vasopressin-induced von Willebrand factor secretion from endothelial cells involves V2 receptors and cAMP. J Clin Invest 2000; 106(1): 107-16. [http://dx.doi.org/10.1172/JCI9516] [PMID: 10880054]

[127] Kimura T, Tanizawa O, Mori K, Brownstein MJ, Okayama H. Structure and expression of a human

oxytocin receptor. Nature 1992; 356(6369): 526-9.
[http://dx.doi.org/10.1038/356526a0] [PMID: 1313946]

[128] Rozen F, Russo C, Banville D, Zingg HH. Structure, characterization, and expression of the rat oxytocin receptor gene. Proc Natl Acad Sci USA 1995; 92(1): 200-4.
[http://dx.doi.org/10.1073/pnas.92.1.200] [PMID: 7816817]

[129] Gimpl G, Fahrenholz F. The oxytocin receptor system: structure, function, and regulation. Physiol Rev 2001; 81(2): 629-83.
[PMID: 11274341]

[130] Sanborn BM, Dodge K, Monga M, Qian A, Wang W, Yue C. Molecular mechanisms regulating the effects of oxytocin on myometrial intracellular calcium. Adv Exp Med Biol 1998; 449: 277-86.
[http://dx.doi.org/10.1007/978-1-4615-4871-3_35] [PMID: 10026815]

[131] Thibonnier M, Conarty DM, Preston JA, Plesnicher CL, Dweik RA, Erzurum SC. Human vascular endothelial cells express oxytocin receptors. Endocrinology 1999; 140(3): 1301-9.
[PMID: 10067857]

[132] Gutkowska J, Jankowski M, Lambert C, Mukaddam-Daher S, Zingg HH, McCann SM. Oxytocin releases atrial natriuretic peptide by combining with oxytocin receptors in the heart. Proc Natl Acad Sci USA 1997; 94(21): 11704-9.
[http://dx.doi.org/10.1073/pnas.94.21.11704] [PMID: 9326674]

[133] Jacob S, Brune CW, Carter CS, Leventhal BL, Lord C, Cook EH Jr. Association of the oxytocin receptor gene (OXTR) in Caucasian children and adolescents with autism. Neurosci Lett 2007; 417(1): 6-9.
[http://dx.doi.org/10.1016/j.neulet.2007.02.001] [PMID: 17383819]

[134] Takayanagi Y, Yoshida M, Bielsky IF, *et al.* Pervasive social deficits, but normal parturition, in oxytocin receptor-deficient mice. Proc Natl Acad Sci USA 2005; 102(44): 16096-101.
[http://dx.doi.org/10.1073/pnas.0505312102] [PMID: 16249339]

[135] Boarder MR, Weisman GA, Turner JT, Wilkinson GF. G protein-coupled P2 purinoceptors: from molecular biology to functional responses. Trends Pharmacol Sci 1995; 16(4): 133-9.
[http://dx.doi.org/10.1016/S0165-6147(00)89001-X] [PMID: 7610499]

[136] Zenteno-Savin T, Sada-Ovalle I, Ceballos G, Rubio R. Effects of arginine vasopressin in the heart are mediated by specific intravascular endothelial receptors. Eur J Pharmacol 2000; 410(1): 15-23.
[http://dx.doi.org/10.1016/S0014-2999(00)00853-0] [PMID: 11134652]

[137] Mei Q, Liang BT. P2 purinergic receptor activation enhances cardiac contractility in isolated rat and mouse hearts. Am J Physiol Heart Circ Physiol 2001; 281(1): H334-41.
[PMID: 11406501]

[138] Knott TK, Marrero HG, Custer EE, Lemos JR. Endogenous ATP potentiates only vasopressin secretion from neurohypophysial terminals. J Cell Physiol 2008; 217(1): 155-61.
[http://dx.doi.org/10.1002/jcp.21485] [PMID: 18481265]

[139] Song Z, Vijayaraghavan S, Sladek CD. ATP increases intracellular calcium in supraoptic neurons by activation of both P2X and P2Y purinergic receptors. Am J Physiol Regul Integr Comp Physiol 2007; 292(1): R423-31.

[http://dx.doi.org/10.1152/ajpregu.00495.2006] [PMID: 16973929]

[140] Kapoor JR, Sladek CD. Purinergic and adrenergic agonists synergize in stimulating vasopressin and oxytocin release. J Neurosci 2000; 20(23): 8868-75. [PMID: 11102496]

[141] Sladek CD, Song Z. Regulation of vasopressin release by co-released neurotransmitters: mechanisms of purinergic and adrenergic synergism. Prog Brain Res 2008; 170: 93-107. [http://dx.doi.org/10.1016/S0079-6123(08)00409-3] [PMID: 18655875]

[142] Cha SH, Sekine T, Endou H. P2 purinoceptor localization along rat nephron and evidence suggesting existence of subtypes P2Y1 and P2Y2. Am J Physiol 1998; 274(6 Pt 2): F1006-14. [PMID: 9841490]

[143] Wildman SS, Boone M, Peppiatt-Wildman CM, *et al.* Nucleotides downregulate aquaporin 2 *via* activation of apical P2 receptors. J Am Soc Nephrol 2009; 20(7): 1480-90. [http://dx.doi.org/10.1681/ASN.2008070686] [PMID: 19423692]

[144] Rieg T, Bundey RA, Chen Y, *et al.* Mice lacking P2Y2 receptors have salt-resistant hypertension and facilitated renal Na+ and water reabsorption. FASEB J 2007; 21(13): 3717-26. [http://dx.doi.org/10.1096/fj.07-8807com] [PMID: 17575258]

[145] Freedman NJ, Lefkowitz RJ. Desensitization of G protein-coupled receptors. Recent Prog Horm Res 1996; 51: 319-51. [PMID: 8701085]

[146] Chuang TT, Iacovelli L, Sallese M, De Blasi A. G protein-coupled receptors: heterologous regulation of homologous desensitization and its implications. Trends Pharmacol Sci 1996; 17(11): 416-21. [http://dx.doi.org/10.1016/S0165-6147(96)10048-1] [PMID: 8990958]

[147] Perry SJ, Baillie GS, Kohout TA, *et al.* Targeting of cyclic AMP degradation to beta 2-adrenergic receptors by beta-arrestins. Science 2002; 298(5594): 834-6. [http://dx.doi.org/10.1126/science.1074683] [PMID: 12399592]

[148] Oakley RH, Laporte SA, Holt JA, Barak LS, Caron MG. Association of beta-arrestin with G protein-coupled receptors during clathrin-mediated endocytosis dictates the profile of receptor resensitization. J Biol Chem 1999; 274(45): 32248-57. [http://dx.doi.org/10.1074/jbc.274.45.32248] [PMID: 10542263]

[149] Innamorati G, Sadeghi H, Birnbaumer M. Phosphorylation and recycling kinetics of G protein-coupled receptors. J Recept Signal Transduct Res 1999; 19(1-4): 315-26. [http://dx.doi.org/10.3109/10799899909036654] [PMID: 10071767]

[150] Roth BL, Spitzer JA. Altered hepatic vasopressin and alpha 1-adrenergic receptors after chronic endotoxin infusion. Am J Physiol 1987; 252(5 Pt 1): E699-702. [PMID: 3034072]

[151] Bucher M, Hobbhahn J, Taeger K, Kurtz A. Cytokine-mediated downregulation of vasopressin V(1A) receptors during acute endotoxemia in rats. Am J Physiol Regul Integr Comp Physiol 2002; 282(4): R979-84. [http://dx.doi.org/10.1152/ajpregu.00520.2001] [PMID: 11893600]

[152] Schmidt C, Höcherl K, Kurt B, Bucher M. Role of nuclear factor-kappaB-dependent induction of

cytokines in the regulation of vasopressin V1A-receptors during cecal ligation and puncture-induced circulatory failure. Crit Care Med 2008; 36(8): 2363-72.
[http://dx.doi.org/10.1097/CCM.0b013e318180b51d] [PMID: 18596633]

[153] Grinevich V, Knepper MA, Verbalis J, Reyes I, Aguilera G. Acute endotoxemia in rats induces down-regulation of V2 vasopressin receptors and aquaporin-2 content in the kidney medulla. Kidney Int 2004; 65(1): 54-62.
[http://dx.doi.org/10.1111/j.1523-1755.2004.00378.x] [PMID: 14675036]

[154] Qahwash IM, Cassar CA, Radcliff RP, Smith GW. Bacterial lipopolysaccharide-induced coordinate downregulation of arginine vasopressin receptor V3 and corticotropin-releasing factor receptor 1 messenger ribonucleic acids in the anterior pituitary of endotoxemic steers. Endocrine 2002; 18(1): 13-20.
[http://dx.doi.org/10.1385/ENDO:18:1:13] [PMID: 12166619]

[155] Indrambarya T, Boyd JH, Wang Y, McConechy M, Walley KR. Low-dose vasopressin infusion results in increased mortality and cardiac dysfunction following ischemia-reperfusion injury in mice. Crit Care 2009; 13(3): R98.
[http://dx.doi.org/10.1186/cc7930] [PMID: 19549333]

[156] Boone M, Deen PM. Physiology and pathophysiology of the vasopressin-regulated renal water reabsorption. Pflugers Arch 2008; 456(6): 1005-24.
[http://dx.doi.org/10.1007/s00424-008-0498-1] [PMID: 18431594]

[157] Patel BM, Chittock DR, Russell JA, Walley KR. Beneficial effects of short-term vasopressin infusion during severe septic shock. Anesthesiology 2002; 96(3): 576-82.
[http://dx.doi.org/10.1097/00000542-200203000-00011] [PMID: 11873030]

[158] Tsuneyoshi I, Yamada H, Kakihana Y, Nakamura M, Nakano Y, Boyle WA III. Hemodynamic and metabolic effects of low-dose vasopressin infusions in vasodilatory septic shock. Crit Care Med 2001; 29(3): 487-93.
[http://dx.doi.org/10.1097/00003246-200103000-00004] [PMID: 11373409]

[159] Eisenman A, Armali Z, Enat R, Bankir L, Baruch Y. Low-dose vasopressin restores diuresis both in patients with hepatorenal syndrome and in anuric patients with end-stage heart failure. J Intern Med 1999; 246(2): 183-90.
[http://dx.doi.org/10.1046/j.1365-2796.1999.00556.x] [PMID: 10447787]

[160] Aiyar N, Nambi P, Crooke ST. Desensitization of vasopressin sensitive adenylate cyclase by vasopressin and phorbol esters. Cell Signal 1990; 2(2): 153-60.
[http://dx.doi.org/10.1016/0898-6568(90)90018-6] [PMID: 2169286]

[161] Morelli A, Rocco M, Conti G, *et al.* Effects of terlipressin on systemic and regional haemodynamics in catecholamine-treated hyperkinetic septic shock. Intensive Care Med 2004; 30(4): 597-604.
[http://dx.doi.org/10.1007/s00134-003-2094-3] [PMID: 14673520]

[162] McVicar AJ. Dose-response effects of pressor doses of arginine vasopressin on renal haemodynamics in the rat. J Physiol 1988; 404: 535-46.
[http://dx.doi.org/10.1113/jphysiol.1988.sp017304] [PMID: 3253442]

[163] Harrison-Bernard LM, Carmines PK. Juxtamedullary microvascular responses to arginine vasopressin in rat kidney. Am J Physiol 1994; 267(2 Pt 2): F249-56.

[PMID: 8067385]

[164] Dünser MW, Mayr AJ, Ulmer H, *et al.* The effects of vasopressin on systemic hemodynamics in catecholamine-resistant septic and postcardiotomy shock: a retrospective analysis. Anesth Analg 2001; 93(1): 7-13.
[http://dx.doi.org/10.1097/00000539-200107000-00003] [PMID: 11429329]

[165] Dünser MW, Mayr AJ, Ulmer H, *et al.* Arginine vasopressin in advanced vasodilatory shock: a prospective, randomized, controlled study. Circulation 2003; 107(18): 2313-9.
[http://dx.doi.org/10.1161/01.CIR.0000066692.71008.BB] [PMID: 12732600]

[166] Johnston CI. Vasopressin in circulatory control and hypertension. J Hypertens 1985; 3(6): 557-69.
[http://dx.doi.org/10.1097/00004872-198512000-00001] [PMID: 2935570]

[167] Schwartz J, Reid IA. Role of vasopressin in blood pressure regulation in conscious water-deprived dogs. Am J Physiol 1983; 244(1): R74-7.
[PMID: 6336915]

[168] Abboud FM, Floras JS, Aylward PE, Guo GB, Gupta BN, Schmid PG. Role of vasopressin in cardiovascular and blood pressure regulation. Blood Vessels 1990; 27(2-5): 106-15.
[PMID: 2242439]

[169] Landry DW, Oliver JA. The pathogenesis of vasodilatory shock. N Engl J Med 2001; 345(8): 588-95.
[http://dx.doi.org/10.1056/NEJMra002709] [PMID: 11529214]

[170] Kusano E, Tian S, Umino T, Tetsuka T, Ando Y, Asano Y. Arginine vasopressin inhibits interleukin-1 beta-stimulated nitric oxide and cyclic guanosine monophosphate production via the V1 receptor in cultured rat vascular smooth muscle cells. J Hypertens 1997; 15(6): 627-32.
[http://dx.doi.org/10.1097/00004872-199715060-00009] [PMID: 9218182]

[171] Wakatsuki T, Nakaya Y, Inoue I. Vasopressin modulates K(+)-channel activities of cultured smooth muscle cells from porcine coronary artery. Am J Physiol 1992; 263(2 Pt 2): H491-6.
[PMID: 1387293]

[172] Standen NB, Quayle JM. K+ channel modulation in arterial smooth muscle. Acta Physiol Scand 1998; 164(4): 549-57.
[http://dx.doi.org/10.1046/j.1365-201X.1998.00433.x] [PMID: 9887977]

[173] Surks HK, Mochizuki N, Kasai Y, *et al.* Regulation of myosin phosphatase by a specific interaction with cGMP- dependent protein kinase Ialpha. Science 1999; 286(5444): 1583-7.
[http://dx.doi.org/10.1126/science.286.5444.1583] [PMID: 10567269]

[174] Jackson WF. Ion channels and vascular tone. Hypertension 2000; 35(1 Pt 2): 173-8.
[http://dx.doi.org/10.1161/01.HYP.35.1.173] [PMID: 10642294]

[175] Reid IA. Role of vasopressin deficiency in the vasodilation of septic shock. Circulation 1997; 95(5): 1108-10.
[http://dx.doi.org/10.1161/01.CIR.95.5.1108] [PMID: 9054835]

[176] Noguera I, Medina P, Segarra G, *et al.* Potentiation by vasopressin of adrenergic vasoconstriction in the rat isolated mesenteric artery. Br J Pharmacol 1997; 122(3): 431-8.
[http://dx.doi.org/10.1038/sj.bjp.0701397] [PMID: 9351498]

[177] Caramelo C, Okada K, Tsai P, Linas SL, Schrier RW. Interaction of arginine vasopressin and angiotensin II on Ca2+ in vascular smooth muscle cells. Kidney Int 1990; 38(1): 47-54.
[http://dx.doi.org/10.1038/ki.1990.165] [PMID: 2385086]

[178] Iversen BM, Arendshorst WJ. ANG II and vasopressin stimulate calcium entry in dispersed smooth muscle cells of preglomerular arterioles. Am J Physiol 1998; 274(3 Pt 2): F498-508.
[PMID: 9530266]

[179] Altura BM. Dose-response relationships for arginine vasopressin and synthetic analogs on three types of rat blood vessels: possible evidence for regional differences in vasopressin receptor sites within a mammal. J Pharmacol Exp Ther 1975; 193(2): 413-23.
[PMID: 167149]

[180] Suzuki Y, Satoh S, Oyama H, Takayasu M, Shibuya M. Regional differences in the vasodilator response to vasopressin in canine cerebral arteries *in vivo*. Stroke 1993; 24(7): 1049-53.
[http://dx.doi.org/10.1161/01.STR.24.7.1049] [PMID: 7686696]

[181] García-Villalón AL, Garcia JL, Fernández N, Monge L, Gómez B, Diéguez G. Regional differences in the arterial response to vasopressin: role of endothelial nitric oxide. Br J Pharmacol 1996; 118(7): 1848-54.
[http://dx.doi.org/10.1111/j.1476-5381.1996.tb15613.x] [PMID: 8842453]

[182] Liard JF. Does vasopressin-induced vasoconstriction persist during prolonged infusion in dogs? Am J Physiol 1987; 252(4 Pt 2): R668-73.
[PMID: 3565599]

[183] Martikainen TJ, Tenhunen JJ, Uusaro A, Ruokonen E. Vasopressin causes selective intestinal hypoperfusion and lactate release in lethal endotoxin shock. Intensive Care Med 2002; 28: S65.

[184] Rudichenko VM, Beierwaltes WH. Arginine vasopressin-induced renal vasodilation mediated by nitric oxide. J Vasc Res 1995; 32(2): 100-5.
[http://dx.doi.org/10.1159/000159082] [PMID: 7734655]

[185] Tamaki T, Kiyomoto K, He H, *et al.* Vasodilation induced by vasopressin V2 receptor stimulation in afferent arterioles. Kidney Int 1996; 49(3): 722-9.
[http://dx.doi.org/10.1038/ki.1996.101] [PMID: 8648913]

[186] Walker BR, Haynes J Jr, Wang HL, Voelkel NF. Vasopressin-induced pulmonary vasodilation in rats. Am J Physiol 1989; 257(2 Pt 2): H415-22.
[PMID: 2764128]

[187] Jin HK, Chen YF, Yang RH, McKenna TM, Jackson RM, Oparil S. Vasopressin lowers pulmonary artery pressure in hypoxic rats by releasing atrial natriuretic peptide. Am J Med Sci 1989; 298(4): 227-36.
[http://dx.doi.org/10.1097/00000441-198910000-00004] [PMID: 2529763]

[188] Eichinger MR, Walker BR. Enhanced pulmonary arterial dilation to arginine vasopressin in chronically hypoxic rats. Am J Physiol 1994; 267(6 Pt 2): H2413-9.
[PMID: 7528996]

[189] Tayama E, Ueda T, Shojima T, *et al.* Arginine vasopressin is an ideal drug after cardiac surgery for the management of low systemic vascular resistant hypotension concomitant with pulmonary

hypertension. Interact Cardiovasc Thorac Surg 2007; 6(6): 715-9.
[http://dx.doi.org/10.1510/icvts.2007.159624] [PMID: 17704123]

[190] Walker BR, Childs ME, Adams EM. Direct cardiac effects of vasopressin: role of V1- and V2-vasopressinergic receptors. Am J Physiol 1988; 255(2 Pt 2): H261-5.
[PMID: 2970231]

[191] Phillips PA, Abrahams JM, Kelly JM, Mooser V, Trinder D, Johnston CI. Localization of vasopressin binding sites in rat tissues using specific V1 and V2 selective ligands. Endocrinology 1990; 126(3): 1478-84.
[http://dx.doi.org/10.1210/endo-126-3-1478] [PMID: 2307115]

[192] Boyle WA III, Segel LD. Direct cardiac effects of vasopressin and their reversal by a vascular antagonist. Am J Physiol 1986; 251(4 Pt 2): H734-41.
[PMID: 3766750]

[193] Fernández N, García JL, García-Villalón AL, Monge L, Gómez B, Diéguez G. Coronary vasoconstriction produced by vasopressin in anesthetized goats. Role of vasopressin V1 and V2 receptors and nitric oxide. Eur J Pharmacol 1998; 342(2-3): 225-33.
[http://dx.doi.org/10.1016/S0014-2999(97)01504-5] [PMID: 9548390]

[194] Dünser MW, Mayr AJ, Stallinger A, *et al.* Cardiac performance during vasopressin infusion in postcardiotomy shock. Intensive Care Med 2002; 28(6): 746-51.
[http://dx.doi.org/10.1007/s00134-002-1265-y] [PMID: 12107681]

[195] Vanhoutte PM, Katusić ZS, Shepherd JT. Vasopressin induces endothelium-dependent relaxations of cerebral and coronary, but not of systemic arteries. J Hypertens Suppl 1984; 2(3): S421-2.
[PMID: 6242563]

[196] Katusic ZS, Shepherd JT, Vanhoutte PM. Vasopressin causes endothelium-dependent relaxations of the canine basilar artery. Circ Res 1984; 55(5): 575-9.
[http://dx.doi.org/10.1161/01.RES.55.5.575] [PMID: 6488482]

[197] Wenzel V, Kern KB, Hilwig RW, *et al.* The left anterior descending coronary artery dilates after arginine vasopressin during normal sinus rhythm, and ventricular fibrillation with cardiopulmonary resuscitation. Circulation 2001; 104: 2974.

[198] Boyle WA III, Segel LD. Attenuation of vasopressin-mediated coronary constriction and myocardial depression in the hypoxic heart. Circ Res 1990; 66(3): 710-21.
[http://dx.doi.org/10.1161/01.RES.66.3.710] [PMID: 2306803]

[199] Wenzel V, Lindner KH, Baubin MA, Voelckel WG. Vasopressin decreases endogenous catecholamine plasma concentrations during cardiopulmonary resuscitation in pigs. Crit Care Med 2000; 28(4): 1096-100.
[http://dx.doi.org/10.1097/00003246-200004000-00031] [PMID: 10809289]

[200] Raedler C, Voelckel WG, Wenzel V, *et al.* Vasopressor response in a porcine model of hypothermic cardiac arrest is improved with active compression-decompression cardiopulmonary resuscitation using the inspiratory impedance threshold valve. Anesth Analg 2002; 95(6): 1496-502.
[http://dx.doi.org/10.1097/00000539-200212000-00007] [PMID: 12456407]

[201] Voelckel WG, Lurie KG, McKnite S, *et al.* Effects of epinephrine and vasopressin in a piglet model of

prolonged ventricular fibrillation and cardiopulmonary resuscitation. Crit Care Med 2002; 30(5): 957-62.
[http://dx.doi.org/10.1097/00003246-200205000-00001] [PMID: 12006787]

[202] Wenzel V, Lindner KH, Krismer AC, Miller EA, Voelckel WG, Lingnau W. Repeated administration of vasopressin but not epinephrine maintains coronary perfusion pressure after early and late administration during prolonged cardiopulmonary resuscitation in pigs. Circulation 1999; 99(10): 1379-84.
[http://dx.doi.org/10.1161/01.CIR.99.10.1379] [PMID: 10077524]

[203] Zenteno-Savin T, Sada-Ovalle I, Ceballos G, Rubio R. Effects of arginine vasopressin in the heart are mediated by specific intravascular endothelial receptors. Eur J Pharmacol 2000; 410(1): 15-23.
[http://dx.doi.org/10.1016/S0014-2999(00)00853-0] [PMID: 11134652]

[204] Cheng CP, Igarashi Y, Klopfenstein HS, Applegate RJ, Shihabi Z, Little WC. Effect of vasopressin on left ventricular performance. Am J Physiol 1993; 264(1 Pt 2): H53-60.
[PMID: 8430861]

[205] Gold J, Cullinane S, Chen J, *et al.* Vasopressin in the treatment of milrinone-induced hypotension in severe heart failure. Am J Cardiol 2000; 85(4): 506-508, A11.
[http://dx.doi.org/10.1016/S0002-9149(99)00783-3] [PMID: 10728962]

[206] Dünser MW, Mayr AJ, Stallinger A, *et al.* Cardiac performance during vasopressin infusion in postcardiotomy shock. Intensive Care Med 2002; 28(6): 746-51.
[http://dx.doi.org/10.1007/s00134-002-1265-y] [PMID: 12107681]

[207] Dünser MW, Hasibeder WR, Wenzel V, *et al.* Endocrinologic response to vasopressin infusion in advanced vasodilatory shock. Crit Care Med 2004; 32(6): 1266-71.
[http://dx.doi.org/10.1097/01.CCM.0000127264.54807.B7] [PMID: 15187504]

[208] Chrousos GP. The hypothalamic-pituitary-adrenal axis and immune-mediated inflammation. N Engl J Med 1995; 332(20): 1351-62.
[http://dx.doi.org/10.1056/NEJM199505183322008] [PMID: 7715646]

[209] Yates FE, Russell SM, Dallman MF, Hodge GA, McCann SM, Dhariwal AP. Potentiation by vasopressin of corticotropin release induced by corticotropin-releasing factor. Endocrinology 1971; 88(1): 3-15.
[http://dx.doi.org/10.1210/endo-88-1-3] [PMID: 4320769]

[210] Antoni FA. Vasopressinergic control of pituitary adrenocorticotropin secretion comes of age. Front Neuroendocrinol 1993; 14(2): 76-122.
[http://dx.doi.org/10.1006/frne.1993.1004] [PMID: 8387436]

[211] Oshikawa S, Tanoue A, Koshimizu TA, Kitagawa Y, Tsujimoto G. Vasopressin stimulates insulin release from islet cells through V1b receptors: a combined pharmacological/knockout approach. Mol Pharmacol 2004; 65(3): 623-9.
[http://dx.doi.org/10.1124/mol.65.3.623] [PMID: 14978240]

[212] Kirk CJ, Rodrigues LM, Hems DA. The influence of vasopressin and related peptides on glycogen phosphorylase activity and phosphatidylinositol metabolism in hepatocytes. Biochem J 1979; 178(2): 493-6.
[http://dx.doi.org/10.1042/bj1780493] [PMID: 444224]

[213] Haslam RJ, Rosson GM. Aggregation of human blood platelets by vasopressin. Am J Physiol 1972; 223(4): 958-67.
[PMID: 4342380]

[214] Cash JD, Gader AM, da Costa J. Proceedings: The release of plasminogen activator and factor VIII to lysine vasopressin, arginine vasopressin, I-desamino-8-d-arginine vasopressin, angiotensin and oxytocin in man. Br J Haematol 1974; 27(2): 363-4.
[PMID: 4367720]

[215] Mannucci PM. Desmopressin (DDAVP) in the treatment of bleeding disorders: the first 20 years. Blood 1997; 90(7): 2515-21.
[PMID: 9326215]

[216] Young LJ, Flanagan-Cato LM. Editorial comment: oxytocin, vasopressin and social behavior. Horm Behav 2012; 61(3): 227-9.
[http://dx.doi.org/10.1016/j.yhbeh.2012.02.019] [PMID: 22443808]

[217] Winslow JT, Hastings N, Carter CS, Harbaugh CR, Insel TR. A role for central vasopressin in pair bonding in monogamous prairie voles. Nature 1993; 365(6446): 545-8.
[http://dx.doi.org/10.1038/365545a0] [PMID: 8413608]

[218] Lim MM, Bielsky IF, Young LJ. Neuropeptides and the social brain: potential rodent models of autism. Int J Dev Neurosci 2005; 23(2-3): 235-43.
[http://dx.doi.org/10.1016/j.ijdevneu.2004.05.006] [PMID: 15749248]

[219] Mavani GP, DeVita MV, Michelis MF. A review of the nonpressor and nonantidiuretic actions of the hormone vasopressin. Front Med (Lausanne) 2015; 2: 19.
[http://dx.doi.org/10.3389/fmed.2015.00019] [PMID: 25853137]

[220] Holt NF, Haspel KL. Vasopressin: a review of therapeutic applications. J Cardiothorac Vasc Anesth 2010; 24(2): 330-47.
[http://dx.doi.org/10.1053/j.jvca.2009.09.006] [PMID: 19945299]

[221] Key DW, Bloom DA, Sanvordenker J. Low-dose DDAVP in nocturnal enuresis. Clin Pediatr (Phila) 1992; 31(5): 299-301.
[http://dx.doi.org/10.1177/000992289203100507] [PMID: 1582097]

[222] Wise-Faberowski L, Soriano SG, Ferrari L, *et al.* Perioperative management of diabetes insipidus in children. J Neurosurg Anesthesiol 2004; 16(3): 220-5.
[http://dx.doi.org/10.1097/00008506-200407000-00006] [PMID: 15211159]

[223] Ozgönenel B, Rajpurkar M, Lusher JM. How do you treat bleeding disorders with desmopressin? Postgrad Med J 2007; 83(977): 159-63.
[http://dx.doi.org/10.1136/pgmj.2006.052118] [PMID: 17344569]

[224] Cochran EB, Phelps SJ, Tolley EA, Stidham GL. Prevalence of, and risk factors for, upper gastrointestinal tract bleeding in critically ill pediatric patients. Crit Care Med 1992; 20(11): 1519-23.
[http://dx.doi.org/10.1097/00003246-199211000-00007] [PMID: 1424693]

[225] Darcy M. Treatment of lower gastrointestinal bleeding: vasopressin infusion *versus* embolization. J Vasc Interv Radiol 2003; 14(5): 535-43.
[http://dx.doi.org/10.1097/01.RVI.0000064862.65229.8A] [PMID: 12761306]

[226] Molleston JP. Variceal bleeding in children. J Pediatr Gastroenterol Nutr 2003; 37(5): 538-45. [http://dx.doi.org/10.1097/00005176-200311000-00006] [PMID: 14581793]

[227] Ioannou GN, Doust J, Rockey DC. Systematic review: terlipressin in acute oesophageal variceal haemorrhage. Aliment Pharmacol Ther 2003; 17(1): 53-64. [http://dx.doi.org/10.1046/j.1365-2036.2003.01356.x] [PMID: 12492732]

[228] Walder AD, Aitkenhead AR. Role of vasopressin in the haemodynamic response to laparoscopic cholecystectomy. Br J Anaesth 1997; 78(3): 264-6. [http://dx.doi.org/10.1093/bja/78.3.264] [PMID: 9135302]

[229] Choong K, Bohn D, Fraser DD, *et al.* Canadian critical care trials group. Vasopressin in pediatric vasodilatory shock: a multicenter randomized controlled trial. Am J Respir Crit Care Med 2009; 180(7): 632-9. [http://dx.doi.org/10.1164/rccm.200902-0221OC] [PMID: 19608718]

[230] Dünser MW, Mayr AJ, Ulmer H, *et al.* Arginine vasopressin in advanced vasodilatory shock: a prospective, randomized, controlled study. Circulation 2003; 107(18): 2313-9. [http://dx.doi.org/10.1161/01.CIR.0000066692.71008.BB] [PMID: 12732600]

[231] Russell JA, Walley KR, Singer J, *et al.* VASST Investigators. Vasopressin *versus* norepinephrine infusion in patients with septic shock. N Engl J Med 2008; 358(9): 877-87. [http://dx.doi.org/10.1056/NEJMoa067373] [PMID: 18305265]

[232] Dellinger RP, Levy MM, Rhodes A, *et al.* Surviving Sepsis Campaign Guidelines Committee including The Pediatric Subgroup. Surviving Sepsis Campaign: international guidelines for management of severe sepsis and septic shock, 2012. Intensive Care Med 2013; 39(2): 165-228. [http://dx.doi.org/10.1007/s00134-012-2769-8] [PMID: 23361625]

[233] Scharte M, Meyer J, Van Aken H, Bone HG. Hemodynamic effects of terlipressin (a synthetic analog of vasopressin) in healthy and endotoxemic sheep. Crit Care Med 2001; 29(9): 1756-60. [http://dx.doi.org/10.1097/00003246-200109000-00017] [PMID: 11546979]

[234] Rivers E, Nguyen B, Havstad S, *et al.* Early Goal-Directed Therapy Collaborative Group. Early goal-directed therapy in the treatment of severe sepsis and septic shock. N Engl J Med 2001; 345(19): 1368-77. [http://dx.doi.org/10.1056/NEJMoa010307] [PMID: 11794169]

[235] Hall LG, Oyen LJ, Taner CB, *et al.* Fixed-dose vasopressin compared with titrated dopamine and norepinephrine as initial vasopressor therapy for septic shock. Pharmacotherapy 2004; 24(8): 1002-12. [http://dx.doi.org/10.1592/phco.24.11.1002.36139] [PMID: 15338849]

[236] Luckner G, Dünser MW, Jochberger S, *et al.* Arginine vasopressin in 316 patients with advanced vasodilatory shock. Crit Care Med 2005; 33(11): 2659-66. [http://dx.doi.org/10.1097/01.CCM.0000186749.34028.40] [PMID: 16276194]

[237] Luckner G, Mayr VD, Jochberger S, *et al.* Comparison of two dose regimens of arginine vasopressin in advanced vasodilatory shock. Crit Care Med 2007; 35(10): 2280-5. [http://dx.doi.org/10.1097/01.CCM.0000281853.50661.23] [PMID: 17944015]

[238] Klinzing S, Simon M, Reinhart K, Bredle DL, Meier-Hellmann A. High-dose vasopressin is not superior to norepinephrine in septic shock. Crit Care Med 2003; 31(11): 2646-50.

[http://dx.doi.org/10.1097/01.CCM.0000094260.05266.F4] [PMID: 14605537]

[239] Morelli A, Ertmer C, Rehberg S, *et al.* Continuous terlipressin *versus* vasopressin infusion in septic shock (TERLIVAP): a randomized, controlled pilot study. Crit Care 2009; 13(4): R130. [http://dx.doi.org/10.1186/cc7990] [PMID: 19664253]

[240] Scarpati G, Piazza O. Vasopressin *vs* terlipressin in treatment of refractory shock. Transl Med UniSa 2013; 5: 22-7. [PMID: 23905079]

[241] Ceneviva G, Paschall JA, Maffei F, Carcillo JA. Hemodynamic support in fluid-refractory pediatric septic shock. Pediatrics 1998; 102(2): e19. [http://dx.doi.org/10.1542/peds.102.2.e19] [PMID: 9685464]

[242] Brierley J, Carcillo JA, Choong K, *et al.* Clinical practice parameters for hemodynamic support of pediatric and neonatal septic shock: 2007 update from the American College of Critical Care Medicine. Crit Care Med 2009; 37(2): 666-88. [http://dx.doi.org/10.1097/CCM.0b013e31819323c6] [PMID: 19325359]

[243] Argenziano M, Chen JM, Choudhri AF, *et al.* Management of vasodilatory shock after cardiac surgery: identification of predisposing factors and use of a novel pressor agent. J Thorac Cardiovasc Surg 1998; 116(6): 973-80. [http://dx.doi.org/10.1016/S0022-5223(98)70049-2] [PMID: 9832689]

[244] Paparella D, Yau TM, Young E. Cardiopulmonary bypass induced inflammation: pathophysiology and treatment. An update. Eur J Cardiothorac Surg 2002; 21(2): 232-44. [http://dx.doi.org/10.1016/S1010-7940(01)01099-5] [PMID: 11825729]

[245] Argenziano M, Choudhri AF, Oz MC, Rose EA, Smith CR, Landry DW. A prospective randomized trial of arginine vasopressin in the treatment of vasodilatory shock after left ventricular assist device placement. Circulation 1997; 96(9 Suppl): II-286-90. [PMID: 9386112]

[246] Morales DL, Gregg D, Helman DN, *et al.* Arginine vasopressin in the treatment of 50 patients with postcardiotomy vasodilatory shock. Ann Thorac Surg 2000; 69(1): 102-6. [http://dx.doi.org/10.1016/S0003-4975(99)01197-2] [PMID: 10654495]

[247] Egi M, Bellomo R, Langenberg C, *et al.* Selecting a vasopressor drug for vasoplegic shock after adult cardiac surgery: a systematic literature review. Ann Thorac Surg 2007; 83(2): 715-23. [http://dx.doi.org/10.1016/j.athoracsur.2006.08.041] [PMID: 17258030]

[248] Stadlbauer KH, Wenzel V, Krismer AC, Voelckel WG, Lindner KH. Vasopressin during uncontrolled hemorrhagic shock: less bleeding below the diaphragm, more perfusion above. Anesth Analg 2005; 101(3): 830-2. [http://dx.doi.org/10.1213/01.ANE.0000175217.55775.1C] [PMID: 16115999]

[249] Voelckel WG, Raedler C, Wenzel V, *et al.* Arginine vasopressin, but not epinephrine, improves survival in uncontrolled hemorrhagic shock after liver trauma in pigs. Crit Care Med 2003; 31(4): 1160-5. [http://dx.doi.org/10.1097/01.CCM.0000060014.75282.69] [PMID: 12682488]

[250] Cossu AP, Mura P, De Giudici LM, *et al.* Vasopressin in hemorrhagic shock: a systematic review and

meta-analysis of randomized animal trials. Biomed Res Int 2014; 2014: 421291. [http://dx.doi.org/10.1155/2014/421291]

[251] Haas T, Voelckel WG, Wiedermann F, Wenzel V, Lindner KH. Successful resuscitation of a traumatic cardiac arrest victim in hemorrhagic shock with vasopressin: a case report and brief review of the literature. J Trauma 2004; 57(1): 177-9. [http://dx.doi.org/10.1097/01.TA.0000044357.25191.1B] [PMID: 15284571]

[252] Erkek N, Senel S, Hizli S, Karacan CD. Terlipressin saved the life of a child with severe nonvariceal upper gastrointestinal bleeding. Am J Emerg Med 2011; 29: 133.e5-6. [http://dx.doi.org/10.1016/j.ajem.2010.02.010]

[253] Lienhart HG, Wenzel V, Braun J, *et al.* Vasopressin for therapy of persistent traumatic hemorrhagic shock: The VITRIS.at study. Anaesthesist 2007; 56(2): 145-148, 150. [http://dx.doi.org/10.1007/s00101-006-1114-4] [PMID: 17265038]

[254] Schummer C, Wirsing M, Schummer W. The pivotal role of vasopressin in refractory anaphylactic shock. Anesth Analg 2008; 107(2): 620-4. [http://dx.doi.org/10.1213/ane.0b013e3181770b42] [PMID: 18633042]

[255] Tsuda A, Tanaka KA, Huraux C, *et al.* The *in vitro* reversal of histamine-induced vasodilation in the human internal mammary artery. Anesth Analg 2001; 93(6): 1453-9. [http://dx.doi.org/10.1097/00000539-200112000-00020] [PMID: 11726422]

[256] Kill C, Wranze E, Wulf H. Successful treatment of severe anaphylactic shock with vasopressin. Two case reports. Int Arch Allergy Immunol 2004; 134(3): 260-1. [http://dx.doi.org/10.1159/000078775] [PMID: 15178897]

[257] Di Chiara L, Stazi GV, Ricci Z, *et al.* Role of vasopressin in the treatment of anaphylactic shock in a child undergoing surgery for congenital heart disease: a case report. J Med Case Reports 2008; 2: 36. [http://dx.doi.org/10.1186/1752-1947-2-36] [PMID: 18252001]

[258] Meng L, Williams EL. Case report: treatment of rocuronium-induced anaphylactic shock with vasopressin. Can J Anaesth 2008; 55(7): 437-40. [http://dx.doi.org/10.1007/BF03016310] [PMID: 18591701]

[259] Woodhouse SP, Cox S, Boyd P, Case C, Weber M. High dose and standard dose adrenaline do not alter survival, compared with placebo, in cardiac arrest. Resuscitation 1995; 30(3): 243-9. [http://dx.doi.org/10.1016/0300-9572(95)00890-X] [PMID: 8867714]

[260] Perondi MB, Reis AG, Paiva EF, Nadkarni VM, Berg RA. A comparison of high-dose and standard-dose epinephrine in children with cardiac arrest. N Engl J Med 2004; 350(17): 1722-30. [http://dx.doi.org/10.1056/NEJMoa032440] [PMID: 15102998]

[261] Lin S, Callaway CW, Shah PS, *et al.* Adrenaline for out-of-hospital cardiac arrest resuscitation: a systematic review and meta-analysis of randomized controlled trials. Resuscitation 2014; 85(6): 732-40. [http://dx.doi.org/10.1016/j.resuscitation.2014.03.008] [PMID: 24642404]

[262] Lindner KH, Haak T, Keller A, Bothner U, Lurie KG. Release of endogenous vasopressors during and after cardiopulmonary resuscitation. Heart 1996; 75(2): 145-50. [http://dx.doi.org/10.1136/hrt.75.2.145] [PMID: 8673752]

[263] Wenzel V, Krismer AC, Arntz HR, Sitter H, Stadlbauer KH, Lindner KH. European Resuscitation Council Vasopressor during Cardiopulmonary Resuscitation Study Group. A comparison of vasopressin and epinephrine for out-of-hospital cardiopulmonary resuscitation. N Engl J Med 2004; 350(2): 105-13.
[http://dx.doi.org/10.1056/NEJMoa025431] [PMID: 14711909]

[264] Stiell IG, Hébert PC, Wells GA, *et al.* Vasopressin *versus* epinephrine for inhospital cardiac arrest: a randomised controlled trial. Lancet 2001; 358(9276): 105-9.
[http://dx.doi.org/10.1016/S0140-6736(01)05328-4] [PMID: 11463411]

[265] Layek A, Maitra S, Pal S, Bhattacharjee S, Baidya DK. Efficacy of vasopressin during cardio-pulmonary resuscitation in adult patients: a meta-analysis. Resuscitation 2014; 85(7): 855-63.
[http://dx.doi.org/10.1016/j.resuscitation.2014.03.303] [PMID: 24704138]

[266] Neumar RW, Otto CW, Link MS, *et al.* Part 8: adult advanced cardiovascular life support: 2010 American Heart Association Guidelines for Cardiopulmonary Resuscitation and Emergency Cardiovascular Care. Circulation 2010; 122(18) (Suppl. 3): S729-67.
[http://dx.doi.org/10.1161/CIRCULATIONAHA.110.970988] [PMID: 20956224]

[267] Deakin CD, Nolan JP, Soar J, *et al.* European Resuscitation Council Guidelines for Resuscitation 2010 Section 4. Adult advanced life support. Resuscitation 2010; 81(10): 1305-52.
[http://dx.doi.org/10.1016/j.resuscitation.2010.08.017] [PMID: 20956049]

[268] Gueugniaud PY, David JS, Chanzy E, *et al.* Vasopressin and epinephrine *vs.* epinephrine alone in cardiopulmonary resuscitation. N Engl J Med 2008; 359(1): 21-30.
[http://dx.doi.org/10.1056/NEJMoa0706873] [PMID: 18596271]

[269] Mentzelopoulos SD, Zakynthinos SG, Tzoufi M, *et al.* Vasopressin, epinephrine, and corticosteroids for in-hospital cardiac arrest. Arch Intern Med 2009; 169(1): 15-24.
[http://dx.doi.org/10.1001/archinternmed.2008.509] [PMID: 19139319]

[270] Mentzelopoulos SD, Malachias S, Chamos C, *et al.* Vasopressin, steroids, and epinephrine and neurologically favorable survival after in-hospital cardiac arrest: a randomized clinical trial. JAMA 2013; 310(3): 270-9.
[http://dx.doi.org/10.1001/jama.2013.7832] [PMID: 23860985]

[271] Mann K, Berg RA, Nadkarni V. Beneficial effects of vasopressin in prolonged pediatric cardiac arrest: a case series. Resuscitation 2002; 52(2): 149-56.
[http://dx.doi.org/10.1016/S0300-9572(01)00470-1] [PMID: 11841882]

[272] Yilidzdaş D, Horoz OO, Erdem S. Beneficial effects of terlipressin in pediatric cardiac arrest. Pediatr Emerg Care 2011; 27(9): 865-8.
[http://dx.doi.org/10.1097/PEC.0b013e31822c286a] [PMID: 21926888]

[273] Gil-Antón J, López-Herce J, Morteruel E, Carrillo A, Rodríguez-Núñez A. Pediatric cardiac arrest refractory to advanced life support: is there a role for terlipressin? Pediatr Crit Care Med 2010; 11(1): 139-41.
[http://dx.doi.org/10.1097/PCC.0b013e3181ae7834] [PMID: 19581820]

[274] Carroll TG, Dimas VV, Raymond TT. Vasopressin rescue for in-pediatric intensive care unit cardiopulmonary arrest refractory to initial epinephrine dosing: a prospective feasibility pilot trial.

Pediatr Crit Care Med 2012; 13(3): 265-72.
[http://dx.doi.org/10.1097/PCC.0b013e31822f1569] [PMID: 21926666]

[275] Duncan JM, Meaney P, Simpson P, Berg RA, Nadkarni V, Schexnayder S. National Registry of CPR Investigators. Vasopressin for in-hospital pediatric cardiac arrest: results from the American Heart Association National Registry of Cardiopulmonary Resuscitation. Pediatr Crit Care Med 2009; 10(2): 191-5.
[http://dx.doi.org/10.1097/PCC.0b013e31819a36f2] [PMID: 19188873]

[276] Kleinman ME, Chameides L, Schexnayder SM, *et al.* Part 14: pediatric advanced life support: 2010 American Heart Association Guidelines for Cardiopulmonary Resuscitation and Emergency Cardiovascular Care. Circulation 2010; 122(18) (Suppl. 3): S876-908.
[http://dx.doi.org/10.1161/CIRCULATIONAHA.110.971101] [PMID: 20956230]

[277] Biarent D, Bingham R, Eich C, *et al.* European resuscitation council guidelines for resuscitation 2010 section 6. paediatric life support. Resuscitation 2010; 81(10): 1364-88.
[http://dx.doi.org/10.1016/j.resuscitation.2010.08.012] [PMID: 20956047]

[278] Hopf HB, Arand D, Peters J. Sympathetic blockade by thoracic epidural anaesthesia suppresses renin release in response to hypotension, but activates the vasopressin system. Eur J Anaesthesiol 1992; 9(1): 63-9.
[PMID: 1735399]

[279] Jochberger S, Dünser MW. Arginine vasopressin as a rescue vasopressor to treat epidural anaesthesia-induced arterial hypotension. Best Pract Res Clin Anaesthesiol 2008; 22(2): 383-91.
[http://dx.doi.org/10.1016/j.bpa.2008.04.002] [PMID: 18683483]

[280] Boccara G, Ouattara A, Godet G, *et al.* Terlipressin *versus* norepinephrine to correct refractory arterial hypotension after general anesthesia in patients chronically treated with renin-angiotensin system inhibitors. Anesthesiology 2003; 98(6): 1338-44.
[http://dx.doi.org/10.1097/00000542-200306000-00007] [PMID: 12766641]

[281] Morelli A, Tritapepe L, Rocco M, *et al.* Terlipressin *versus* norepinephrine to counteract anesthesia-induced hypotension in patients treated with renin-angiotensin system inhibitors: effects on systemic and regional hemodynamics. Anesthesiology 2005; 102(1): 12-9.
[http://dx.doi.org/10.1097/00000542-200501000-00006] [PMID: 15618781]

[282] Meersschaert K, Brun L, Gourdin M, *et al.* Terlipressin-ephedrine *versus* ephedrine to treat hypotension at the induction of anesthesia in patients chronically treated with angiotensin converting-enzyme inhibitors: a prospective, randomized, double-blinded, crossover study. Anesth Analg 2002; 94(4): 835-40.
[http://dx.doi.org/10.1097/00000539-200204000-00011] [PMID: 11916781]

[283] De Kock M, Laterre PF, Andruetto P, *et al.* Ornipressin (Por 8): An efficient alternative to counteract hypotension during combined general/epidural anesthesia. Anesth Analg 2000; 90(6): 1301-7.
[http://dx.doi.org/10.1097/00000539-200006000-00008] [PMID: 10825311]

[284] Baldasso E, Garcia PC, Piva JP, Branco RG, Tasker RC. Pilot safety study of low-dose vasopressin in non-septic critically ill children. Intensive Care Med 2009; 35(2): 355-9.
[http://dx.doi.org/10.1007/s00134-008-1392-1] [PMID: 19132338]

[285] Yeh CC, Wu CT, Lu CH, Yang CP, Wong CS. Early use of small-dose vasopressin for unstable

hemodynamics in an acute brain injury patient refractory to catecholamine treatment: a case report. Anesth Analg 2003; 97(2): 577-9.
[http://dx.doi.org/10.1213/01.ANE.0000070231.16378.A6] [PMID: 12873956]

[286] Bradley PG, Allen EK, Menon DK. Terlipressin for cerebral perfusion pressure support in a patient with septic shock. Anaesthesia 2004; 59(6): 619-20.
[http://dx.doi.org/10.1111/j.1365-2044.2004.03816.x] [PMID: 15144312]

[287] Chen JM, Cullinane S, Spanier TB, *et al.* Vasopressin deficiency and pressor hypersensitivity in hemodynamically unstable organ donors. Circulation 1999; 100(19 Suppl.): II244-6.
[PMID: 10567311]

[288] Katz K, Lawler J, Wax J, O'Connor R, Nadkarni V. Vasopressin pressor effects in critically ill children during evaluation for brain death and organ recovery. Resuscitation 2000; 47(1): 33-40.
[http://dx.doi.org/10.1016/S0300-9572(00)00196-9] [PMID: 11004379]

[289] Augoustides JG, Abrams M, Berkowitz D, Fraker D. Vasopressin for hemodynamic rescue in catecholamine-resistant vasoplegic shock after resection of massive pheochromocytoma. Anesthesiology 2004; 101(4): 1022-4.
[http://dx.doi.org/10.1097/00000542-200410000-00031] [PMID: 15448539]

[290] Veall GR, Peacock JE, Bax ND, Reilly CS. Review of the anaesthetic management of 21 patients undergoing laparotomy for carcinoid syndrome. Br J Anaesth 1994; 72(3): 335-41.
[http://dx.doi.org/10.1093/bja/72.3.335] [PMID: 8130054]

[291] Papoff P, Caresta E, Versacci P, Grossi R, Midulla F, Moretti C. The role of terlipressin in the management of severe pulmonary hypertension in congenital diaphragmatic hernia. Paediatr Anaesth 2009; 19(8): 805-6.
[http://dx.doi.org/10.1111/j.1460-9592.2009.03078.x] [PMID: 19624374]

[292] Stathopoulos L, Nicaise C, Michel F, *et al.* Terlipressin as rescue therapy for refractory pulmonary hypertension in a neonate with a congenital diaphragmatic hernia. J Pediatr Surg 2011; 46(2): e19-21.
[http://dx.doi.org/10.1016/j.jpedsurg.2010.10.006] [PMID: 21292065]

[293] Filippi L, Gozzini E, Daniotti M, Pagliai F, Catarzi S, Fiorini P. Rescue treatment with terlipressin in different scenarios of refractory hypotension in newborns and infants. Pediatr Crit Care Med 2011; 12(6): e237-41.
[http://dx.doi.org/10.1097/PCC.0b013e3181fe304c] [PMID: 21057354]

[294] Scheurer MA, Bradley SM, Atz AM. Vasopressin to attenuate pulmonary hypertension and improve systemic blood pressure after correction of obstructed total anomalous pulmonary venous return. J Thorac Cardiovasc Surg 2005; 129(2): 464-6.
[http://dx.doi.org/10.1016/j.jtcvs.2004.06.043] [PMID: 15678072]

[295] Kahn JM, Kress JP, Hall JB. Skin necrosis after extravasation of low-dose vasopressin administered for septic shock. Crit Care Med 2002; 30(8): 1899-901.
[http://dx.doi.org/10.1097/00003246-200208000-00038] [PMID: 12163813]

[296] Asfar P, Bracht H, Radermacher P. Impact of vasopressin analogues on the gut mucosal microcirculation. Best Pract Res Clin Anaesthesiol 2008; 22(2): 351-8.
[http://dx.doi.org/10.1016/j.bpa.2008.02.009] [PMID: 18683480]

[297] Dünser MW, Mayr AJ, Tür A, *et al.* Ischemic skin lesions as a complication of continuous vasopressin infusion in catecholamine-resistant vasodilatory shock: incidence and risk factors. Crit Care Med 2003; 31(5): 1394-8.
[http://dx.doi.org/10.1097/01.CCM.0000059722.94182.79] [PMID: 12771608]

CHAPTER 4

Cerebral Small Vessel Disease: A Clinical Review Focusing on Therapeutic Strategies

Francisco José Álvarez-Pérez[*]

Medicine Department, Health Sciences Research Center, Sciences Faculty, Beira Interior University, Stroke Unit, Hospital of Covilha, Covilha, Portugal

Abstract: The term cerebral small vessel disease (CSVD) or microangiopathy includes several pathological processes of different aetiologies which cause an increase of wall thickness (basically the basement membrane), a narrowing of the lumen, and a weakening of walls in arterioles, capillaries and venules. These vascular modifications cause a loss of proteins towards the interstice and a slowness of blood flow, increasing the risk of ischemia and tissue bleeding.

The CSVD may be aetiopathogenically classified in 6 types. The CSVD type 1, called arteriolosclerosis, is the most prevalent form and has a 6 to 10 times higher prevalence than stroke. It is related to aging and classical vascular risk factors, like arterial hypertension and diabetes mellitus. This review will focus on type 1 CSVD.

In the brain, the main pathological findings are loss of smooth muscle cells in the media, accumulation of fibrohyaline material, fibrinoid necrosis, and development of microatheromas and Charcot-Bouchard microaneurysms. The parenchymatous consequences of these vessel modifications are both ischemic (white matter lesions, lacunes) and haemorrhagic (microhaemorrhages, intracerebral haemorrhages). The clinical manifestations of arteriolosclerosis include cognitive deterioration, dementia, mood disorders, gait and motor disturbances, lacunar strokes, and disability. *In vivo*, the diagnosis of CSVD is supported by neuroimaging findings (lacunes, leukoaraiosis, white matter lesions, microhaemorrhages), especially by use of magnetic resonance techniques. The role of other biomarkers (plasma and cerebrospinal fluid biochemical parameters, resistance indexes in transcranial Doppler study) is not completely defined.

[*] **Corresponding author Francisco J. Álvarez-Pérez:** Medicine Department, Health Sciences Research Center, Sciences Faculty, Beira Interior University, Stroke Unit, Hospital of Covilha, Covilha, Portugal; Tel: +351275329002; Fax: +351275329099; E-mails: fjalvarez@fcsaude.ubi.pt, franciscoplus@hotmail.com

Atta-ur-Rahman and M. Iqbal Choudhary (Eds.)

In patients with diagnosis of microangiopathy there are three main therapeutic considerations. First, there are specific risks in these patients during standard clinical management of acute ischemic stroke. Several studies showed an increased risk of intracranial bleeding related to thrombolytic therapy for acute stroke and anticoagulant treatment for secondary prevention. Indeed, the presence of leukoaraiosis raised the probability of peri-operative stroke or death in patients who underwent carotid endarterectomy. Second, the symptomatic management of patients with cognitive impairment related to CSVD, which is currently based on memantine and acetylcholinesterase inhibitors used in Alzheimer's disease. Third, the specific therapy directed to vessel pathology and parenchymatous consequences (secondary prevention). Available data support the use of antiaggregant drugs to reduce the risk of recurrence of lacunar strokes. Aspirin, ticlopidine, aspirin plus clopidogrel, dipiridamol plus aspirin, and cilostazol showed efficacy in this subtype of stroke. The optimal control of arterial pressure and cholesterol level also reduces the risk of stroke, independently if mechanism of disease was macro or microvascular. However, the specific drugs and the optimal goals are not defined and ongoing trials are trying to evaluate different drugs and preventive strategies (cilostazol plus aspirin, aggressive versus standard blood pressure control). Considering the specific treatment of vascular pathology, there are few available data. Experimental studies showed that relaxin may increase the arterial distensibility. In humans, one ongoing trial is investigating the efficacy and safety of an anti-amyloid beta monoclonal antibody in patients with probable cerebral amyloid angiopathy (CSVD type 2).

Keywords: Acetylcholinesterase Inhibitors, Antiaggregants, Cerebral Amyloid Angiopathy, Cerebral Microangiopathy, Cerebral Microhaemorrhages, Cerebral Small Vessel Disease, Deep Brain Infarcts, Deep Intracerebral Haemorrhages, Enlarged Perivascular Spaces, Lacunar Stroke, Memantine, Vascular Dementia, White Matter Lesions.

CONCEPT OF CEREBRAL SMALL VESSEL DISEASE

The small vessel diseases are mainly systemic disorders that may affect different organs and areas of the body. In some conditions, the brain can be the main or only target of the disease, but in other disorders the nervous system might not be affected at all. The term cerebral small vessel disease (CSVD) includes the pathological processes affecting small arteries, arterioles, capillaries, and small veins of the brain. These processes increase the wall thickness, reduce the vascular lumen, and cause structural weakness. The parenchymatous results are both ischemia and haemorrhage [1]. Therefore, the presence of CSVD is associated with a higher risk of developing ischemic and haemorrhagic stroke, cognitive decline, gait disturbances and dementia. Because the small vessels cannot be visualized *in vivo* and only indirect manifestations may be assessed, the most accepted biomarker of CSVD is the presence of white matter lesions, lacunar infarcts, subcortical atrophy, and haemorrhagic lesions on magnetic resonance imaging (MRI) [2].

The extremely high prevalence of CSVD implies that all disorders associated with this pathology represent an important issue for health systems. Cerebral small vessel disease is the basis for nearly 30% of all ischaemic strokes, it is the first cause of vascular dementia, and it probably is the second cause of dementia syndrome and age-related cognitive decline [3].

Currently, the therapeutic approaches to CSVD are a preventive strategy, based on control of some modifiable risk factors, and a symptomatic control of some clinical manifestations. More specific or "curative" treatments are not available.

ANATOMY OF CEREBRAL SMALL VESSELS

The small vessels are penetrating vessels which vascularise the cerebral and cerebellar cortices, deep white matter, basal nuclei, and brain stem. These vessels originate from the circle of Willis, the system formed by the middle, anterior, and posterior cerebral arteries, the basilar artery, and the anterior and posterior communicating arteries. Classically, two kind of penetrating arteries originate from the circle of Willis: central, ganglionic or deep, and cortical, circumference or superficial [4].

Central System

The vessels of the central system emerge from the own circle and the first segment of main cerebral arteries to penetrate perpendicularly into the parenchyma. They consist of: (1) lenticulostriate arteries, originated from the middle and anterior cerebral arteries to irrigate diencephalon, striate and anterior arm of the internal capsule; (2) thalamo-perforating branches, originated from the posterior cerebral artery to irrigate the thalamus. The anterior and posterior choroid arteries may be also included in this central system. The penetrating branches have a diameter of 100-400 microns, have no collaterals, and suffer an intense blood pressure due to their radical reduction of luminal diameter. Because these vessels establish low efficacy precapilar anastomosis, they may be considered terminal arteries [5 - 7].

Cortical System

The vessels of the cortical system originate from the pial branches of the anterior, middle and posterior cerebral arteries over the surface of the brain, cerebellum and brain stem. The cortical perforators are of variable length; shorter ones supply the cerebral and cerebellar cortices and longer ones (called medullary arteries) supply the deep white matter. Short penetrators in the brain stem originate as paramedian branches of the basilar artery [8]. The arteries of the cortical system may be classified as conducting and distributing.

Conducting Arteries

Conducting arteries run for long distances along the pial surface and are about 700 microns in diameter. They run along the sulci that demarcate adjacent gyri or run directly across the gyral surface. Distributing arteries are smaller, about 150 to 200 microns in diameter, and branch from the conducting arteries. As described by several researchers, it is probable that focal constrictions where the distributing arteries emerge from larger arteries represent muscular sphincters. Because the small arteries on the pial surface have a high resistance, they are called "resistance vessels". This is a basic mechanism to transform the pulsatile ejection of blood from the heart into a regular flow. By the reduction of blood pressure it is possible to avoid the loss of blood volume through the thin capillary wall [9].

Distributing Arteries

The distributing arteries continue to ramify on the cortical surface, originating smaller precortical arteries or arterioles with a diameter of 50-70 microns. Anastomoses between these arterioles constitute plexuses which allow the establishment of effective communications among the main arteries. A distributing artery supplies a 2-by-3.5 mm area on the cortical surface and each precortical artery supplies a 1-by-1-mm area of cortical surface [10, 11]. From the cortical plexuses and precortical arteries emerge smaller arterioles of about 30-40 microns in diameter that penetrate the cortical surface at right angles and go across a variable distance. The shorter vessels ramify in the cortex and the longer ones reach deep brain matter.

Duvernoy and colleagues classified these intracortical arterioles into six categories [12]. The first five categories vascularise different cortical levels. Characteristically, the diameter of these vessels increases for those that vascularise deeper layers. The density of vascularisation is not uniform across cortical layers and the nourishment is more intense where there are the highest concentrations of neuronal somas. Some of these intracortical vessels have been described as resembling a "fountain" or "candelabra", with dense ramifications ascending into more superficial layers. Vascularisation of the first 3-4 mm of subcortical white matter depends on these "candelabra" vessels of pial origin. The vessels of the sixth category of intracortical arterioles present the largest diameter and penetrate straight through the cortex to vascularise the white matter below. They go centripetally to converge in the outer surface of lateral ventricles, where they give right angle distribution vessels. The vascularisation of white matter is less dense than the one of gray matter.

Because the cortical perforators have very limited collateral connections until they divide into capillaries, they are also considered terminal arteries. The central and cortical perforators do not anastomose deep in the brain but meet in a junctional zone. Finally, after arterioles originate the capillary network, the venous return follows nearly parallel with the arterial supply described.

CLASSIFICATION OF CEREBRAL SMALL VESSEL DISEASES

Following Pantoni [13], CSVD may be classified aetiopathogenically in 6 categories, summarised in Table **1**. The frequency of the 6 types of CSVD is very different, with types 1 (arteriolosclerosis) and 2 (sporadic and hereditary cerebral amyloid angiopathy) being the most prevalent. Type 1 CSVD is a systemic disorder affecting the vascular beds of brain, retina, kidney, heart and lung. Probably, it is one of the most frequent neurological disorders, with a prevalence

6 to 10 times higher than stroke. Therefore, this review will be focused on types 1 and 2 of vascular microangiopathy, more specifically on the type 1 CSVD.

Table 1. Aetiopathogenic classification of cerebral small vessel diseases. (Adapted from reference [13]).

Type 1: Arteriolosclerosis (age and vascular risk factors related small vessel disease) - Fibrinoid necrosis - Lipohyalinosis - Microatheroma - Microaneurysms (saccular, lipohyalinotic, asymmetric fusiform, bleeding globe) - Segmental arterial disorganization
Type 2: Sporadic and hereditary cerebral amyloid angiopathy
Type 3: Inherited or genetic small vessel diseases distinct from cerebral amyloid angiopathy - Cerebral autosomal dominant arteriopathy with subcortical ischaemic strokes and leukoencephalopathy (CADASIL) - Cerebral autosomal recessive arteriopathy with subcortical ischaemic strokes and leukoencephalopathy (CARASIL) - Mitochondrial encephalopathy with lactic acidosis and stroke-like episodes (MELAS) - Hereditary multi-infarct dementia of the Swedish type - Fabry's disease - Hereditary cerebroretinal vasculopathy - Hereditary endotheliopathy with retinopathy, nephropathy and stroke - Small vessel diseases caused by COL4A1 mutations
Type 4: Inflammatory and immunologically mediated small vessel diseases - Systemic necrotizing vasculitis: Churg-Strauss syndrome, classic polyarteritis nodosa - Hypersensitivity vasculitis: Henoch-Schönlein purpura, nervous system vasculitis secondary to infections, nervous system vasculitis associated with connective tissue disorders such as systemic lupus erythematosus, vasculitis associated with neoplasm - Wegener's granulomatosis - Giant cell arteritis: temporal arteritis, Takayasu's arteritis - Other vasculitic syndromes: cryoglobulinaemic vasculitis, cutaneous leukocytoclastic angiitis, primary angiitis of the CNS, Sneddon's syndrome, Sjögren's syndrome, rheumatoid vasculitis, scleroderma, dermatomyositis
Type 5: Venous collagenosis
Type 6: Other small vessel diseases. For example, post-radiation angiopathy and non-amyloid microvessel degeneration in Alzheimer's disease

PATHOLOGY OF TYPES 1 AND 2 CEREBRAL SMALL VESSEL DISEASES

Type 1 Cerebral Small Vessel Disease (Arteriolosclerosis)

Vascular Changes

The main pathological changes appear in the small perforating arteries with diameters from 40 to 900 microns which emerge from the leptomeningeal arteries and enter a variable depth into the parenchyma, previously called deep and superficial penetrators.

The pathological changes start in the arteries of basal ganglia (first putamen and pallidus), followed by small arteries of white matter, leptomeninges, cerebellum and, finally, brain stem. Usually the cortical vessels are spared [8, 14, 15].

Four main changes were described in the wall of small penetrating arteries in type 1 CSVD: (1) atherosclerosis; (2) fibrinoid necrosis (lipohyalinosis); (3) arteriolosclerosis; (4) microaneurysms.

Atherosclerosis (Microatheroma)

This process affects leptomeningeal and intracerebral arteries with a diameter of 200-900 microns. The main findings are plaques formed by accumulations of plasma proteins, lymphocytes, and macrophages (microatheromas) located in the proximal segments of branching and parent vessels. They are associated with endothelial proliferation and breaking of the lamina elastica interna.

Fibrinoid Necrosis and Lipohyalinosis

This disorder affects basically arteries with a diameter of 40-300 microns. Initially, the arterial walls are thickened by eosinophilic fibrinoid material. This material is rich in plasma proteins (mainly fibrin which crosses through a disrupted blood-brain barrier) and fragments of smooth muscle cells. The weakened blood-brain barrier increases the risk of rupture in the affected arteries. In advanced stages, the fibrinoid material is replaced by collagen produced by fibroblasts (phenomenon of acellular fibrosis), foam cells, and plasma proteins, like ApoE, alpha-2-macroglobulin, and G immunoglobulin. These changes give the arterial wall a thickened and disorganized appearance. Probably, this is the stage called "lipohyalinosis" or "segmental arterial disorganization" by Fisher [16 - 18]. Figs. (**1** and **2**) show the typical histological aspect of fibrinoid necrosis and lipohyalinosis, respectively.

Arteriolosclerosis

The pathological changes appear in arterioles of 40-150 microns in diameter. The walls present a hyaline thickening without fibrinoid necrosis which reduces the arterial lumen. This arteriolar thickening is similar to the one observed in cerebral amyloid angiopathy and CADASIL. In arteriolosclerosis, the changes are different from the previously mentioned lipohyalinosis, in which the walls are thickened and fibrotic. Clinically, arteriolosclerosis is associated with vascular dementia rather than lacunar infarcts. Due to the thickening of the arteriolar walls the vascular rupture is rare [8].

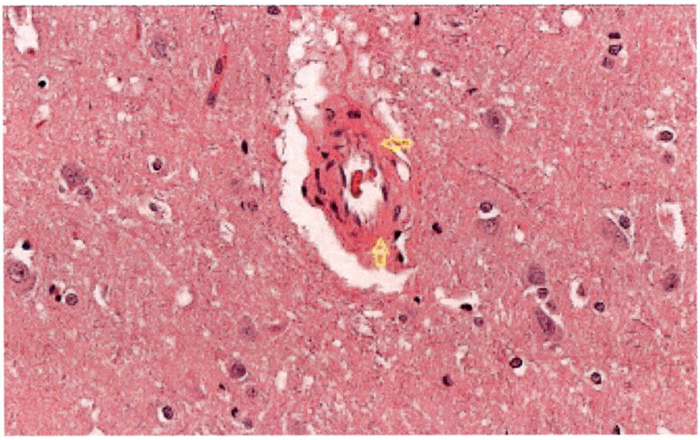

Fig. (1). Haematoxylin and eosin stained sections of small cerebellar arterioles showing fibrinoid necrosis (yellow arrows). Image courtesy of Dr. Javier Muñoz.

Microaneurysms

Charcot–Bouchard or miliary microaneurysms originate as 0.3-2mm protrusions from arteries of 100–300 microns in diameter at sites of wall weakening. The walls of the aneurysms show an accumulation of hyaline connective tissue and a destruction of smooth muscle cells and elastica interna layers. The rupture of microaneurysms causes intraparenchymatous haemorrhages, but if they suffer thrombosis and fibrosis they transform into fibrocollagenous tissue. Although microaneurysms are classically related to hypertension, this association was questioned by some authors [8, 19].

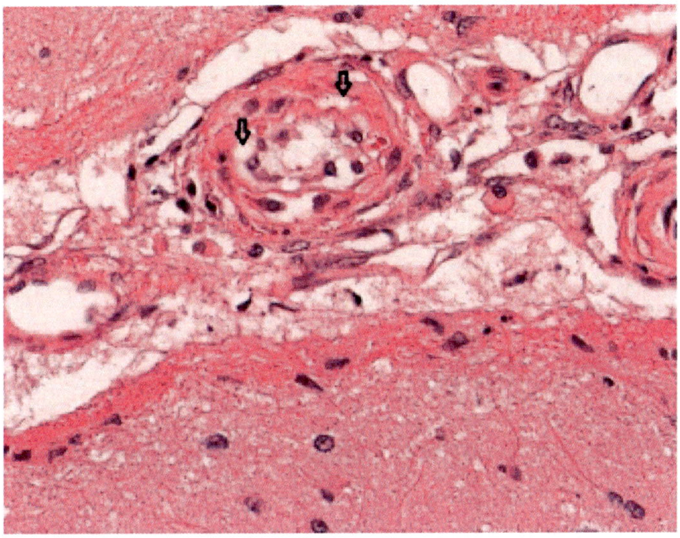

Fig. (2). Haematoxylin and eosin stained sections of small cerebellar arterioles. Black arrows mark lipohyalinotic material. Image courtesy of Dr. Javier Muñoz.

Parenchymatous Changes

The parenchymatous consequences of type 1 CSVD are: (1) deep brain infarcts; (2) white matter lesions; (3) deep intracerebral haemorrhages; (4) cerebral microhaemorrhages; (5) enlarged perivascular spaces.

Deep Brain Infarcts

Deep brain infarcts (DBI), also called lacunar infarcts, appear as irregular 3-20 mm in diameter cavities with surrounding gliosis, lipid-rich and haemosiderin-rich macrophages, and fragmented blood vessels. The presence of haemosiderin-rich macrophages may be related to microhaemorrhages due to endothelial damage. The works of Fisher are still a reference to understand the pathology and mechanism of DBI. In an autopsy examination of 4 patients, Fisher described 50 lacunes and the artery proximal to the infarction. In 45 of these lacunes he found a total occlusion of the perforating artery, habitually caused by "segmental arterial disorganization". Probably, this change represents fibrinoid necrosis and lipohyalinosis, similar to that observed in larger vessels of patients with poorly controlled hypertension [18].

White Matter Lesions

The pathological substrates of white matter lesions (WML) are myelin pallor, enlarged perivascular spaces, tissue infarction, gliosis, and axonal loss. Perivascular infiltration of foam cells, presence of inflammatory mediators (apolipoprotein E, alpha2-macroglobulin, immunoglobulin G), reactive astrocytosis and microglial activation have been reported. Probably, these changes are due to the disruption of blood-brain barrier and the loss of integrity of small vessel endothelium [20].

Deep Intracerebral Haemorrhages

The pathological findings in broken vessels causing deep intracerebral haemorrhages (DIH) are similar to the changes found in occluded vessels causing lacunar infarcts: fibrinoid necrosis, lipohyalinosis and degeneration of media layer. It is not clear why this common pathology may be associated with both DIH and small deep infarcts. The association between DIH and rupture of Charcot–Bouchard microaneurysms is still controversial [8, 16, 17].

Cerebral Microbleeds

Cerebral microbleeds (CMB) or microhaemorrhages include acute microhaemorrhages, haemosiderin residua of old bleedings, and lacunes encircled by haemosiderin. Other lesions which are frequently associated with CMB are wall amyloid pathology and WML [21].

Enlarged Perivascular Spaces

Enlarged perivascular or Virchow–Robin spaces (EPVS) are common findings on brain magnetic resonance imaging in older people. They are cavities filled by cerebrospinal fluid which surround small penetrating cerebral arterioles. Usually EPVS are 2 mm in diameter, although they may be larger. Their prevalence increases with aging and they are associated with greater volumes of WML and

DBI. Because this association with DBI is stronger than with cortical infarcts, it has been suggested that they are a form of CSVD. The possible mechanisms for development of EPVS are impairment of the blood-brain barrier permeability and amyloid deposition on the vessel wall [22].

Type 2 Cerebral Small Vessel Disease (Sporadic and Hereditary Cerebral Amyloid Angiopathy)

Cerebral amyloid angiopathy (CAA) is characterised by the progressive accumulation of congophilic and Aβ (especially Aβ40) immunoreactive amyloid protein in the walls of small to medium size arteries and arterioles. It may be found less intensely in the walls of capillaries and veins. The specific histological markers of CAA are a green birefringent appearance under polarised light with Congo red stain and a fluorescent appearance under ultraviolet light with thioflavin S stain. The arterial walls are thickened by this deposition in the tunica media and adventitia, causing the vessels to become more rigid and fragile, with a round contour in cross-section. In more severe forms of CAA the vessels are dilated and disrupted, with focal fragmentation of the wall and blood extravasation. In these severe cases, the concentric separation of the media and adventitia often causes an appearance of a "lumen within a lumen".

There is a topographic pattern for CAA, with the vessels in the occipital and parietal cortex and meninges being the most affected. On the other hand, the hippocampus, white matter and basal ganglia are rarely affected [8, 23, 24].

The type 2 CSVD is very frequent in the general elderly population and the prevalence increases with age. It is also a pathological hallmark of Alzheimer's disease and it may appear in rare genetically transmitted diseases and other disorders such as Down's syndrome. Clinically, CAA is related to lobar haemorrhages, cortical petechial haemorrhages, small infarcts, cognitive impairment, and focal and diffuse white matter ischaemic lesions [24].

CLINICAL MANIFESTATIONS OF CEREBRAL SMALL VESSEL DISEASE

The main clinical manifestations of CSVD depend on the pathological changes which prevail in each patient. Therefore, a different phenotype may be found when dominant lesions are small deep brain infarcts, white matter lesions, deep intracerebral haemorrhages, or cerebral microbleeds.

Deep Brain Infarcts

These small subcortical infarcts may be associated with acute focal deficits or may be an incidental finding on brain imaging studies performed in patients without symptomatology (then called subclinical or "silent" infarcts). The prevalence of "silent" DBI ranges from 8% to 28%, depending on the type of population studied and the imaging test used. This prevalence is higher than the prevalence of lacunar infarcts associated with clinical strokes [25, 26]. Deep brain infarcts represent approximately 20% of all ischemic strokes. Conceptually, DBI are similar to lacunar infarcts and, in most cases, both are related to lacunar syndromes. However, the clinical manifestations of a lacunar syndrome may be occasionally caused by an ischemic stroke due to large artery pathology or cardiac embolism, or may be caused by a deep intracerebral haemorrhage in 4-10% of patients. Globally, a mechanism and aetiology different from CSVD were reported in nearly 20% of patients with a clinical lacunar syndrome [27 - 30].

Usually, patients with a lacunar syndrome present one of the 5 classical syndromes initially described, although infrequent atypical syndromes have also been reported. The classical syndromes include: (1) pure motor hemiparesis, due to an infarct in the posterior limb of the internal capsule or basis pontis; (2) pure sensory syndrome, secondary to an infarct in the ventral thalamus; (3) sensory-motor syndrome, caused by an infarct in the posterior limb of the internal capsule; (4) ataxic hemiparesis, due to an infarct in the ventral pons or internal capsule; (5) and dysarthria and clumsy hand, due to an infarction in the ventral pons or in the genu of the internal capsule. Atypical syndromes include pure motor hemiparesis with transient internuclear ophtalmoplegia, dysarthria-facial paresis, isolate dysarthria, isolated hemiataxia, pure motor hemiparesis with transient subcortical aphasia, unilateral or bilateral paramedian thalamic infarct syndrome, and hemichorea-hemiballismus [31, 32].

The recovery from lacunar syndromes due to DBI is generally more rapid and complete than recovery from ischemic stroke of other aetiology. The mortality rate reported for symptomatic DBI is less than 1% at 1 month and 2-10% at 1 year. However, some patients may present a severe and permanent disability, depending on the number and topography of lesions [33].

Lacunar infarcts, both clinical and silent, may also be associated with cognitive impairment. In a community study, the presence and number of silent infarcts were related to worse performance in executive and global cognitive functions. The risk of developing cognitive impairment is related to the number and location of lacunes [34 - 36]. Indeed, a single lacunar infarct may be associated with specific cognitive deficits if the topography is strategic. Thalamic infarcts were associated with low scores on the Mini-Mental State Examination (MMSE), less motor speed and executive dysfunction. Lacunes located in putamen or pallidus were associated with impairment of memory and motor speed [37, 38]. These clinical presentations, both cognitive and motor, show that clinical and silent DBI are associated with an increased risk of developing cognitive decline, dementia, depression, and functional impairment over time [39 - 41].

White Matter Lesions

White matter lesions appear as hyperintensities in the subcortical white matter on T2 MRI sequences and hypodensities in computed tomography (CT) scans (called leukoaraiosis) [42]. The topography of WML is typically periventricular in the frontal white matter, but they may be more peripheral (so called “deep”). These lesions are extremely frequent in the normal population and can be found in nearly 80% of Caucasians older than 60 years. As a marker of CSVD, WML coexist commonly with DBI [43, 44].

Initially, WML were considered a neuroimaging finding of unclear clinical significance. However, the evidence from cross-sectional studies showed that these lesions are associated with cognitive impairment, mood disorders, falls, gait disturbances, and bladder instability. The cognitive impairment manifests as a subcortical deterioration, including impairment of executive functions, deficits of attention, reduced processing speed, depressive mood, and apathy [45, 46]. Because WML are not associated with global cognitive decline unless other lesions are also present, they should not be considered a marker of dementia in cross-sectional studies. However, the data from longitudinal studies confirmed a positive association between WML and cognitive impairment and dementia. A meta-analysis of 46 longitudinal studies showed that WML were related to a greater risk of stroke, dementia, and death during follow-up. A correlation between the progression of WML load and the decline in cognitive functions was reported [47 - 51].

Deep Intracerebral Haemorrhages

Deep intracerebral haemorrhages are the most common type of intracranial haemorrhage and frequently coexist with others markers of this disease such as DBI and WML. Approximately, they represent 10% of all strokes and near 50% of all intracerebral haemorrhages. Because DIH are associated with causes of CSVD, especially hypertension, they are frequently called hypertensive haemorrhages. Although hypertensive haemorrhages are mainly DIH, they may be also pontine, cerebellar, and, less frequently, lobar [8, 16].

The haemorrhage generally presents as a sudden onset focal neurologic deficit which worsens over 30–90 minutes and is associated with a diminishing level of consciousness and others signs of raised intracranial pressure, as headache and vomiting. The putamen is the most common topography of DIH (19-53%), followed by thalamus (4-26%) and caudate nucleus (1-5%) [34].

Putaminal haemorrhage causes contralateral hemiparesis with dysarthria. If the bleeding is mild, hemiparesis develops gradually over 30-90 minutes, and the eyes deviate away from the side of the motor deficit. The paralysis may worsen until hemiplegia, but the level of consciousness is spared. When the haemorrhage is large it causes drowsiness and may lead to stupor and coma with signs of upper brainstem compression (central respiratory pattern, III cranial nerve paresis homolateral to stroke, and decerebrate rigidity).

Thalamic haemorrhage causes a sensory deficit involving all modalities in the contralateral side of the body. If the bleeding causes oedema or dissection into the adjacent internal capsule, it produces a contralateral hemiplegia or hemiparesis. After the acute phase, patients may develop a chronic contralateral neurogenic pain syndrome called Dejerine-Roussy syndrome. When the bleeding occurs into the dominant thalamus a thalamic aphasia (anomic with preserved understanding and verbal repetition) may be observed. If the non-dominant thalamus is affected, constructional apraxia or mutism may be found. Homonymous hemianopsia may be present and several pupillary and oculomotor disturbances appear when there is an inferior dissection into the upper midbrain. The ocular disorders include deviation of the eyes downward and inward, absence of convergence, pupilar asymmetry without light response, skew deviation, homolateral Horner's syndrome, and others.

Pontine bleedings cause coma, tetraplegia and decerebrate rigidity, usually over minutes. Pupils are small (approximately 1 mm) but react to light. Reflex horizontal eye movements evoked by head or caloric tests are impaired. Autonomic signs like hyperpnoea, severe hypertension, and hyperhidrosis may be present. Excepting very small haemorrhages, the prognosis of pontine bleedings is ominous in a short period of time. Globally, DIH are associated with a 50% fatality rate and severe disability in survivors [52, 53].

Cerebral Microbleeds

Cerebral microbleeds, also known as microhaemorrhages or lacunar haemorrhages, have been defined as multiple ovoid 2-5 mm in diameter foci of marked loss of signal intensity on T2-weighted gradient-echo (GRE-T2) or susceptibility weighted (SW) MRI. These foci represent deposits of hemosiderin that can remain in macrophages for years after acute microhemorrhage and they must be differentiated in MRI studies from vascular flow voids and cerebral calcifications [54 - 56]. Cerebral microhaemorrhages are particularly common in individuals with CSVD. There is a positive correlation between CMB and severity of leukoaraiosis and lacunar infarct count [57].

Microhaemorrhages may be classified as deep (related to vascular risk factors and a greater load of DBI and WML) and lobar (associated with the genotype ApoE4) [58]. Microbleeds may be also related to congophilic amyloid or hypertensive cerebral angiopathy. Less common causes of CMB are diffuse axonal injury, vasculitis, cerebral cavernous malformations, micrometastasis and external radiotherapy for lymphoblastic leukaemia [59].

In a systematic review, the prevalence of microbleeds in GRE-T2 MRI studies was approximately 5% in healthy adults, 34% in patients with ischaemic stroke, and 60% in patients with intracerebral haemorrhages. The prevalence is higher in patients with recurrent stroke, both ischaemic and haemorrhagic [59]. A 5.5 years follow-up study showed that in patients with ischemic stroke or transient ischemic attack the development of new CMB was related to systolic blood pressure, independently of the clinical state. The authors conclude that optimal control of hypertension may help prevent new CMB [60].

Clinically, the presence of CMB is related to increased risk of developing intracranial haemorrhage, cognitive impairment, and dementia, especially in patients who suffered a previous stroke. Although this association may suggest a cumulative effect of bleeding lesions, the real clinical significance of CMB is not clearly defined [61, 62].

Others Markers of Cerebral Small Vessel Disease: Brain Atrophy and Enlarged Perivascular Spaces

The presence of brain atrophy in CSVD patients has been correlated with cognitive impairment and disability. In patients with lacunar stroke and leukoaraiosis, brain volume was related to executive function and global cognitive function. This association persisted after controlling for other markers of CSVD, like WML load and number of DBI. Probably, EPVS have no clinical significance and should only be considered markers of incipient CSVD [51].

In summary, CSVD may cause clinical stroke syndromes and progressive cognitive impairment and dementia, depending on the presence and extension of the different lesions in the patient.

DIAGNOSIS OF CEREBRAL SMALL VESSEL DISEASE

The diagnosis of CSVD is not possible *in vivo* and only histopathology gives the definitive confirmation. The surrogate markers used to support the diagnosis are specially imaging studies. The role of biochemical parameters and transcranial Doppler is not defined.

Imaging Studies

Neuroimaging studies, mainly MRI, are fundamental for clinical diagnosis of CSVD. Indeed, the progression of lesions in resonance is associated with the clinical evolution of disease. Therefore, MRI is considered a surrogate marker to assess the effects of treatment and it has been applied in some clinical trials [63 - 65].

Computed Tomography

The computed tomography was the first technique used to study CSVD. The parenchymatous areas suffering CSVD appear hypodense, an aspect called leukoaraiosis by Hachinski more than 20 years ago [42]. This concept described the hypodense aspect of periventricular or subcortical white matter due to chronic ischemia. These lesions should not be adjacent to focal areas of cortical damage or ventricular enlargement, to distinguish them from large infarcts on white matter.

Lacunar infarcts may be seen on CT as small hypodense areas in basal nuclei and internal capsule, but this technique is less sensitive than magnetic resonance and a differentiation between acute and chronic ischemia is not possible. Fig. (**3**) shows lacunar infarcts and periventricular leukoaraiosis in a CT scan of a hypertensive male.

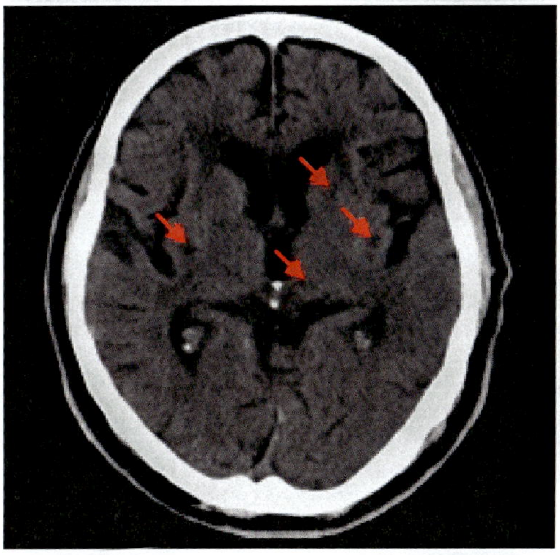

Fig. (3). Axial CT scan of a hypertense 80-years old male showing bilateral periventricular leukoaraiosis and deep infarcts (red arrows).

Acute deep intracerebral haemorrhages appear as hyperdense lesions on non-contrast CT. These haemorrhages are usually located in the basal ganglia or external capsule.

Microbleeds and EPVS may be seen occasionally in CT as small hypodense areas similar to lacunar infarcts. This low discrimination limits the usefulness of CT in the diagnosis and management of CSVD.

Magnetic Resonance Imaging

Standard Magnetic Resonance Imaging

Conventional MRI sequences are essential for diagnosis of CSVD by identification of the 5 main pathological changes distinctive of the condition: (1) deep brain infarcts; (2) white matter lesions; (3) deep intracerebral haemorrhages; (4) cerebral microbleedings; (5) other findings: enlarged perivascular spaces and brain atrophy.

Deep Brain Infarcts (Lacunar Infarcts)

Chronic lacunar infarcts causing tissue loss and cavitations are seen as regions of hypointensity on T1-weighted and FLuid Attenuated Inversion Recovery (FLAIR) sequences, and as hyperintense areas on T2-weighted images. Lacunar infarcts are predominantly located in basal ganglia, internal capsule, thalamus, and pons [66]. Because these hypodensities may be caused by other disorders, several limits for lacunes have been proposed. A lower limit of 3-5 mm in diameter has been used to differentiate lacunes from smaller perivascular spaces and an upper limit of 15-20 mm has been used to differentiate lacunes from subcortical infarcts of other aetiologies, basically embolic. It is possible to quantify the volume of individual infarcts with accuracy by using segmented T1-weighted images, as was reported in a study of 147 patients with CADASIL. A relevant question in the assessment of chronic lacunar infarcts on MRI is the differentiation between these lesions and EPVS.

Acute lacunar infarcts appear as hyperintense lesions, first on diffusion-weighted imaging (DWI) and later on T2 and FLAIR sequences [67, 68].

White Matter Lesions

White matter lesions are seen as bilateral, symmetric and more or less confluent areas of hyperintensity. They are located preferentially in the hemispheric white matter, but an infratentorial (pontine leukoaraiosis) location is possible. Leukoaraiosis is best seen on T2-weighted and FLAIR sequences. The last suppresses the cerebrospinal fluid (CSF) signal and increases the contrast between leukoaraiosis areas and normal parenchyma. Both sequences allow the quantification of lesion burden. The correlation between histological micro-angiopathy and confluent WML has been confirmed in studies comparing MRI with post-mortem samples [69]. Fig. (**4**) shows WML and DBI in a MRI of a hypertensive patient.

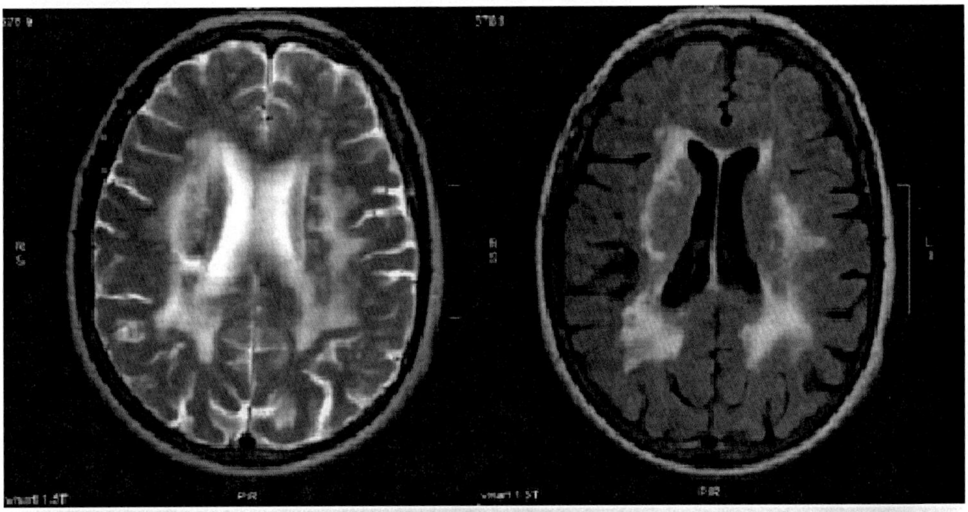

Fig. (4). Axial MRI scans of a 78 years old hypertense woman showing intense WML and some DBI. Left imaging T2 weighted sequence, right imaging FLAIR sequence.

Longitudinal cohort studies showed the progression of WML over a period of few years. The main factors associated with greater progression are age and baseline lesion volume. The secondary factors related to progression are the vascular risk factors, especially hypertension [70, 71]. Because WML changes are relatively quick and may be assessed over short periods, it has been suggested that MRI could be used as a surrogate marker to evaluate the effects of potential therapies [63 - 65].

Deep Intracerebral Haemorrhages

The best sequences to identify haemorrhages are T2-weighted gradient echo (GRE-T2) and susceptibility weighted imaging (SWI). These sequences detect the susceptibility artefact induced by iron in haemoglobin, which creates a bloom of hypointense signal drop-out in the haematoma. Calcium has a similar susceptibility effect and CT scan may help to distinguish between both causes if clinically indicated.

The products of haemoglobin degradation and its evolution may be seen on T1 and T2 images. In the first few hours, the haematoma has predominantly oxyhaemoglobin, which appears iso/hypointense on T1 and hyperintense on T2. The formation of deoxyhaemoglobin starts at the haematoma rim, appearing hypointense on T1 and T2. After the first 1 or 2 days intracellular methaemoglobin appears. The haematoma shows an aspect hyperintense on T1 and hypointense on T2. Approximately after 1 week, the methaemoglobin is extracellular and the bleeding is hyperintense on T2 and T1. Later, the liquefaction of the haematoma creates a central area hypointense on T1 sequences and hyperintense on T2. In this stage, a hypointense rim remains due to the generation of ferritin and haemosiderin [72].

Cerebral Microbleedings

The most sensitive MRI sequence for detection of CMB is GRE-T2. These lesions appear as small foci of black signal voids [21, 73]. Fig. (**5**) shows a GRE-T2 sequence of a 78 years old hypertensive woman with diffuse CMB.

In patients with CSVD, the predominant topography of CMB is the white matter, deep grey matter nuclei, and infratentorial regions. Cerebral microbleeds may be classified by size using different cut-off points, being 5-10 mm the maximum diameter and 2 mm the minimum. The hypointense areas of CMB on GRE-MRI appear larger than the actual haemosiderin deposits ("blooming effect"), a phenomenon that depends on several MRI parameters. This is a limitation when a direct comparison between sizes in different studies needs to be done. The use of three-dimensional GRE-MRI at submillimetre spatial resolution allows the detection of more CMB than the conventional two-dimensional study [21, 74].

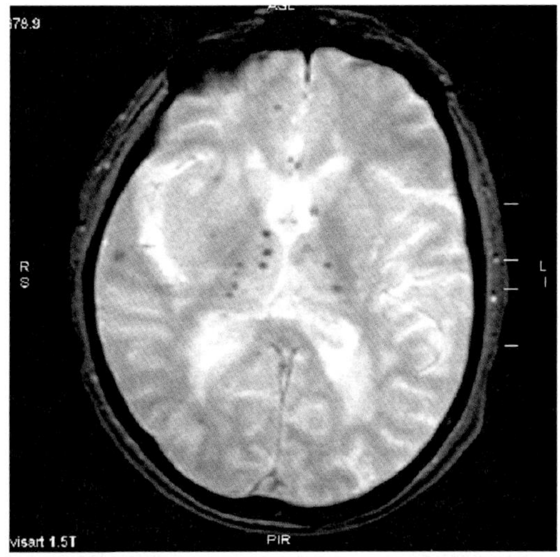

Fig. (5). Axial GRE-T2 weighted MRI of a 78 years old hypertense woman showing CMB.

Other Findings: Enlarged Perivascular Spaces and Brain Atrophy

Enlarged perivascular spaces appear as punctate hyperintensities surrounding the perforating arteries and arterioles in T2-weighted MRI. The Virchow-Robin spaces are related to aging and risk factors for CSVD, but their association with cognition is still unclear. However, because EPVS share the same risk factor profile as lacunar infarcts, they are considered by some investigators to be another expression of small vessel disease in the brain [75].

The Topography and size of EPVS help to differentiate them from DBI. Enlarged perivascular spaces may be found in the centrum semiovale, anterior commissure, basal ganglia, and hippocampus. Virchow-Robin spaces are usually smaller (less than 1-2 mm in diameter) and more isointense relative to CSF on proton density sequences [76 - 78].

The brain volume is best measured on T1-weighted sequences. This data may be automatically calculated by programmes which showed high reproducibility. Most studies used normalised brain volume or brain parenchymal fraction relative to the intracranial volume. Several studies showed that brain volume reduces with age and the presence of vascular risk factors. Longitudinal studies in normal middle-aged and elderly subjects with follow-up periods of up to 6 years showed a decline in brain volume of 0.4-0.5% per year. This rate is higher in patients with lacunar stroke and leukoaraiosis (0.4-0.9% per year). Brain atrophy was related to deterioration of executive function in patients with symptomatic CSVD [51, 79 - 82]. Recent papers suggest that 7 Tesla MRI could have higher sensibility than conventional magnetic fields to detect CSVD markers [83].

New Magnetic Resonance Imaging Sequences

Newer MRI sequences allow the assessment of brain perfusion, metabolism, blood-brain barrier permeability, microhaemorrhages and the analysis of white matter tracts. This information may contribute to clarify the pathophysiology of CSVD [66].

Brain Perfusion

Cerebral blood flow (CBF) and perfusion studies using xenon clearance, positron emission tomography, and perfusion MRI have shown a reduction of CBF in the white matter of patients with CSVD [84, 85]. Perfusion MRI studies assessing CBF in patients with diagnosis of lacunar stroke and leukoaraiosis showed a reduction of flow in all white matter regions, but not in grey matter. This reduction in CBF has been also demonstrated in normal appearing white matter of patients with CSVD and patients with sporadic lacunar stroke and CADASIL, suggesting that white matter is particularly vulnerable to hypoperfusion [86].

Blood-brain Barrier Permeability

Contrast-enhanced MRI may be used to study the blood-brain barrier permeability. This technique uses a T1-weighted sequence done before and after a bolus of a gadolinium-based contrast agent. The increased postcontrast enhancement of brain parenchyma and the increased signal intensity in the CSF are considered markers of raised blood-brain barrier permeability. The increase of permeability was associated with diabetes mellitus, vascular dementia, lacunar stroke, and normal appearance white matter in patients with CSVD [87 - 89]. These findings suggest that patients with CSVD present an increase in blood-brain barrier permeability. This phenomenon may be caused by endothelial dysfunction, which allows the leakage of plasma components into the vessel wall and surrounding brain tissue. This could be one of the mechanisms for damage of vessel wall and adjacent parenchyma [90, 91].

Analysis of White Matter Tissue Structure

Diffusion tensor imaging (DTI) techniques are based in the application of diffusion gradients in more than six different directions to measure the translational motion of water molecules and later produce bidimensional images. This MRI method gives quantitative data on white matter ultrastructure and allows track the fibres. In the white matter tracts the diffusion is greater along, rather than perpendicular (anisotropic), whereas in the CSF the diffusion is equal in all directions (isotropic). As axonal membranes and myelin limit the diffusion, the damage to these structures within the white matter interferes with the directionality of diffusion. Conventionally, two parameters are obtained: (1) fractional anisotropy (FA), a measure of the directionality of diffusion which gives information about the integrity of white matter tracts; (2) mean diffusivity (MD), a measure of the extent of diffusion which is sensitive to white matter ultrastructural damage.

It is probable that the pathological processes underlying DTI changes include axonal degeneration and ischaemic demyelination, but there are limited data correlating DTI and histology in CSVD patients.

The DTI studies showed damage in white matter of patients with CSVD, including abnormalities in apparently normal white matter. Indeed, areas of leukoaraiosis which appear similar on T2-weighted sequences may have different characteristics on DTI. Diffusion tensor imaging may be complementary to standard sequences and may differentiate between areas of severely damaged white matter tracts and areas of only limited disruption [66, 92, 93]. A recent study assessed the differential sensitivity of DTI markers to evaluate the progression of CSVD. The change in DTI histogram parameters using linear mixed effect models were investigated in 99 patients with symptomatic CSVD (defined as clinical lacunar syndrome with MRI as well as confluent WML). Over a 3 year follow-up period it was observed a decline in FA and an increase in MD in white matter, suggesting that the progression of disease can be monitored sensitively using DTI histogram analysis [94]. Other work of the same group showed that DTI parameters and WML volume were more sensitive markers of CSVD progression over short time periods than neuropsychologic assessment. The application of these markers could be useful to reduce the size of clinical trials to investigate the efficacy of treatments for CSVD [95].

Probably, patients with CSVD present cognitive impairment due to the disruption of cortical–cortical and cortical–subcortical white matter tracts. Therefore, it is not surprising that DTI abnormalities (both MD and FA parameters) are strongly correlated with cognition, especially executive function, information processing speed, and working memory. This correlation appears to be independent of other lesions found in MRI, such as WML burden on T2 sequences and brain volume. More sophisticated techniques to study the spatial pattern of DTI changes may provide further understanding of the relationship between damage to specific white matter tracts and cognitive deficits. These techniques include voxel-based and tract-based statistical approaches and tractography to assess a specific white matter tract [96 - 98].

The magnetisation transfer ratio (MTR) evaluates the exchange of magnetisation between protons bound to macro-molecules and protons of free water inside tissue. A low MTR indicates a reduction in the capacity of macro-molecules to exchange magnetisation with tissue water molecules, reflecting damage to myelin or axonal membrane. Magnetisation transfer ratio was exhaustively studied in multiple sclerosis, but data in CSVD are still limited. One study showed a correlation between reduced MTR and aging and impairment of executive function. Recently, a research evaluating 355 participants of the Austrian Stroke Prevention Study found that the whole brain and the lobar cortical MTR were significantly related to performance on tests of memory, executive function, and motor skills [99 - 102].

Transcranial Doppler Study

The transcranial Doppler (TCD) examination allows the assessment of the velocity of blood flow in the main intracerebral arteries, mostly the vessels which integrate the Circle of Willis. From the measured systolic and diastolic velocities, the mean velocity and the pulsatility and resistance indexes may be calculated.

Both indexes are considered markers of arterial resistance due to reduced elasticity of their walls and the capillary bed. However, the use of TCD is controversial because the study of arterioles and capillars is indirect and the resistance indexes are calculated from velocities, which may be affected by different variables (*e.g.* proximal cervical or intracranial atherosclerosis, anaemia, thyroid disorders).

A study found that pulsatility and resistance indexes were higher in diabetic patients, suggesting that there was an increased resistance in capillary bed related to microangiopathy [103]. Another TCD study explored the association between pulsatility index with other measures of CSVD assessed by MRI (WML, lacunes, CMB) in the community. The multiple logistic regression found that pulsatility index of middle cerebral artery was associated with severe load of WML (odds ratio, 1.33 per 0.1 increase in PI; 95% CI 1.04-1.70; P=0.02). The authors defined a pulsatility index cut-off, positive predictive value, and negative predictive value of 0.70 (95% confidence interval, 0.60-0.80), 34.9%, and 85.6%, respectively, for detection of severe WML. They did not find an association between pulsatility and number of lacunes and microbleeds [104].

Recently, a TCD study which included 56 patients with CSVD diagnosed by MRI and 48 controls found that increased pulsatility index was related to CSVD, specifically periventricular and deep white matter hyperintensities. These results suggested that TCD could be used as a non-invasive method for diagnosing CSVD [105]. However, other study assessed the reliability of cerebral pulsatility indexes to identify candidates for MRI screening in population-based samples. Seventy subjects were included, with mean age 70.6 ± 4.6 years, 57% were women and 40% had moderate-to-severe WML in MRI. The multivariate models showed no differences across categories of WML in the mean pulsatility index of middle cerebral arteries. The authors concluded that cerebral pulsatility index should not be used to identify candidates for MRI screening [106].

It has been suggested that impaired cerebral autoregulation and vasodilatory capacity may play a role in the pathogenesis of the WML. The autoregulation of cerebral vessels may be assessed with techniques based on TCD examination. A study compared 24 h ambulatory blood pressure measurement, quantitative volumetric MRI analysis of WML volume, and CO_2 vasoreactivity in response to hypercapnia and dynamic cerebral autoregulatory index by TCD in 64 patients with CSVD. The results showed that cerebral autoregulation and CO_2 reactivity were not related to WML volume but they were related to blood pressure levels and duration of hypertension [107].

In summary, although the current standard for diagnosing CSVD is neuroimaging, the usefulness of TCD as a guide to select candidates for MRI examination in the community in controversial. Additional studies including more patients and new MRI sequences could help to define the role of TCD.

Biomarkers as In-vivo Markers of Small Vessel Disease

It has been proposed that CSF biomarkers could be used as surrogate markers for CSVD pathology and could be used to evaluate the course and effects of therapies. In a cohort of patients with dementia, the authors found 2 different profiles of CSF. Patients with "pure" vascular dementia showed elevated albumin ratio suggesting an impairment of blood-brain barrier function and normal beta-amyloid ratio. Patients with Alzheimer's disease showed typical beta-amyloid ratio and normal albumin ratio. The results support the role of blood-brain barrier dysfunction in the development of cognitive decline in CSVD [108].

A study compared the association between genes and plasma levels of C-reactive protein and interleukin-6 and CSVD defined by MRI (WML and DBI). The results showed a relationship between the levels of both inflammatory markers and the presence of WML and DBI, suggesting that inflammation has a role in pathophysiology of CSVD. Additionally, an association between CSVD and some haplotypes was reported [109].

A recent study did not find a significant association between plasma biomarkers of inflammation and lacunar and cortical strokes. Only plasma t-PA level was significantly lower in lacunar stroke subtype [110].

A lack of association between serum fibrosis markers (transforming growth factor-β and procollagen type III N-terminal propeptide) and CSVD was reported [111].

A study performed with 210 patients with CSVD and 207 controls found that serum levels of protein S100B and asymmetric dimethylarginine were elevated in patients with CSVD and were significantly correlated with cognitive decline [112].

An increase in serum levels of endothelial activation markers (including von Willebrand factor antigen and homocysteine) and high-sensitivity C-reactive protein, but not of platelet activation markers (activated glycoprotein IIb/IIIa, P-selectin and platelet microparticles) was found in 74 consecutive patients with recent DBI [113].

Finally, an association between albuminuria and oxidized low density lipoprotein (ox-LDL) levels and higher risk of progression in patients with lacunar stroke (defined as initial NIHSS score worsening ≥4 points within the first 72 h) was reported with adjusted OR for ox-LDL=1.03 (95% CI: 1.01-1.07, p=0.019) and for albuminuria=2.07 (95% CI: 1.04-4.13, p=0.039) [114].

In conclusion, the published data suggest a role for inflammatory and blood-brain barrier impairment markers in pathophysiology of CSVD. However, these data are limited and currently CSF and plasma biomarkers have no a defined role in the diagnosis of CSVD.

TREATMENT OF CEREBRAL SMALL VESSEL DISEASE

The therapeutic management of type 1 CSVD is a relevant topic because this disorder causes approximately 25% of all acute ischaemic strokes and represents the second aetiology of dementia syndrome and the first cause of vascular cognitive impairment. However, there is not a specific curative treatment for the vascular and brain changes related to CSVD and the patients receive the standard treatment for dementia (symptomatic) and stroke (symptomatic and primary and secondary prevention), with limited evidence about its effectivity in this particular setting. The next section will focus on the habitual strategies for the management of stroke and dementia in these patients and some novel approaches to specific treatment will be summarised.

The type 2 CSVD does not have any specific treatment. The usual management includes: (1) standard care for patients with brain haemorrhage, considering surgery of hematoma in selected cases due to the risk of new bleeding during perioperative period; (2) to avoid the use of antiaggregants and anticoagulants due to the haemorrhagic risk. An anti-amyloid beta monoclonal antibody is currently under research (see below).

Ischemic Stroke Caused by Small Vessel Disease: Acute Treatment and Secondary Prevention

The presence of small vessel disease is a marker of worse outcome during some therapies, like acute phase thrombolysis, and anticoagulation and carotid endarterectomy for secondary prevention. In these settings, CSVD was related to increased risk of symptomatic haemorrhage (patients treated with intravenous thrombolysis or chronic anticoagulants) and raised risk of perioperative stroke (patients who underwent carotid surgery). However, the presence of leukoaraiosis is not a contraindication to these treatments and it should be regarded as an indication for more intensive care in this group of patients. Other strategies for secondary prevention, such as treatment of vascular risk factors and antiaggregant therapy, are used with relatively little evidences about the efficacy and goals to achieve.

Thrombolysis

Currently, intravenous thrombolysis with recombinant tissue plasminogen activator is the acute phase treatment approved for less than 4.5 hours ischaemic stroke. The most dangerous complication of this treatment is symptomatic intracranial haemorrhage, which may occur in approximately 6.4% of patients. Some factors associated with an increased risk of bleeding are advanced age, hyperglycaemia, increased blood pressure, and neuroimaging evidence of leukoaraiosis. A study reported a significantly higher rate of symptomatic cerebral haemorrhage in patients with moderate-severe leukoaraiosis in deep white matter compared with those with mild or no leukoaraiosis (10.5 *vs*. 3.8%, respectively; OR 2.9 [95% CI; 1.29–6.59]). This association was independent of age, stroke severity, and type of thrombolytic treatment (intravenous, intraarterial, combined). A recent review summarised the results of thrombolysis in patients with CSVD and concluded that fibrinolysis is an effective treatment in acute lacunar stroke, and that the presence of CSVD increases the risk of intracranial haemorrhage during this treatment, but it does not represent an absolute exclusion criterion [115 - 119].

Secondary Prevention of Ischemic Stroke in Patients with Cerebral Small Vessel Disease

Anticoagulation

Several studies showed that the presence of leukoaraiosis is an independent risk factor for major intracranial haemorrhage in patients treated with warfarin for secondary prevention of ischemic stroke of cardioembolic origin. The results of the Stroke Prevention in Reversible Ischemia Trial (SPIRIT) and European Atrial Fibrillation Trial (EAFT) studies showed that leukoaraiosis (hazard ratio 2.7, 95% confidence interval 1.4-5.3) and age older than 65 years (hazard ratio 1.9, 95% confidence interval 1.0-3.4) were independent predictors of all anticoagulation-related haemorrhages. The incidence of intracranial bleeding in SPIRIT was 3.7% per year; this incidence increased by a factor of 1.37 for each 0.5 unit in the international normalized ratio [120].

A case-control study showed that the presence and severity of leukoaraiosis on CT scan had a strong correlation with the incidence of intracerebral haemorrhage. Leukoaraiosis was present in 24 of 26 cases (92%), compared with 27 of 56 controls (48%). The odds ratio was 12.9 (95% confidence interval 2.8 to 59.8). Other clinical factors associated with bleeding were an international normalized ratio >3.0, history of multiple previous strokes, and presence of carotid artery stenosis. The association between leukoaraiosis and haemorrhage persisted after multivariate analysis [121].

A recent study on 69 patients with atrial fibrillation and CSVD treated with new anticoagulants during 1 year showed that these drugs do not increase CMB. Because the sample was small and the follow-up was only 1 year, further research with a longer follow-up and larger samples is needed [122].

In summary, the presence of CSVD is an independent risk factor for intracerebral haemorrhage related to chronic anticoagulant therapy in survivors of ischemic stroke, including those in the commonly used range of anticoagulation. Chronic anticoagulation is not indicated as secondary prevention of stroke caused by CSVD, but if there is other indication (*e.g*. atrial fibrillation), the microangiopathy does not represent a contraindication. An exhaustive control of anticoagulant parameters and risk factors must be emphasised. The risk of new anticoagulant drugs seems to be lower, but more evidence is necessary.

Carotid Endarterectomy

Among the 2618 patients included in the North American Symptomatic Carotid Endarterectomy Trial (NASCET), 493 had leukoaraiosis: 354 restricted and 139 widespread. The patients with leukoaraiosis were older, had a history of hypertension, had more hemispheric ischemic events, and had more DBI. The 30-day perioperative risks of any stroke or death for surgical patients were 5.3% (no leukoaraiosis), 10.6% (restricted leukoaraiosis), and 13.9% (widespread leukoaraiosis). The 3-year risk of stroke for patients in the medical treatment group were 20.2% (no leukoaraiosis), 27.3% (restricted leukoaraiosis), and 37.2% (widespread leukoaraiosis) ($p=0.01$). In the surgical arm the risks were 14.2%, 25.4%, and 33.6%, respectively ($p<0.001$). Despite a higher perioperative risk, endarterectomy significantly reduced the absolute 3-year risk of ipsilateral stroke by 11.6% ($p=0.46$), 7.6% ($p=0.39$), and 10.9% ($p<0.001$) for patients with widespread leukoaraiosis, restricted leukoaraiosis, and no leukoaraiosis, respectively. Thus, the presence of leukoaraiosis in CT reduces the benefit from endarterectomy, but it still remains and WML are not a contraindication for surgery [123].

Antiaggregation

Although the strokes related to CSVD have aetiopathogenic characteristics different from strokes due to large vessel atherosclerosis or cardiac disorders, no randomised trial has independently assessed the usefulness of currently used antiplatelet agents in this group of patients. Some clinical trials evaluating antiaggregant drugs in secondary prevention of stroke assessed subgroups of patients with stroke caused by CSVD. The analysis of subgroups of patients with

DBI in four randomised trials supports the use of antiplatelet therapy in lacunar stroke, suggesting that antiaggregation may be effective for secondary prevention. Aspirin, aspirin plus dipyridamole, ticlopidine, and cilostazol were more effective than placebo in randomised clinical trials of secondary prevention of ischemic stroke in these patients. There were no significant differences among drugs and there was no evidence of an increased risk of intracranial haemorrhage. Ongoing studies could give additional information about the most convenient antiaggregant drug for patients with CSVD [124 - 127].

A phase 4, double-blind, randomised clinical trial comparing aspirin (100 mg daily) and cilostazol (200 mg daily) is currently recruiting patients. The primary objective of this study is to compare the efficacy of aspirin and cilostazol on the volume of WML changes assessed by MRI in patients with CSVD. The secondary objectives are to compare the impact of aspirin and cilostazol on diffusion tensor imaging parameters (mean diffusivity and fractional anisotropy), the number of new lacunes and microbleeds, brain atrophy, cognition, depression, neurologic signs, gait and urinary disturbances, and activities of daily living [128].

A randomised phase 2, dose escalation, open label, blinded intermediary end-point trial, will be conducted in two hospital centres in the United Kingdom. It will evaluate the tolerability and safety of cilostazol, isosorbide mononitrate, both or neither in 60 patients with CSVD with symptomatic DBI. The primary outcome measure is the proportion of patients able to tolerate the target dose. The secondary outcome measures are safety (systemic or intracranial bleeding, recurrent stroke, recurrent vascular events, death, reduction in blood pressure, effect on platelet function assessed using p-selectin), efficacy (effect on cerebrovascular reactivity assessed using carbon dioxide challenge in magnetic resonance imaging, effect on systemic large artery stiffness assessed with pulse wave velocity measurement), and tolerability (proportion of patients with headache that interferes with daily activities, proportion with dizziness that interferes with daily activities, proportion of patients with nausea that interferes with daily activities, proportion of patients with palpitations, proportion of patients with loose stools, and tablet count) [129].

The effect of cilostazol compared with placebo on pulsatility index in the middle cerebral artery (evaluated by serial TCD) and WML burden was studied in a 90 days multicenter, randomized, double-blind, placebo-controlled trial which included 130 patients with acute lacunar infarction. Cilostazol was given to 63 patients and placebo to 67 patients. All baseline characteristics were similar in the two groups, and there were no significant differences. There was a significant decrease of TCD pulsatility index at 90-day study from baseline in the cilostazol group ($p = 0.02$). The mean WML volume was 11.57 cm^3 (0.13-68.45, median 4.86) and the mean pulsatility index in the middle cerebral artery was 0.95 (0.62-1.50). There were no significant correlations between WML volume and changes in pulsatility index, but a trend of inverse correlation was observed from the baseline to the day 90. For analysis, the WML volume was dichotomized based on its median value (4.90 cm^3). At 90-days, cilostazol reduced significantly the pulsatility index in patients with WML volumes $\leq$ 4.9 cm^3 ($p = 0.002$). The authors concluded that the study showed that cilostazol decreased brain artery pulsatility in patients with WML, especially in those with mild WML changes [130].

Control of Arterial Hypertension

Arterial hypertension is the most prevalent vascular risk factor in patients with CSVD. A pooled analysis of trials on hypertension control in secondary prevention of stroke in patients with previous stroke or transient ischemic attack showed that the reduction of blood pressure with antihypertensive drugs decreased in approximately 28% the recurrence of stroke. However, there is no definitive guidance about the optimal target level of blood pressure control or about a specific antihypertensive drug [131].

The Perindopril Protection Against Recurrent Stroke Study (PROGRESS) showed that an average reduction of 9 mmHg in systolic blood pressure decreased in 28% the recurrence of stroke. The result was similar for the approximately 30% of patients with lacunar stroke. Additionally, cognitive outcome in PROGRESS showed that the risk of dementia in patients treated with perindopril was non-significantly reduced, although the risk of cognitive impairment related to recurrent stroke was significantly less in the active treatment group. These results support the necessity of optimal blood pressure control to reduce the cognitive decline in the elderly [132 - 134].

The Action to Control Cardiovascular Risk in Diabetics (ACCORD) trial tested intensive (systolic blood pressure < 120 mmHg) vs standard (systolic blood pressure < 140 mmHg) blood pressure control in 4733 adults with type 2 diabetes and at least one vascular risk factor or diagnosed vascular disease. The mean systolic blood pressures after one year were 119 and 134 mmHg, respectively. After a mean follow-up of 4.7 years, the primary composite outcome (nonfatal myocardial infarction, nonfatal stroke or death from cardiovascular causes) was not significantly different between both groups. The annual rates of stroke, a prespecified secondary outcome, were 0.32% and 0.53% in the two groups, respectively (hazard ratio, 0.59; 95% CI, 0.39 to 0.89; p=0.01). The authors concluded that in patients with type 2 diabetes at high risk for cardiovascular events the intensive control of blood pressure did not reduce the rate of a composite outcome of fatal and nonfatal major cardiovascular events compared with the standard control [135].

A multicenter clinical trial included 2977 participants without baseline clinical evidence of cognitive impairment or dementia and with haemoglobin A1c (HbA1c) levels under 7.5%. The aim was to examine whether intensive therapy for hypertension (goal of less than 120 mmHg vs less than 140 mmHg) and combination therapy with a statin plus a fibrate versus placebo reduced the risk of cognitive decline and the total brain volume. Cognition was assessed at baseline and 20 and 40 months. A subgroup of 503 patients underwent baseline and 40-month brain MRI to assess changes in whole brain volume. At 40 months, no differences in cognitive function were found in the intensive blood pressure-lowering trial or in the fibrate trial. At 40 months, the total brain volume had declined more in the intensive vs standard blood pressure lowering group (difference, −4.4 [95% CI, −7.8 to −1.1] cm^3; p= 0.01). Compared with placebo, fibrate therapy had no effect on brain volume. The authors concluded that intensive blood pressure control and fibrate therapy did not produce a measurable effect on cognitive decline at 40 months of follow-up. Indeed, intensive blood pressure control was associated with greater decline in total brain volume at 40 months [136].

A phase 4, parallel, open label, safety/efficacy clinical trial is currently recruiting hypertensive patients with a recent diagnosis of lacunar stroke due to CSVD defined by MRI. The patients are randomised to regular blood pressure control (systolic pressure in the range of 130-139 mmHg) or intensive blood pressure control (systolic pressure below 130 mmHg). The drugs used for treatment are azelnidipine (8 or 16 mg daily) plus perindopril (4 or 8 mg daily) with or without hydroclorothiazide (12.5 or 25 mg daily). The primary outcome measure is the progression of CSVD measured as area of WML and number of CMB [137].

The Secondary Prevention of Small Subcortical Strokes (SPS3) trial was specifically designed to evaluate the secondary prevention of stroke in patients with CSVD. This was an interventional phase 3 study for which 3020 patients with symptomatic DBI within the previous 6 months and an eligible lesion on MRI were enrolled. The patients were randomized, in a factorial design, to therapy with aspirin (325 mg daily) plus clopidogrel (75 mg daily) *vs* aspirin (325 mg daily) plus placebo and to one of two levels of systolic blood pressure control (intensive, <130 mmHg; standard, 130-149 mmHg). The primary outcomes of the study were the prevention of recurrent stroke and the reduction in cognitive decline. The patients with DBI were defined on the basis of criteria from the Trial of ORG 10172 in Acute Stroke Treatment (TOAST) supplemented by MRI data [138]. Data about racial and ethnic differences among the participants were published [139]. After a mean 3.7 years follow-up, an analysis of recurrence of ischemic stroke among the 3020 participants in the SPS3 trial showed that new ischemic event occurred at a rate of 4.3%/year in patients with prior symptomatic lacunar stroke or TIA, 3.1%/year in those with >1 of the defined 3 risk factors (diabetes, black race, male sex), and 1.3%/year in those with 0 to 1 risk factors. There were no significant interactions between treatment effects and stroke risk. The results showed that prior symptomatic lacunar ischemia, diabetes, black race, and male sex were independently related to development of new lacunar stroke. The effects of blood pressure goals and dual antiaggregant treatment were similar across the spectrum of risk factors and recurrence [140].

In summary, the evidence supports the control of blood pressure for the prevention of stroke. However, there are still questions without a definitive response which need to be assessed in future randomised trials. First, if clinical effects observed in previous clinical trials can be obtained in patients with CSVD. Second, whether an intensive versus a standard blood pressure control is optimal. Third, which specific drug or class may be preferentially used.

Control of Cholesterol Level

The results from the Stroke Prevention by Aggressive Reduction of Cholesterol Levels (SPARCL) showed that patients with CSVD benefit from statin therapy, similarly to patients with stroke caused by large vessel disease. In this trial, the effect of 80 mg daily of atorvastatin on the reduction of stroke recurrence was similar among all subgroups of stroke [141].

In a double-blind, placebo-controlled, 33 months trial which included 535 patients, pravastatin treatment (40 mg daily) was ineffective in preventing worsening of WML measured by repeated MRI [142].

A post-hoc analysis of the 2 years, double-blind, placebo-controlled Regression of Cerebral Artery Stenosis (ROCAS) trial showed that the treatment with 20 mg daily of simvastatin was not associated with a significant reduction in the increase of WML volume in the group of 208 individuals without stroke and asymptomatic stenosis of middle cerebral artery. However, the treatment was effective when the subgroup of subjects with severe baseline WML was analysed, suggesting that statins may delay the progression of cerebral WML only in individuals with severe damage at baseline [143].

In a 3-month, double-blind trial, 94 adults with recent lacunar stroke were randomly allocated to receive 80 mg of atorvastatin daily or placebo. The primary end point was the change in cerebrovascular reactivity after 3 months of treatment. The secondary outcomes were the changes in brachial and carotid artery endothelial-dependent vasodilatations. Compared with placebo, the patients in the active arm reduced in 55% and 30% the low-density lipoprotein cholesterol and high-sensitivity C-reactive protein levels, respectively. However, the active drug did not improve vasomotor reactivity or endothelial dysfunction of carotid and brachial arteries. This result excluded a significant effect of atorvastatin in endothelial dysfunction of microvasculature in patients with lacunar stroke [144].

Symptomatic Treatment of Cognitive Impairment in Patients with Cerebral Small Vessel Disease

The available information about the effects of drugs used in the treatment of cognitive manifestations derives from the trials carried in patients with Alzheimer's disease with CSVD and vascular dementia. The vascular dementia spectrum includes dementia associated with CSVD, multi-stroke dementia, dementia due to strategic infarct and others.

Memantine

Memantine, an uncompetitive antagonist of N-methyl-D-aspartate (NMDA) glutamate receptors used in Alzheimer's disease, was tested in a 28-week, double-blind, randomised controlled trial in 579 patients with probable vascular dementia. Compared with placebo, memantine 20 mg daily modestly improved cognition, assessed by the Alzheimer's Disease Assessment Scale-Cognitive Subscale (ADAS-cog) score (mean change of ADAS-cog from baseline of -1.75 points [95% confidence intervals -3.023 to -0.49]). There was no difference in the Clinical Global Impression of Change (CGI-C) score. The study drug was generally well tolerated [145].

Acetylcholinesterase Inhibitors

The acetylcholinesterase inhibitors commonly used to treat Alzheimer's disease symptoms (galantamine, donepezil, and rivastigmine) were also studied in vascular dementia trials.

Galantamine

Galantamine is a cholinesterase inhibitor that also modulates central nicotinic receptors. A multicenter, double-blind, placebo-controlled, 6-month, randomized clinical trial included patients with diagnosis of probable vascular dementia or Alzheimer's disease combined with CSVD to receive galantamine or placebo. The primary end points were cognition (ADAS-cog) and global function (Clinician's Interview-Based Impression of Change-plus caregiver input, CIBIC-plus). The secondary end points included assessment of behavioural symptoms (Neuropsychiatric Inventory, NPI) and activities of daily living (Disability

Assessment in Dementia, DAD) score. The analysis of both groups as a whole showed that galantamine was effective on all outcome measures. However, the changes in the "pure" vascular dementia subgroup did not achieve significance [146].

In a multinational, randomized, double-blind, parallel-group trial, 788 patients with probable vascular dementia were randomised to receive galantamine or placebo during 26 weeks. The efficacy was evaluated using measures of cognition (ADAS-cog), daily function (Alzheimer's Disease Cooperative Study-Activities of Daily Living Inventory, ADCS-ADL), and behaviour (NPI). Patients treated with galantamine had a modest improvement in ADAS-cog compared with placebo, including executive function, but there was no difference between galantamine and placebo on the ADCS-ADL score. In both studies galantamine showed good safety and tolerability [147].

Donepezil

Donepezil was assessed in vascular dementia in three main randomised clinical trials. Two 24-weeks randomized, placebo-controlled, trials enrolled 1219 patients with probable or possible vascular cognitive impairment diagnosed according to the National Institute of Neurological Disorders and Stroke and the Association International pour la Recherche et l'Enseignement en Neurosciences (NINCDS-AIREN) criteria. The patients were randomized to placebo, donepezil 5 mg per day, or donepezil 10 mg per day. From week 6 through week 24 both active treatment groups showed a statistically significant improvement in cognitive measures, global function, and activities of daily living when compared with placebo. Although side effects were more pronounced in the donepezil group, the drug was generally well tolerated, both with 5 mg and 10 mg daily. However, the study did not entirely rule out the possibility of including patients with Alzheimer's dementia rather than vascular dementia [148, 149].

This drug was also studied in 168 patients with CADASIL and cognitive impairment. The patients were followed for 18 weeks after randomisation to donepezil or placebo. There was a non significant difference between donepezil (n=84) and placebo (n=77) in the primary endpoint (change in Vascular

Alzheimer's Disease Assessment Scale-cognitive subscale). There was a significant treatment effect favouring donepezil on secondary outcomes measuring executive function (Trail Making Test B and A times, Executive Interview [p=0.022]) [150].

Rivastigmine

Rivastigmine is a non-specific inhibitor of acetylcholinesterase and butyryl-cholinesterase. A 22 months open study with 16 patients (8 rivastigmine 3-6 mg/day; 8 cardioaspirin) diagnosed with probable vascular dementia, showed that patients treated with rivastigmine had significant improvements in executive function and behavioural symptoms. Later, a randomized, open label, one year study, with 208 patients diagnosed with probable vascular dementia evaluated the effects of rivastigmine. The results showed a slight improvement in executive function (clock drawing tests) and behaviour [151, 152].

The Vascular Dementia trial studying Exelon (VANTAGE) was a large international trial which included more than 700 patients with "pure" vascular dementia. Patients were randomised to receive rivastigmine (3–12 mg per day) or placebo. After the 24 weeks of blinded follow-up the patients continued in the study in an open phase of 12 months. Near three-quarters of the patients included had CSVD, defined by clinical and neuroimaging criteria. Rivastigmine demonstrated superiority over placebo on three measures of cognitive performance (Vascular Dementia Assessment Scale, ADAS-cog, and MMSE), but not on other outcomes. The authors considered that rivastigmine, like others acetylcholinesterase inhibitors, did not provide consistent efficacy in patients with probable vascular dementia and the positive results on cognitive outcomes derived from effects in older patients who probably had concomitant Alzheimer pathology [153].

A meta-analysis of clinical effects in patients with vascular dementia including all drugs currently used to treat Alzheimer's disease concluded that cholinesterase inhibitors and memantine produce small benefits in cognition of uncertain clinical significance in patients with mild to moderate vascular dementia. The conclusion was that current data are insufficient to support the widespread use of these drugs in patients with vascular dementia [154].

Other Drugs

Several drugs were assessed to treat cognitive symptoms in patients with vascular dementia. Because the results were modest and these trials had methodological limitations, the use of following drugs is not recommended in clinical guidelines.

Hydergine

Hydergine is a derivative of ergotoxine used to treat patients with either dementia or "age-related" cognitive symptoms in some countries. The results of Cochrane database meta-analysis showed 11 hydergine clinical trials on over 200 patients. The diagnoses of patients included Alzheimer's disease, vascular dementia, "cerebral insufficiency" and thromboembolic stroke. The combined analyses indicated that hydergine had statistically significant benefits on global measures. However, the number of patients in vascular dementia trials was small, losing the statistic significance. Due to the positive dose-dependent effects observed and the reduced number of patients studied in vascular dementia group, new clinical trials with higher doses in bigger samples of patients with clinical and radiological definition of CSVD may be useful [155].

Nicergoline

Nicergoline is another ergot derivative used in the treatment of cognitive, affective and behavioural disorders in the elderly. The Cochrane database meta-analysis included data from 11 nicergoline clinical trials. Approximately 1300 patients were included, with one half receiving nicergoline and the other half placebo. Diagnoses of the patients were relatively confusing, including "senile cognitive deterioration," "cerebral metabolic and nutritional disturbances", "hypertension and leukoaraiosis", "senile cerebral insufficiency", "senile dementia", "senile dementia of Alzheimer's type" and "multi-infarct dementia". The review of one mixed-group of data of three studies including 261 patients with multi-infarct dementia showed that there was a significant effect of nicergoline on MMSE scores. The duration of the studies ranged from 3 to 12 months. In conclusion, nicergoline may have a beneficial effect in vascular dementia but further studies with more patients recruited using current diagnostic criteria are needed to confirm the previous findings [156].

Nimodipine

Nimodipine is an L-type voltage-dependent calcium channel antagonist. Theoretically, an excessive opening of these voltage-dependent channels could contribute to toxicity induced by stimulation of NMDA receptors. Then, the blockade of L-type calcium channels by nimodipine could reduce the damage. Additionally, nimodipine has antihypertensive properties as a calcium channel blocker in smooth muscle cells. This effect could further reduce the vascular and parenchymatous damage in hypertense patients.

A systematic review of the Cochrane database included 14 trials which tested two treatment regimes, 90 and 180 mg/day of nimodipine, for 12 and 24 weeks. Two trials included patients with Alzheimer's disease, 9 trials included patients with vascular dementia, and 3 trials included patients with Alzheimer's disease and vascular dementia. The outcome measures from 9 trials (2492 patients) showed a benefit associated with nimodipine (90 mg/day at 12 weeks) compared with placebo on clinical global impression and cognitive function, assessed by the Sandoz Clinical Assessment Geriatric scale, but not on activities of daily living. Globally, nimodipine was well tolerated and showed a low rate of adverse effects, similar to placebo. The review concludes that nimodipine can be of some benefit in the treatment of patients with dementia due to unclassified disease or to Alzheimer's disease, cerebrovascular disease, or mixed dementia, but short-term benefits demonstrated in the trials do not justify its use as a long-term treatment [157].

A 12-month, randomised, placebo-controlled clinical trial specifically focused on dementia related to CSVD. The results showed positive findings only for secondary outcome measures (lexical production and a deterioration of three or more points on the mini-mental state examination), but the results for the main outcome (a measure of global cognitive status) were negative [158].

Cytidine-5-diphosphate Choline (CDP-choline, Citicoline)

Citicoline is a precursor essential for the synthesis of phosphatidylcholine, one of the components of the cell membrane that is degraded during cerebral ischemia to free fatty acids and free radicals. Animal studies suggested that CDP-choline may protect the cell membranes by accelerating resynthesis of phospholipids and may also reduce the ischaemic cell damage by suppressing the release of free fatty acids. The Cochrane review included 14 studies. The diagnosis of participants varied over the years and ranged from aged individuals with subjective memory disorders to patients with vascular cognitive impairment (mild to moderate), vascular dementia, or senile dementia (mild to moderate). Similarly, the follow-up of the patients studied was very variable, ranging from 20 days to 12 months. The results showed an evidence of benefit of CDP-choline on memory function, behaviour, and global impression, but there was no a beneficial effect on attention. Citicoline was well tolerated [159].

Cerebrolysin®

Cerebrolysin® is a peptide product derived from pig brain with potential neurotrophic (including nerve growth factor activity) and neuroprotective activities. The Cochrane systematic review found 6 randomized controlled trials with a total of 597 patients. The meta-analysis revealed a beneficial effect of Cerebrolysin® on general cognitive function measured by MMSE (weighted mean difference 1.10; 95% confidence interval 0.37 to 1.82) or ADAS-cog (weighted mean difference -4.01; 95% confidence interval -5.36 to -2.66). The product also improved the global clinical function of patients. The peptide was only associated with non-serious adverse events. The conclusion of the meta-analysis is that Cerebrolysin® may have positive effects on cognitive function and global function in patients with mild-moderate vascular dementia, but there is still insufficient evidence to recommend it as a routine treatment for this condition. Further clinical trials in CSVD patients are needed [160].

Folic Acid

Folic acid is a fundamental vitamin in central nervous system development. Its deficiency is associated with high homocysteine levels, which is related to risk of developing depression, dementia and stroke. The Cochrane database meta-analysis included 4 double-blind, controlled trials with participants ranging from healthy subjects to patients with mild-moderate cognitive decline and dementia. The results showed no benefit for improving cognition. One trial showed that treatment with 2 mg folic acid plus 1 mg vitamin B12 daily significantly lowered serum homocysteine level. Because the trials were considered short (35 to 90 days) and specific groups of participants were not subanalysed, further research with longer trials and differentiation of diseases may be necessary to delineate the role of folic acid in vascular dementia [161].

Vitamin B_{12}

The association between baseline vitamin B_{12} level and progression of WML over 2 years of follow-up was studied in 107 patients with first-ever lacunar stroke. The brain MRI assessed the progression of periventricular and deep WML using a visual scale of change. The results showed that vitamin B_{12} level was lower in patients with progression of periventricular WML compared to those without progression, but B_{12} was not associated with progression of deep WML [162].

Because elevated concentrations of homocysteine are associated with CSVD and supplementation with folate and vitamins B_{12} and B_6 reduces plasma homocysteine, a substudy of the vitamins TO Prevent Stroke (VITATOPS) trial assessed if the addition of these supplements could reduce the progression of CSVD. A total of 359 patients with recent stroke or transient ischemic attack were randomly allocated to placebo or B vitamins. Patients underwent brain MRI at randomization and after 2 years to assess the progression of WML and incidence of lacunes. After 2 years of treatment, there were no significant differences in WML volume change and incidence of lacunes between both groups. In a subanalysis of patients with severe CSVD at baseline MRI, B-vitamin supplementation was associated with a significant reduction in WML volume change (0.3 *vs.* 1.7 cm^3; P=0.039). Therefore, it is possible that in this subgroup of patients with recent stroke or transient ischemic attack and severe CSVD B-vitamin supplementation reduces the increase in WML volume [163].

Due to contradictory results, the real benefit of vitamin B_{12} supplementation in patients with CSVD is unclear and further investigation is required.

Novel Approaches For Treatment of Cerebral Small Vessel Disease

Novel therapeutic strategies to reduce the burden of vascular and parenchymatous damage need to be designed. This section summarises some ongoing trials and experimental studies. A comprehensive review of potential new ways for treatment of CSVD was recently published [164].

Ponezumab

Ponezumab (PF-04360365) is a humanized anti-amyloid beta monoclonal antibody designed to treat Alzheimer disease. A phase 2, double-blind, placebo-controlled study will examine the safety and efficacy of ponezumab *versus* placebo in patients diagnosed with probable cerebral amyloid angiopathy following Boston criteria (probability requires clinical data and MRI or CT demostrating multiple lobar/cortical/subcortical hemorrhages or a single hemorrhage with brain siderosis in a patient older than 55 years without other cause of bleeding) without clinical cognitive impairment [165, 166]. The drug will be administered 3 times: day 1, an initial dose of 10 mg/kg; days 30 and 60, a maintenance dose of 7.5mg/kg. Subjects will be followed for 6 months after receiving the last dose of study medication. The primary outcome measures will be the change from baseline to day 2 or day 90 in cerebrovascular reactivity measured by the slope (amplitude over time to peak) from visual task-evoked functional MRI. The secondary outcome measures will be the change from baseline to day 2 or day 90 in cerebrovascular reactivity measured by the time to peak, magnitude, and time to baseline from visual task-evoked functional MRI, and the change from baseline of total plasma amyloid beta species.

Hyperbaric Oxygen

An ongoing trial is currently recruiting patients with CSVD to be treated with 10 hyperbaric oxygen sessions for 1 hour at 2 atmospheres absolute over the course of 2 weeks. The main goal is to assess the internal and cross network connectivity by functional MRI. Secondarily, the change in the National Institute of Health Neurobehavioral scale will be assessed [167].

Tadalafil

Tadalafil is a phosphodiesterase type 5 inhibitor in the vascular smooth muscle cells used to treat erectile dysfunction and pulmonary arterial hypertension. A phase 2, double-blind, placebo-controlled trial will compare the effects of tadalafil (20 mg single dose) versus placebo on deep brain blood flow (measured by MRI-arterial spin labelling), cortical grey matter blood flow, and neuropsychological parameters in patients with clinical and MRI evidence of CSVD. The study may help define if this drug can improve cerebral blood flow and cognition [168].

Fasudil

The blood-brain barrier function is impaired in CSVD. In experimental models of acute stroke, fasudil, a selective rho-kinase inhibitor, increases the integrity of the blood-brain barrier and reduces the small muscle cell proliferation. A multicenter, double-blind, placebo-controlled study was conducted to assess the efficacy and safety of fasudil in 160 patients with less than 48 hours ischemic stroke. Patients received 60 mg fasudil or placebo by intravenous injection over 60 min, twice daily for 14 days. The primary end points were the neurological status at 2 weeks and the clinical outcome 1 month after the onset of symptoms. The patients treated with fasudil showed significantly greater improvements in both neurological functions and clinical outcome. There were no serious adverse events reported in the fasudil group. The authors concluded that fasudil was effective and safe in patients with acute stroke, but there are no specific data for patients with CSVD. Further evaluations in specific stroke categories are needed [169].

Vitamin D

A study was conducted to determine the association between 25-hydroxyvitamin D (25(OH)D) and neuroimaging correlates of CSVD. Lacunes, WML, and CMB were assessed by MRI in 759 consecutive patients with acute ischemic stroke or transient ischemic attack. On bivariate analysis, both 25-nmol/L decrease in 25(OH)D and 25(OH)D deficiency (defined as level $\leq$ 25 nmol/L) were associated with lacunes, severe WML, and CMB. The association remained significant after multivariable adjustment. The authors concluded that 25(OH)D is inversely associated with lacunes, WML, and CMB, suggesting that 25(OH)D is linked to

CSVD. This may justify future trials testing 25(OH)D supplementation to prevent CSVD [170].

Relaxin

Relaxin is a peptide hormone that exerts specific effects on the cardiovascular system and brain, leading to the hypothesis that it may have protective properties in vascular disease. An experimental study investigated the effect of hypertension on the function and structure of cerebral parenchymal arterioles of spontaneously hypertensive Wistar-Kyoto rats. The study tried to determine the effects of relaxin treatment on CSVD during hypertension. The results suggested that relaxin crosses the blood-brain barrier and increases the distensibility of parenchymal arterioles [171].

The information about clinical effects in patients with stroke is limited. A Italian study was performed to demonstrate the efficacy of relaxin on functional recovery of 36 post-stroke patients admitted in a Rehabilitation Unit. Eighteen patients were randomized to relaxin (40 mcg/d) plus rehabilitation and 18 patients (control) underwent only rehabilitation. The variables assessed were the modified Rankin scale, the Functional Independent Measure (FIM), and the Trail Making Test (TMT) at 20 and 40 days. After 20 days there were not differences between the two groups. After 40 days, patients treated with relaxin + rehabilitation showed a significantly better recovery (FIM 96 *vs*. 75; $p=0.001$) and better performance of cognitive functions (TMT 3.5 *vs*. 2; $p=0.002$). The authors concluded that relaxin showed positive effects on recovery of stroke patients [172].

CONCLUSIONS

The prevalence of CSVD is extremely high, and due to its association with aging, it will probably be greater in the future. Although CSVD is a spectrum of disorders, the types 1 and 2 of CSVD are the most frequent. Clinically, type 1 CSVD is related to cognitive impairment, dementia, progressive motor disturbances, and stroke.

The *in vivo* diagnosis is based on MRI findings, both ischaemic and haemorrhagic. Biochemical parameters assessed in plasma and CSF and resistance indexes on transcranial Doppler could be useful, but their role is not defined yet.

The strategy for management of patients with CSVD implies preventive therapies to control classical vascular risk factors and symptomatic treatment of dementia, mood disorders, and motor disability. However, adequate drugs and the optimal goals for control of risk factors are not defined yet. Different approaches to reduce the progression of brain damage due to small vessel disease are under research.

CONFLICT OF INTEREST

The author confirms that he has no conflict of interest to declare for this publication.

ACKNOWLEDGEMENTS

I thank my colleagues Dr. Joana Infante (Health Sciences Faculty, Beira Interior University), for her valuable commentaries and grammar review of the final text, and Dr. Javier Muñoz (Health Sciences Faculty, Beira Interior University), for the excellent and high quality images gived up.

REFERENCES

[1] Thompson CS, Hakim AM. Living beyond our physiological means: small vessel disease of the brain is an expression of a systemic failure in arteriolar function: a unifying hypothesis. Stroke 2009; 40(5): e322-30.
[http://dx.doi.org/10.1161/STROKEAHA.108.542266] [PMID: 19228835]

[2] Vermeer SE, Longstreth WT Jr, Koudstaal PJ. Silent brain infarcts: a systematic review. Lancet Neurol 2007; 6(7): 611-9.
[http://dx.doi.org/10.1016/S1474-4422(07)70170-9] [PMID: 17582361]

[3] Vermeer SE, Prins ND, den Heijer T, Hofman A, Koudstaal PJ, Breteler MM. Silent brain infarcts and the risk of dementia and cognitive decline. N Engl J Med 2003; 348(13): 1215-22.
[http://dx.doi.org/10.1056/NEJMoa022066] [PMID: 12660385]

[4] Carpenter M, Sutin J. Blood supply of the central nervous system. Human Neuroanatomy. 8th ed. Baltimore: Williams & Wilkins 1983; pp. 707-41.

[5] Reina-De La Torre F, Rodríguez-Baeza A, Sahuquillo-Barris J. Morphological characteristics and distribution pattern of the arterial vessels in human cerebral cortex: a scanning electron microscope study. Anat Rec 1998; 251(1): 87-96.
[http://dx.doi.org/10.1002/(SICI)1097-0185(199805)251:1<87::AID-AR14>3.0.CO;2-7] [PMID: 9605225]

[6] Rowbotham GF, Little E. Circulations of the cerebral hemispheres. Br J Surg 1965; 52: 8-21. [http://dx.doi.org/10.1002/bjs.1800520104] [PMID: 14251345]

[7] Rodriguez-Baeza A, Reina-De La Torre F, Ortega-Sanchez M, Sahuquillo-Barris J. Perivascular structures in corrosion casts of the human central nervous system: a confocal laser and scanning electron microscope study. Anat Rec 1998; 252(2): 176-84. [http://dx.doi.org/10.1002/(SICI)1097-0185(199810)252:2<176::AID-AR3>3.0.CO;2-1] [PMID: 9776072]

[8] Ferrer I, Kaste M, Kalimo H. Vascular diseases. Greenfield's Neuropathology. 8th ed. London: Hodder Arnold 2008; pp. 121-241.

[9] Iadecola C. Intrinsic signals and functional brain mapping: caution, blood vessels at work. Cereb Cortex 2002; 12(3): 223-4. [http://dx.doi.org/10.1093/cercor/12.3.223] [PMID: 11839596]

[10] Nonaka H, Akima M, Hatori T, Nagayama T, Zhang Z, Ihara F. The microvasculature of the human cerebellar meninges. Acta Neuropathol 2002; 104(6): 608-14. [PMID: 12410382]

[11] Nonaka H, Akima M, Nagayama T, Hatori T, Zhang Z, Ihara F. Microvasculature of the human cerebral meninges. Neuropathology 2003; 23(2): 129-35. [http://dx.doi.org/10.1046/j.1440-1789.2003.00487.x] [PMID: 12777101]

[12] Duvernoy HM, Delon S, Vannson JL. Cortical blood vessels of the human brain. Brain Res Bull 1981; 7(5): 519-79. [http://dx.doi.org/10.1016/0361-9230(81)90007-1] [PMID: 7317796]

[13] Pantoni L. Cerebral small vessel disease: from pathogenesis and clinical characteristics to therapeutic challenges. Lancet Neurol 2010; 9(7): 689-701. [http://dx.doi.org/10.1016/S1474-4422(10)70104-6] [PMID: 20610345]

[14] Thal DR, Ghebremedhin E, Orantes M, Wiestler OD. Vascular pathology in Alzheimer disease: correlation of cerebral amyloid angiopathy and arteriosclerosis/lipohyalinosis with cognitive decline. J Neuropathol Exp Neurol 2003; 62(12): 1287-301. [http://dx.doi.org/10.1093/jnen/62.12.1287] [PMID: 14692704]

[15] Grinberg LT, Thal DR. Vascular pathology in the aged human brain. Acta Neuropathol 2010; 119(3): 277-90. [http://dx.doi.org/10.1007/s00401-010-0652-7] [PMID: 20155424]

[16] Fisher CM. Pathological observations in hypertensive cerebral hemorrhage. J Neuropathol Exp Neurol 1971; 30(3): 536-50. [http://dx.doi.org/10.1097/00005072-197107000-00015] [PMID: 4105427]

[17] Fisher CM. Cerebral miliary aneurysms in hypertension. Am J Pathol 1972; 66(2): 313-30. [PMID: 5009976]

[18] Fisher CM. Lacunar infarcts: a review. Cerebrovasc Dis 1991; 1: 311-20. [http://dx.doi.org/10.1159/000108861]

[19] Rosenblum WI. Miliary aneurysms and "fibrinoid" degeneration of cerebral blood vessels. Hum Pathol 1977; 8(2): 133-9.

[http://dx.doi.org/10.1016/S0046-8177(77)80076-2] [PMID: 856713]

[20] Fazekas F, Kleinert R, Offenbacher H, *et al.* Pathologic correlates of incidental MRI white matter signal hyperintensities. Neurology 1993; 43(9): 1683-9. [http://dx.doi.org/10.1212/WNL.43.9.1683] [PMID: 8414012]

[21] Greenberg SM, Vernooij MW, Cordonnier C, *et al.* Cerebral microbleeds: a guide to detection and interpretation. Lancet Neurol 2009; 8(2): 165-74. [http://dx.doi.org/10.1016/S1474-4422(09)70013-4] [PMID: 19161908]

[22] Doubal FN, MacLullich AM, Ferguson KJ, Dennis MS, Wardlaw JM. Enlarged perivascular spaces on MRI are a feature of cerebral small vessel disease. Stroke 2010; 41(3): 450-4. [http://dx.doi.org/10.1161/STROKEAHA.109.564914] [PMID: 20056930]

[23] Vinters HV. Cerebral amyloid angiopathy. A critical review. Stroke 1987; 18(2): 311-24. [http://dx.doi.org/10.1161/01.STR.18.2.311] [PMID: 3551211]

[24] Vinters HV, Gilbert JJ. Cerebral amyloid angiopathy: incidence and complications in the aging brain. II. The distribution of amyloid vascular changes. Stroke 1983; 14(6): 924-8. [http://dx.doi.org/10.1161/01.STR.14.6.924] [PMID: 6658996]

[25] Vermeer SE, Longstreth WT Jr, Koudstaal PJ. Silent brain infarcts: a systematic review. Lancet Neurol 2007; 6(7): 611-9. [http://dx.doi.org/10.1016/S1474-4422(07)70170-9] [PMID: 17582361]

[26] Vermeer SE, Den Heijer T, Koudstaal PJ, Oudkerk M, Hofman A, Breteler MM. Incidence and risk factors of silent brain infarcts in the population-based Rotterdam Scan Study. Stroke 2003; 34(2): 392-6. [http://dx.doi.org/10.1161/01.STR.0000052631.98405.15] [PMID: 12574548]

[27] Gan R, Sacco RL, Kargman DE, Roberts JK, Boden-Albala B, Gu Q. Testing the validity of the lacunar hypothesis: the Northern Manhattan Stroke Study experience. Neurology 1997; 48(5): 1204-11. [http://dx.doi.org/10.1212/WNL.48.5.1204] [PMID: 9153444]

[28] Arboix A, Massons J, García-Eroles L, Targa C, Comes E, Parra O. Clinical predictors of lacunar syndrome not due to lacunar infarction. BMC Neurol 2010; 10: 31. [http://dx.doi.org/10.1186/1471-2377-10-31] [PMID: 20482763]

[29] Arboix A, García-Eroles L, Massons J, Oliveres M, Targa C. Hemorrhagic lacunar stroke. Cerebrovasc Dis 2000; 10(3): 229-34. [http://dx.doi.org/10.1159/000016061] [PMID: 10773650]

[30] Anzalone N, Landi G. Non ischaemic causes of lacunar syndromes: prevalence and clinical findings. J Neurol Neurosurg Psychiatry 1989; 52(10): 1188-90. [http://dx.doi.org/10.1136/jnnp.52.10.1188] [PMID: 2795047]

[31] Donnan GA, Norrving B. Lacunes and lacunar syndromes. Handb Clin Neurol 2009; 93: 559-75. [http://dx.doi.org/10.1016/S0072-9752(08)93027-X] [PMID: 18804668]

[32] Arboix A, López-Grau M, Casasnovas C, García-Eroles L, Massons J, Balcells M. Clinical study of 39 patients with atypical lacunar syndrome. J Neurol Neurosurg Psychiatry 2006; 77(3): 381-4. [http://dx.doi.org/10.1136/jnnp.2005.071860] [PMID: 16484649]

[33] Bamford J, Sandercock P, Jones L, Warlow C. The natural history of lacunar infarction: the Oxfordshire Community Stroke Project. Stroke 1987; 18(3): 545-51. [http://dx.doi.org/10.1161/01.STR.18.3.545] [PMID: 3590244]

[34] Wright CB, Festa JR, Paik MC, *et al.* White matter hyperintensities and subclinical infarction: associations with psychomotor speed and cognitive flexibility. Stroke 2008; 39(3): 800-5. [http://dx.doi.org/10.1161/STROKEAHA.107.484147] [PMID: 18258844]

[35] Carey CL, Kramer JH, Josephson SA, *et al.* Subcortical lacunes are associated with executive dysfunction in cognitively normal elderly. Stroke 2008; 39(2): 397-402. [http://dx.doi.org/10.1161/STROKEAHA.107.491795] [PMID: 18096844]

[36] Tatemichi TK, Desmond DW, Prohovnik I, *et al.* Confusion and memory loss from capsular genu infarction: a thalamocortical disconnection syndrome? Neurology 1992; 42(10): 1966-79. [http://dx.doi.org/10.1212/WNL.42.10.1966] [PMID: 1407580]

[37] Wardlaw JM. Differing risk factors and outcomes in ischemic stroke subtypes: focus on lacunar stroke. Future Neurol 2011; 6: 201-22. [http://dx.doi.org/10.2217/fnl.11.1]

[38] Benisty S, Gouw AA, Porcher R, *et al.* Location of lacunar infarcts correlates with cognition in a sample of non-disabled subjects with age-related white-matter changes: the LADIS study. J Neurol Neurosurg Psychiatry 2009; 80(5): 478-83. [http://dx.doi.org/10.1136/jnnp.2008.160440] [PMID: 19211595]

[39] Miyao S, Takano A, Teramoto J, Takahashi A. Leukoaraiosis in relation to prognosis for patients with lacunar infarction. Stroke 1992; 23(10): 1434-8. [http://dx.doi.org/10.1161/01.STR.23.10.1434] [PMID: 1412580]

[40] Samuelsson M, Söderfeldt B, Olsson GB. Functional outcome in patients with lacunar infarction. Stroke 1996; 27(5): 842-6. [http://dx.doi.org/10.1161/01.STR.27.5.842] [PMID: 8623103]

[41] Vermeer SE, Prins ND, den Heijer T, Hofman A, Koudstaal PJ, Breteler MM. Silent brain infarcts and the risk of dementia and cognitive decline. N Engl J Med 2003; 348(13): 1215-22. [http://dx.doi.org/10.1056/NEJMoa022066] [PMID: 12660385]

[42] Hachinski VC, Potter P, Merskey H. Leuko-araiosis. Arch Neurol 1987; 44(1): 21-3. [http://dx.doi.org/10.1001/archneur.1987.00520130013009] [PMID: 3800716]

[43] de Leeuw FE, de Groot JC, Achten E, *et al.* Prevalence of cerebral white matter lesions in elderly people: a population based magnetic resonance imaging study. The Rotterdam Scan Study. J Neurol Neurosurg Psychiatry 2001; 70(1): 9-14. [http://dx.doi.org/10.1136/jnnp.70.1.9] [PMID: 11118240]

[44] Pullicino P, Ostrow P, Miller L, Snyder W, Munschauer F. Pontine ischemic rarefaction. Ann Neurol 1995; 37(4): 460-6. [http://dx.doi.org/10.1002/ana.410370408] [PMID: 7717682]

[45] Pantoni L, Poggesi A, Inzitari D. The relation between white-matter lesions and cognition. Curr Opin Neurol 2007; 20(4): 390-7. [http://dx.doi.org/10.1097/WCO.0b013e328172d661] [PMID: 17620872]

[46] Pantoni L. Leukoaraiosis: from an ancient term to an actual marker of poor prognosis. Stroke 2008; 39(5): 1401-3.
[http://dx.doi.org/10.1161/STROKEAHA.107.505602] [PMID: 18340098]

[47] Frisoni GB, Galluzzi S, Pantoni L, Filippi M. The effect on cognition of white matter lesions in the elderly: small but detectable. Nat Clin Pract Neurol 2007; 3: 620-7.
[http://dx.doi.org/10.1038/ncpneuro0638] [PMID: 17982432]

[48] Wright CB, Festa JR, Paik MC, *et al.* White matter hyperintensities and subclinical infarction: associations with psychomotor speed and cognitive flexibility. Stroke 2008; 39(3): 800-5.
[http://dx.doi.org/10.1161/STROKEAHA.107.484147] [PMID: 18258844]

[49] Carey CL, Kramer JH, Josephson SA, *et al.* Subcortical lacunes are associated with executive dysfunction in cognitively normal elderly. Stroke 2008; 39(2): 397-402.
[http://dx.doi.org/10.1161/STROKEAHA.107.491795] [PMID: 18096844]

[50] O'Sullivan M, Morris RG, Huckstep B, Jones DK, Williams SC, Markus HS. Diffusion tensor MRI correlates with executive dysfunction in patients with ischaemic leukoaraiosis. J Neurol Neurosurg Psychiatry 2004; 75(3): 441-7.
[http://dx.doi.org/10.1136/jnnp.2003.014910] [PMID: 14966162]

[51] Nitkunan A, Barrick TR, Charlton RA, Clark CA, Markus HS. Multimodal MRI in cerebral small vessel disease: its relationship with cognition and sensitivity to change over time. Stroke 2008; 39(7): 1999-2005.
[http://dx.doi.org/10.1161/STROKEAHA.107.507475] [PMID: 18436880]

[52] Kase CS. Vascular diseases of the nervous system. Intracerebral hemorrhage. In: Daroff RB, Fenichel GM, Jankovic J, Manzziotta JC, Eds. Bradley's Neurology in clinical practice. 6th ed. Philadelphia: Elsevier 2012; pp. 1054-69.
[http://dx.doi.org/10.1016/B978-1-4377-0434-1.00063-3]

[53] Xi G, Keep RF, Hoff JT. Mechanisms of brain injury after intracerebral haemorrhage. Lancet Neurol 2006; 5(1): 53-63.
[http://dx.doi.org/10.1016/S1474-4422(05)70283-0] [PMID: 16361023]

[54] Koennecke HC. Cerebral microbleeds on MRI: prevalence, associations, and potential clinical implications. Neurology 2006; 66(2): 165-71.
[http://dx.doi.org/10.1212/01.wnl.0000194266.55694.1e] [PMID: 16434647]

[55] Tsushima Y, Tanizaki Y, Aoki J, Endo K. MR detection of microhemorrhages in neurologically healthy adults. Neuroradiology 2002; 44(1): 31-6.
[http://dx.doi.org/10.1007/s002340100649] [PMID: 11942497]

[56] Blitstein MK, Tung GA. MRI of cerebral microhemorrhages. AJR Am J Roentgenol 2007; 189(3): 720-5.
[http://dx.doi.org/10.2214/AJR.07.2249] [PMID: 17715122]

[57] Kato H, Izumiyama M, Izumiyama K, Takahashi A, Itoyama Y. Silent cerebral microbleeds on T2*-weighted MRI: correlation with stroke subtype, stroke recurrence, and leukoaraiosis. Stroke 2002; 33(6): 1536-40.
[http://dx.doi.org/10.1161/01.STR.0000018012.65108.86] [PMID: 12052987]

[58] Vernooij MW, van der Lugt A, Ikram MA, *et al.* Prevalence and risk factors of cerebral microbleeds: the Rotterdam Scan Study. Neurology 2008; 70(14): 1208-14. [http://dx.doi.org/10.1212/01.wnl.0000307750.41970.d9] [PMID: 18378884]

[59] Cordonnier C, Al-Shahi Salman R, Wardlaw J. Spontaneous brain microbleeds: systematic review, subgroup analyses and standards for study design and reporting. Brain 2007; 130(Pt 8): 1988-2003. [http://dx.doi.org/10.1093/brain/awl387] [PMID: 17322562]

[60] Gregoire SM, Brown MM, Kallis C, Jäger HR, Yousry TA, Werring DJ. MRI detection of new microbleeds in patients with ischemic stroke: five-year cohort follow-up study. Stroke 2010; 41(1): 184-6. [http://dx.doi.org/10.1161/STROKEAHA.109.568469] [PMID: 19892991]

[61] Yakushiji Y, Nishiyama M, Yakushiji S, *et al.* Brain microbleeds and global cognitive function in adults without neurological disorder. Stroke 2008; 39(12): 3323-8. [http://dx.doi.org/10.1161/STROKEAHA.108.516112] [PMID: 18688000]

[62] Werring DJ, Frazer DW, Coward LJ, *et al.* Cognitive dysfunction in patients with cerebral microbleeds on T2*-weighted gradient-echo MRI. Brain 2004; 127(Pt 10): 2265-75. [http://dx.doi.org/10.1093/brain/awh253] [PMID: 15282216]

[63] Schmidt R, Scheltens P, Erkinjuntti T, *et al.* White matter lesion progression: a surrogate endpoint for trials in cerebral small-vessel disease. Neurology 2004; 63(1): 139-44. [http://dx.doi.org/10.1212/01.WNL.0000132635.75819.E5] [PMID: 15249623]

[64] Schmidt R, Enzinger C, Ropele S, Schmidt H, Fazekas F. Progression of cerebral white matter lesions: 6-year results of the Austrian Stroke Prevention Study. Lancet 2003; 361(9374): 2046-8. [http://dx.doi.org/10.1016/S0140-6736(03)13616-1] [PMID: 12814718]

[65] Longstreth WT Jr, Arnold AM, Beauchamp NJ Jr, *et al.* Incidence, manifestations, and predictors of worsening white matter on serial cranial magnetic resonance imaging in the elderly: the Cardiovascular Health Study. Stroke 2005; 36(1): 56-61. [http://dx.doi.org/10.1161/01.STR.0000149625.99732.69] [PMID: 15569873]

[66] Patel B, Markus HS. Magnetic resonance imaging in cerebral small vessel disease and its use as a surrogate disease marker. Int J Stroke 2011; 6(1): 47-59. [http://dx.doi.org/10.1111/j.1747-4949.2010.00552.x] [PMID: 21205241]

[67] El-Koussy M, Schroth G, Brekenfeld C, Arnold M. Imaging of acute ischemic stroke. Eur Neurol 2014; 72(5-6): 309-16. [http://dx.doi.org/10.1159/000362719] [PMID: 25323674]

[68] Viswanathan A, Godin O, Jouvent E, *et al.* Impact of MRI markers in subcortical vascular dementia: a multi-modal analysis in CADASIL. Neurobiol Aging 2010; 31(9): 1629-36. [http://dx.doi.org/10.1016/j.neurobiolaging.2008.09.001] [PMID: 18926602]

[69] Sabri O, Ringelstein EB, Hellwig D, *et al.* Neuropsychological impairment correlates with hypoperfusion and hypometabolism but not with severity of white matter lesions on MRI in patients with cerebral microangiopathy. Stroke 1999; 30(3): 556-66. [http://dx.doi.org/10.1161/01.STR.30.3.556] [PMID: 10066852]

[70] Firbank MJ, Wiseman RM, Burton EJ, Saxby BK, O'Brien JT, Ford GA. Brain atrophy and white

matter hyperintensity change in older adults and relationship to blood pressure. Brain atrophy, WMH change and blood pressure. J Neurol 2007; 254(6): 713-21. [http://dx.doi.org/10.1007/s00415-006-0238-4] [PMID: 17446997]

[71] Jeerakathil T, Wolf PA, Beiser A, *et al.* Stroke risk profile predicts white matter hyperintensity volume: the Framingham Study. Stroke 2004; 35(8): 1857-61. [http://dx.doi.org/10.1161/01.STR.0000135226.53499.85] [PMID: 15218158]

[72] Bradley WG Jr. MR appearance of hemorrhage in the brain. Radiology 1993; 189(1): 15-26. [http://dx.doi.org/10.1148/radiology.189.1.8372185] [PMID: 8372185]

[73] Werring DJ. Cerebral microbleeds: clinical and pathophysiological significance. J Neuroimaging 2007; 17(3): 193-203. [http://dx.doi.org/10.1111/j.1552-6569.2006.00070.x] [PMID: 17608904]

[74] Vernooij MW, Ikram MA, Wielopolski PA, Krestin GP, Breteler MM, van der Lugt A. Cerebral microbleeds: accelerated 3D T2*-weighted GRE MR imaging versus conventional 2D T2*-weighted GRE MR imaging for detection. Radiology 2008; 248(1): 272-7. [http://dx.doi.org/10.1148/radiol.2481071158] [PMID: 18490493]

[75] Rouhl RP, van Oostenbrugge RJ, Knottnerus IL, Staals JE, Lodder J. Virchow-Robin spaces relate to cerebral small vessel disease severity. J Neurol 2008; 255(5): 692-6. [http://dx.doi.org/10.1007/s00415-008-0777-y] [PMID: 18286319]

[76] van Swieten JC, van den Hout JH, van Ketel BA, Hijdra A, Wokke JH, van Gijn J. Periventricular lesions in the white matter on magnetic resonance imaging in the elderly. A morphometric correlation with arteriolosclerosis and dilated perivascular spaces. Brain 1991; 114(Pt 2): 761-74. [http://dx.doi.org/10.1093/brain/114.2.761] [PMID: 2043948]

[77] Bokura H, Kobayashi S, Yamaguchi S. Distinguishing silent lacunar infarction from enlarged Virchow-Robin spaces: a magnetic resonance imaging and pathological study. J Neurol 1998; 245(2): 116-22. [http://dx.doi.org/10.1007/s004150050189] [PMID: 9507419]

[78] Maclullich AM, Wardlaw JM, Ferguson KJ, Starr JM, Seckl JR, Deary IJ. Enlarged perivascular spaces are associated with cognitive function in healthy elderly men. J Neurol Neurosurg Psychiatry 2004; 75(11): 1519-23. [http://dx.doi.org/10.1136/jnnp.2003.030858] [PMID: 15489380]

[79] Enzinger C, Fazekas F, Matthews PM, *et al.* Risk factors for progression of brain atrophy in aging: six-year follow-up of normal subjects. Neurology 2005; 64(10): 1704-11. [http://dx.doi.org/10.1212/01.WNL.0000161871.83614.BB] [PMID: 15911795]

[80] Smith SM, Rao A, De Stefano N, *et al.* Longitudinal and cross-sectional analysis of atrophy in Alzheimer's disease: cross-validation of BSI, SIENA and SIENAX. Neuroimage 2007; 36(4): 1200-6. [http://dx.doi.org/10.1016/j.neuroimage.2007.04.035] [PMID: 17537648]

[81] Christiansen P, Larsson HB, Thomsen C, Wieslander SB, Henriksen O. Age dependent white matter lesions and brain volume changes in healthy volunteers. Acta Radiol 1994; 35(2): 117-22. [http://dx.doi.org/10.3109/02841859409172347] [PMID: 8172734]

[82] Wiseman RM, Saxby BK, Burton EJ, Barber R, Ford GA, O'Brien JT. Hippocampal atrophy, whole

brain volume, and white matter lesions in older hypertensive subjects. Neurology 2004; 63(10): 1892-7.
[http://dx.doi.org/10.1212/01.WNL.0000144280.59178.78] [PMID: 15557507]

[83] Bouvy WH, Zwanenburg JJ, Reinink R, *et al.* Perivascular spaces on 7 Tesla brain MRI are related to markers of small vessel disease but not to age or cardiovascular risk factors. J Cereb Blood Flow Metab 2016; 6

[84] Yao H, Sadoshima S, Kuwabara Y, Ichiya Y, Fujishima M. Cerebral blood flow and oxygen metabolism in patients with vascular dementia of the Binswanger type. Stroke 1990; 21(12): 1694-9.
[http://dx.doi.org/10.1161/01.STR.21.12.1694] [PMID: 2264076]

[85] De Reuck JL. Evidence for chronic ischaemia in the pathogenesis of vascular dementia: from neuroPATH to neuroPET. Acta Neurol Belg 1996; 96(3): 228-31.
[PMID: 8886109]

[86] Markus HS, Lythgoe DJ, Ostegaard L, O'Sullivan M, Williams SC. Reduced cerebral blood flow in white matter in ischaemic leukoaraiosis demonstrated using quantitative exogenous contrast based perfusion MRI. J Neurol Neurosurg Psychiatry 2000; 69(1): 48-53.
[http://dx.doi.org/10.1136/jnnp.69.1.48] [PMID: 10864603]

[87] Starr JM, Wardlaw J, Ferguson K, MacLullich A, Deary IJ, Marshall I. Increased blood-brain barrier permeability in type II diabetes demonstrated by gadolinium magnetic resonance imaging. J Neurol Neurosurg Psychiatry 2003; 74(1): 70-6.
[http://dx.doi.org/10.1136/jnnp.74.1.70] [PMID: 12486269]

[88] Wardlaw JM, Farrall A, Armitage PA, *et al.* Changes in background blood-brain barrier integrity between lacunar and cortical ischemic stroke subtypes. Stroke 2008; 39(4): 1327-32.
[http://dx.doi.org/10.1161/STROKEAHA.107.500124] [PMID: 18309161]

[89] Topakian R, Barrick TR, Howe FA, Markus HS. Blood-brain barrier permeability is increased in normal-appearing white matter in patients with lacunar stroke and leucoaraiosis. J Neurol Neurosurg Psychiatry 2010; 81(2): 192-7.
[http://dx.doi.org/10.1136/jnnp.2009.172072] [PMID: 19710048]

[90] Wardlaw JM, Sandercock PA, Dennis MS, Starr J. Is breakdown of the blood-brain barrier responsible for lacunar stroke, leukoaraiosis, and dementia? Stroke 2003; 34(3): 806-12.
[http://dx.doi.org/10.1161/01.STR.0000058480.77236.B3] [PMID: 12624314]

[91] Blood-brain barrier quantification in cerebral small vessel disease. Available from: https://www.clinicaltrials.gov/ct2/show/NCT02033291?titles=small+vessel+disease&rank=2 2015.

[92] Jones DK, Lythgoe D, Horsfield MA, Simmons A, Williams SC, Markus HS. Characterization of white matter damage in ischemic leukoaraiosis with diffusion tensor MRI. Stroke 1999; 30(2): 393-7.
[http://dx.doi.org/10.1161/01.STR.30.2.393] [PMID: 9933277]

[93] O'Sullivan M, Summers PE, Jones DK, Jarosz JM, Williams SC, Markus HS. Normal-appearing white matter in ischemic leukoaraiosis: a diffusion tensor MRI study. Neurology 2001; 57(12): 2307-10.
[http://dx.doi.org/10.1212/WNL.57.12.2307] [PMID: 11756617]

[94] Zeestraten EA, Benjamin P, Lambert C, *et al.* Application of diffusion tensor imaging parameters to detect change in longitudinal studies in cerebral small vessel disease. PLoS One 2016; 11(1):

e0147836.
[http://dx.doi.org/10.1371/journal.pone.0147836] [PMID: 26808982]

[95] Benjamin P, Zeestraten E, Lambert C, *et al.* Progression of MRI markers in cerebral small vessel disease: Sample size considerations for clinical trials. J Cereb Blood Flow Metab 2016; 36(1): 228-40. [PMID: 26036939]

[96] Cook IA, Leuchter AF, Morgan ML, *et al.* Cognitive and physiologic correlates of subclinical structural brain disease in elderly healthy control subjects. Arch Neurol 2002; 59(10): 1612-20.
[http://dx.doi.org/10.1001/archneur.59.10.1612] [PMID: 12374500]

[97] Charlton RA, Barrick TR, McIntyre DJ, *et al.* White matter damage on diffusion tensor imaging correlates with age-related cognitive decline. Neurology 2006; 66(2): 217-22.
[http://dx.doi.org/10.1212/01.wnl.0000194256.15247.83] [PMID: 16434657]

[98] Smith SM, Jenkinson M, Johansen-Berg H, *et al.* Tract-based spatial statistics: voxelwise analysis of multi-subject diffusion data. Neuroimage 2006; 31(4): 1487-505.
[http://dx.doi.org/10.1016/j.neuroimage.2006.02.024] [PMID: 16624579]

[99] Schiavone F, Charlton RA, Barrick TR, Morris RG, Markus HS. Imaging age-related cognitive decline: A comparison of diffusion tensor and magnetization transfer MRI. J Magn Reson Imaging 2009; 29(1): 23-30.
[http://dx.doi.org/10.1002/jmri.21572] [PMID: 19097099]

[100] Seiler S, Pirpamer L, Hofer E, *et al.* Magnetization transfer ratio relates to cognitive impairment in normal elderly. Front Aging Neurosci 2014; 6: 263.
[http://dx.doi.org/10.3389/fnagi.2014.00263] [PMID: 25309438]

[101] O'Sullivan M. Imaging small vessel disease: lesion topography, networks, and cognitive deficits investigated with MRI. Stroke 2010; 41(10) (Suppl.): S154-8.
[http://dx.doi.org/10.1161/STROKEAHA.110.595314] [PMID: 20876494]

[102] Bastin ME, Clayden JD, Pattie A, Gerrish IF, Wardlaw JM, Deary IJ. Diffusion tensor and magnetization transfer MRI measurements of periventricular white matter hyperintensities in old age. Neurobiol Aging 2009; 30(1): 125-36.
[http://dx.doi.org/10.1016/j.neurobiolaging.2007.05.013] [PMID: 17624630]

[103] Lee KY, Sohn YH, Baik JS, Kim GW, Kim JS. Arterial pulsatility as an index of cerebral microangiopathy in diabetes. Stroke 2000; 31(5): 1111-5.
[http://dx.doi.org/10.1161/01.STR.31.5.1111] [PMID: 10797173]

[104] Ghorbani A, Ahmadi MJ, Shemshaki H. The value of transcranial Doppler derived pulsatility index for diagnosing cerebral small-vessel disease. Adv Biomed Res 2015; 4: 54.
[http://dx.doi.org/10.4103/2277-9175.151574] [PMID: 25802823]

[105] Mok V, Ding D, Fu J, *et al.* Transcranial Doppler ultrasound for screening cerebral small vessel disease: a community study. Stroke 2012; 43(10): 2791-3.
[http://dx.doi.org/10.1161/STROKEAHA.112.665711] [PMID: 22949475]

[106] Del Brutto OH, Mera RM, Andrade MdeL, Castillo PR, Zambrano M, Nader JA. Disappointing reliability of pulsatility indices to identify candidates for magnetic resonance imaging screening in population-based studies assessing prevalence of cerebral small vessel disease. J Neurosci Rural Pract

2015; 6(3): 336-8.
[http://dx.doi.org/10.4103/0976-3147.158760] [PMID: 26167015]

[107] Birns J, Jarosz J, Markus HS, Kalra L. Cerebrovascular reactivity and dynamic autoregulation in ischaemic subcortical white matter disease. J Neurol Neurosurg Psychiatry 2009; 80(10): 1093-8. [http://dx.doi.org/10.1136/jnnp.2009.174607] [PMID: 19535355]

[108] Hermann P, Romero C, Schmidt C, Reis C, Zerr I. CSF biomarkers and neuropsychological profiles in patients with cerebral small-vessel disease. PLoS One 2014; 9(8): e105000. [http://dx.doi.org/10.1371/journal.pone.0105000] [PMID: 25147945]

[109] Fornage M, Chiang YA, O'Meara ES, *et al.* Biomarkers of Inflammation and MRI-Defined Small Vessel Disease of the Brain: The Cardiovascular Health Study. Stroke 2008; 39(7): 1952-9. [http://dx.doi.org/10.1161/STROKEAHA.107.508135] [PMID: 18436879]

[110] Wiseman SJ, Doubal FN, Chappell FM, *et al.* Plasma biomarkers of inflammation, endothelial function and hemostasis in cerebral small vessel Disease. Cerebrovasc Dis 2015; 40(3-4): 157-64. [http://dx.doi.org/10.1159/000438494] [PMID: 26279056]

[111] Agarwal I, Arnold A, Glazer NL, *et al.* Fibrosis-related biomarkers and large and small vessel disease: the Cardiovascular Health Study. Atherosclerosis 2015; 239(2): 539-46. [http://dx.doi.org/10.1016/j.atherosclerosis.2015.02.020] [PMID: 25725316]

[112] Gao Q, Fan Y, Mu LY, Ma L, Song ZQ, Zhang YN. S100B and ADMA in cerebral small vessel disease and cognitive dysfunction. J Neurol Sci 2015; 354(1-2): 27-32. [http://dx.doi.org/10.1016/j.jns.2015.04.031] [PMID: 25990800]

[113] Lavallée PC, Labreuche J, Faille D, *et al.* Circulating markers of endothelial dysfunction and platelet activation in patients with severe symptomatic cerebral small vessel disease. Cerebrovasc Dis 2013; 36(2): 131-8.
[http://dx.doi.org/10.1159/000353671] [PMID: 24029712]

[114] Cuadrado-Godia E, Ois A, Garcia-Ramallo E, *et al.* Biomarkers to predict clinical progression in small vessel disease strokes: prognostic role of albuminuria and oxidized LDL cholesterol. Atherosclerosis 2011; 219(1): 368-72.
[http://dx.doi.org/10.1016/j.atherosclerosis.2011.07.114] [PMID: 21862014]

[115] Adams HP Jr, del Zoppo G, Alberts MJ, *et al.* American Heart Association/American Stroke Association Clinical Cardiology Council; American Heart Association/American Stroke Association Cardiovascular Radiology and Intervention Council; Atherosclerotic Peripheral Vascular Disease Working Group; Quality of Care Outcomes in Research Interdisciplinary Working Group. Guidelines for the early management of adults with ischemic stroke: a guideline from the American Heart Association/American Stroke Association Stroke Council, Clinical Cardiology Council, Cardiovascular Radiology and Intervention Council, and the Atherosclerotic Peripheral Vascular Disease and Quality of Care Outcomes in Research Interdisciplinary Working Groups: The American Academy of Neurology affirms the value of this guideline as an educational tool for neurologists. Circulation 2007; 115: 478-534.
[http://dx.doi.org/10.1161/CIRCULATIONAHA.107.181486]

[116] The National Institute of Neurological Disorders and Stroke rtPA Stroke Study Group. Tissue plasminogen activator for acute ischemic stroke. N Engl J Med 1995; 333: 1581-7.

[http://dx.doi.org/10.1056/NEJM199512143332401] [PMID: 7477192]

[117] Neumann-Haefelin T, Hoelig S, Berkefeld J, *et al.* Leukoaraiosis is a risk factor for symptomatic intracerebral hemorrhage after thrombolysis for acute stroke. Stroke 2006; 37(10): 2463-6. [http://dx.doi.org/10.1161/01.STR.0000239321.53203.ea] [PMID: 16931786]

[118] Palumbo V, Boulanger JM, Hill MD, Inzitari D, Buchan AM. Leukoaraiosis and intracerebral hemorrhage after thrombolysis in acute stroke. Neurology 2007; 68(13): 1020-4. [http://dx.doi.org/10.1212/01.wnl.0000257817.29883.48] [PMID: 17389306]

[119] Pantoni L, Fierini F, Poggesi A. Thrombolysis in acute stroke patients with cerebral small vessel disease. Cerebrovasc Dis 2014; 37(1): 5-13. [http://dx.doi.org/10.1159/000356796] [PMID: 24355873]

[120] Gorter JW. Major bleeding during anticoagulation after cerebral ischemia: patterns and risk factors. Stroke Prevention In Reversible Ischemia Trial (SPIRIT). European Atrial Fibrillation Trial (EAFT) study groups. Neurology 1999; 53(6): 1319-27. [http://dx.doi.org/10.1212/WNL.53.6.1319] [PMID: 10522891]

[121] Smith EE, Rosand J, Knudsen KA, Hylek EM, Greenberg SM. Leukoaraiosis is associated with warfarin-related hemorrhage following ischemic stroke. Neurology 2002; 59(2): 193-7. [http://dx.doi.org/10.1212/WNL.59.2.193] [PMID: 12136056]

[122] Saito T, Kawamura Y, Sato N, *et al.* Non-vitamin k antagonist oral anticoagulants do not increase cerebral microbleeds. J Stroke Cerebrovasc Dis 2015; 24(6): 1373-7. [http://dx.doi.org/10.1016/j.jstrokecerebrovasdis.2015.02.018] [PMID: 25847305]

[123] Streifler JY, Eliasziw M, Benavente OR, *et al.* Prognostic importance of leukoaraiosis in patients with symptomatic internal carotid artery stenosis. Stroke 2002; 33(6): 1651-5. [http://dx.doi.org/10.1161/01.STR.0000018010.38749.08] [PMID: 12053006]

[124] Bousser MG, Eschwege E, Haguenau M, *et al.* "AICLA" controlled trial of aspirin and dipyridamole in the secondary prevention of athero-thrombotic cerebral ischemia. Stroke 1983; 14(1): 5-14. [http://dx.doi.org/10.1161/01.STR.14.1.5] [PMID: 6401878]

[125] CAST (Chinese Acute Stroke Trial). Randomised placebo-controlled trial of early aspirin use in 20,000 patients with acute ischaemic stroke. Lancet 1997; 349(9066): 1641-9. [http://dx.doi.org/10.1016/S0140-6736(97)04010-5] [PMID: 9186381]

[126] Gent M, Blakely JA, Easton JD, *et al.* The Canadian American Ticlopidine Study (CATS) in thromboembolic stroke. Lancet 1989; 1(8649): 1215-20. [http://dx.doi.org/10.1016/S0140-6736(89)92327-1] [PMID: 2566778]

[127] Gotoh F, Tohgi H, Hirai S, *et al.* Cilostazol stroke prevention study: A placebo-controlled double-blind trial for secondary prevention of cerebral infarction. J Stroke Cerebrovasc Dis 2000; 9(4): 147-57. [http://dx.doi.org/10.1053/jscd.2000.7216] [PMID: 24192020]

[128] Efficacy study of cilostazol and aspirin on cerebral small vessel disease (Challenge). Available from: https://www.clinicaltrials.gov/ct2/show/NCT01932203?titles=small+vessel+disease&rank=4 2015.

[129] Lacunar intervention trial 1 (LACI-1) (Prevent-SVD). Available from: https://www.clinicaltrials.gov/ct2/show/ NCT02481323?titles=small+vessel+disease&rank=10 2015.

[130] Han SW, Song TJ, Bushnell CD, *et al.* Cilostazol decreases cerebral arterial pulsatility in patients with mild white matter hyperintensities: subgroup analysis from the Effect of Cilostazol in Acute Lacunar Infarction Based on Pulsatility Index of Transcranial Doppler (ECLIPse) study. Cerebrovasc Dis 2014; 38(3): 197-203.
[http://dx.doi.org/10.1159/000365840] [PMID: 25300977]

[131] Rashid P, Leonardi-Bee J, Bath P. Blood pressure reduction and secondary prevention of stroke and other vascular events: a systematic review. Stroke 2003; 34(11): 2741-8.
[http://dx.doi.org/10.1161/01.STR.0000092488.40085.15] [PMID: 14576382]

[132] Chapman N, Huxley R, Anderson C, *et al.* Effects of a perindopril-based blood pressure-lowering regimen on the risk of recurrent stroke according to stroke subtype and medical history: the PROGRESS Trial. Stroke 2004; 35(1): 116-21.
[http://dx.doi.org/10.1161/01.STR.0000106480.76217.6F] [PMID: 14671247]

[133] Tzourio C, Anderson C, Chapman N, *et al.* Effects of blood pressure lowering with perindopril and indapamide therapy on dementia and cognitive decline in patients with cerebrovascular disease. Arch Intern Med 2003; 163(9): 1069-75.
[http://dx.doi.org/10.1001/archinte.163.9.1069] [PMID: 12742805]

[134] Tzourio C, Dufouil C, Ducimetière P, Alpérovitch A. Cognitive decline in individuals with high blood pressure: a longitudinal study in the elderly. EVA Study Group. Epidemiology of Vascular Aging. Neurology 1999; 53(9): 1948-52.
[http://dx.doi.org/10.1212/WNL.53.9.1948] [PMID: 10599763]

[135] Cushman WC, Evans GW, Byington RP, *et al.* Effects of intensive blood-pressure control in type 2 diabetes mellitus. N Engl J Med 2010; 362(17): 1575-85.
[http://dx.doi.org/10.1056/NEJMoa1001286] [PMID: 20228401]

[136] Williamson JD, Launer LJ, Bryan RN, *et al.* Cognitive function and brain structure in persons with type 2 diabetes mellitus after intensive lowering of blood pressure and lipid levels: a randomized clinical trial. JAMA Intern Med 2014; 174(3): 324-33.
[http://dx.doi.org/10.1001/jamainternmed.2013.13656] [PMID: 24493100]

[137] Stratification of blood pressure control against progress of cerebral small vessel diseases in poststroke patients (APPROVE). Available from: https://www.clinicaltrials. gov/ct2/show/ NCT01819441? titles=small+vessel+disease&rank=8 2015.

[138] Benavente OR, White CL, Pearce L, *et al.* The Secondary Prevention of Small Subcortical Strokes (SPS3) study. Int J Stroke 2011; 6(2): 164-75.
[http://dx.doi.org/10.1111/j.1747-4949.2010.00573.x] [PMID: 21371282]

[139] White CL, Szychowski JM, Roldan A, *et al.* Clinical features and racial/ethnic differences among the 3020 participants in the Secondary Prevention of Small Subcortical Strokes (SPS3) trial. J Stroke Cerebrovasc Dis 2013; 22(6): 764-74.
[http://dx.doi.org/10.1016/j.jstrokecerebrovasdis.2012.03.002] [PMID: 22516427]

[140] Hart RG, Pearce LA, Bakheet MF, *et al.* Predictors of stroke recurrence in patients with recent lacunar stroke and response to interventions according to risk status: secondary prevention of small subcortical strokes trial. J Stroke Cerebrovasc Dis 2014; 23(4): 618-24.
[http://dx.doi.org/10.1016/j.jstrokecerebrovasdis.2013.05.021] [PMID: 23800503]

[141] Amarenco P, Benavente O, Goldstein LB, *et al.* Results of the Stroke Prevention by Aggressive Reduction in Cholesterol Levels (SPARCL) trial by stroke subtypes. Stroke 2009; 40(4): 1405-9. [http://dx.doi.org/10.1161/STROKEAHA.108.534107] [PMID: 19228842]

[142] ten Dam VH, van den Heuvel DM, van Buchem MA, *et al.* Effect of pravastatin on cerebral infarcts and white matter lesions. Neurology 2005; 64(10): 1807-9. [http://dx.doi.org/10.1212/01.WNL.0000161844.00797.73] [PMID: 15911821]

[143] Mok VC, Lam WW, Fan YH, *et al.* Effects of statins on the progression of cerebral white matter lesion: Post hoc analysis of the ROCAS (Regression of Cerebral Artery Stenosis) study. J Neurol 2009; 256(5): 750-7. [http://dx.doi.org/10.1007/s00415-009-5008-7] [PMID: 19252811]

[144] Lavallée PC, Labreuche J, Gongora-Rivera F, *et al.* Placebo-controlled trial of high-dose atorvastatin in patients with severe cerebral small vessel disease. Stroke 2009; 40(5): 1721-8. [http://dx.doi.org/10.1161/STROKEAHA.108.540088] [PMID: 19286582]

[145] Wilcock G, Möbius HJ, Stöffler A. A double-blind, placebo-controlled multicentre study of memantine in mild to moderate vascular dementia (MMM500). Int Clin Psychopharmacol 2002; 17(6): 297-305. [http://dx.doi.org/10.1097/00004850-200211000-00005] [PMID: 12409683]

[146] Erkinjuntti T, Kurz A, Gauthier S, Bullock R, Lilienfeld S, Damaraju CV. Efficacy of galantamine in probable vascular dementia and Alzheimer's disease combined with cerebrovascular disease: a randomised trial. Lancet 2002; 359(9314): 1283-90. [http://dx.doi.org/10.1016/S0140-6736(02)08267-3] [PMID: 11965273]

[147] Auchus AP, Brashear HR, Salloway S, Korczyn AD, De Deyn PP, Gassmann-Mayer C. Galantamine treatment of vascular dementia: a randomized trial. Neurology 2007; 69(5): 448-58. [http://dx.doi.org/10.1212/01.wnl.0000266625.31615.f6] [PMID: 17664404]

[148] Black S, Román GC, Geldmacher DS, *et al.* Efficacy and tolerability of donepezil in vascular dementia: positive results of a 24-week, multicenter, international, randomized, placebo-controlled clinical trial. Stroke 2003; 34(10): 2323-30. [http://dx.doi.org/10.1161/01.STR.0000091396.95360.E1] [PMID: 12970516]

[149] Wilkinson D, Doody R, Helme R, *et al.* Donepezil in vascular dementia: a randomized, placebo-controlled study. Neurology 2003; 61(4): 479-86. [http://dx.doi.org/10.1212/01.WNL.0000078943.50032.FC] [PMID: 12939421]

[150] Dichgans M, Markus HS, Salloway S, *et al.* Donepezil in patients with subcortical vascular cognitive impairment: a randomised double-blind trial in CADASIL. Lancet Neurol 2008; 7(4): 310-8. [http://dx.doi.org/10.1016/S1474-4422(08)70046-2] [PMID: 18296124]

[151] Moretti R, Torre P, Antonello RM, Cazzato G, Bava A. Rivastigmine in subcortical vascular dementia: an open 22-month study. J Neurol Sci 2002; 203-204: 141-6. [http://dx.doi.org/10.1016/S0022-510X(02)00280-0] [PMID: 12417373]

[152] Moretti R, Torre P, Antonello RM, Cazzato G, Bava A. Rivastigmine in subcortical vascular dementia: a randomized, controlled, open 12-month study in 208 patients. Am J Alzheimers Dis Other Demen 2003; 18(5): 265-72.

[http://dx.doi.org/10.1177/153331750301800508] [PMID: 14569643]

[153] Ballard C, Sauter M, Scheltens P, *et al.* Efficacy, safety and tolerability of rivastigmine capsules in patients with probable vascular dementia: the VantagE study. Curr Med Res Opin 2008; 24(9): 2561-74.
[http://dx.doi.org/10.1185/03007990802328142] [PMID: 18674411]

[154] Kavirajan H, Schneider LS. Efficacy and adverse effects of cholinesterase inhibitors and memantine in vascular dementia: a meta-analysis of randomised controlled trials. Lancet Neurol 2007; 6(9): 782-92.
[http://dx.doi.org/10.1016/S1474-4422(07)70195-3] [PMID: 17689146]

[155] Olin J, Schneider L, Novit A, Luczak S. Hydergine for dementia. Cochrane Database Syst Rev 2001; 2: CD000359.
[PMID: 11405961]

[156] Fioravanti M, Flicker L. Efficacy of nicergoline in dementia and other age associated forms of cognitive impairment. Cochrane Database Syst Rev 2001; 4: CD003159.
[PMID: 11687175]

[157] López-Arrieta JM, Birks J. Nimodipine for primary degenerative, mixed and vascular dementia. Cochrane Database Syst Rev 2002; 3: CD000147.
[PMID: 12137606]

[158] Pantoni L, del Ser T, Soglian AG, *et al.* Efficacy and safety of nimodipine in subcortical vascular dementia: a randomized placebo-controlled trial. Stroke 2005; 36(3): 619-24.
[http://dx.doi.org/10.1161/01.STR.0000155686.73908.3e] [PMID: 15692125]

[159] Fioravanti M, Yanagi M. Cytidinediphosphocholine (CDP-choline) for cognitive and behavioural disturbances associated with chronic cerebral disorders in the elderly. Cochrane Database Syst Rev 2005; 2: CD000269.
[PMID: 15846601]

[160] Chen N, Yang M, Guo J, Zhou M, Zhu C, He L. Cerebrolysin for vascular dementia. Cochrane Database Syst Rev 2013; 1(1): CD008900.
[PMID: 23440834]

[161] Malouf M, Grimley EJ, Areosa SA. Folic acid with or without vitamin B12 for cognition and dementia. Cochrane Database Syst Rev 2003; 4(4): CD004514.
[PMID: 14584018]

[162] van Overbeek EC, Staals J, van Oostenbrugge RJ. Vitamin B12 and progression of white matter lesions. A 2-year follow-up study in first-ever lacunar stroke patients. PLoS One 2013; 8(10): e78100.
[http://dx.doi.org/10.1371/journal.pone.0078100] [PMID: 24155983]

[163] Cavalieri M, Schmidt R, Chen C, *et al.* B vitamins and magnetic resonance imaging-detected ischemic brain lesions in patients with recent transient ischemic attack or stroke: the vitamins TO Prevent Stroke (VITATOPS) MRI-substudy. Stroke 2012; 43(12): 3266-70.
[http://dx.doi.org/10.1161/STROKEAHA.112.665703] [PMID: 23093615]

[164] Bath PM, Wardlaw JM. Pharmacological treatment and prevention of cerebral small vessel disease: a review of potential interventions. Int J Stroke 2015; 10(4): 469-78.
[http://dx.doi.org/10.1111/ijs.12466] [PMID: 25727737]

[165] Study evaluating the safety, tolerability and efficacy of PF-04360365 in adults with probable cerebral amyloid angiopathy. Available from: https://www.clinicaltrials.gov/ ct2/show/ NCT01821118? term=amyloid+angiopathy&rank=3 2015.

[166] Knudsen KA, Rosand J, Karluk D, Greenberg SM. Clinical diagnosis of cerebral amyloid angiopathy: validation of the Boston criteria. Neurology 2001; 56(4): 537-9.
[http://dx.doi.org/10.1212/WNL.56.4.537] [PMID: 11222803]

[167] Effect of HBO on functional connectivity of resting state networks in patients with cerebral small vessel disease. Available from: https://www.clinicaltrials.gov/ ct2/show/ NCT02232958? titles=small+vessel+disease&rank=6 2015.

[168] Perfusion by arterial spin labelling following single dose tadalafil in small vessel disease (PASTIS) trial. Available from: https://www.clinicaltrials.gov/ct2/show/NCT02450253?titles=small+vessel+ disease&rank=5 2015.

[169] Shibuya M, Hirai S, Seto M, Satoh S, Ohtomo E. Effects of fasudil in acute ischemic stroke: results of a prospective placebo-controlled double-blind trial. J Neurol Sci 2005; 238(1-2): 31-9.
[http://dx.doi.org/10.1016/j.jns.2005.06.003] [PMID: 16005902]

[170] Chung PW, Park KY, Kim JM, *et al.* 25-hydroxyvitamin D status is associated with chronic cerebral small vessel disease. Stroke 2015; 46(1): 248-51.
[http://dx.doi.org/10.1161/STROKEAHA.114.007706] [PMID: 25424481]

[171] Chan SL, Sweet JG, Cipolla MJ. Treatment for cerebral small vessel disease: effect of relaxin on the function and structure of cerebral parenchymal arterioles during hypertension. FASEB J 2013; 27(10): 3917-27.
[http://dx.doi.org/10.1096/fj.13-230797] [PMID: 23783073]

[172] Milia P, Caserio M, Bani D, *et al.* Efficacy of relaxin on functional recovery of post stroke patients. Ital J Anat Embryol 2013; 118(1) (Suppl.): 92-7.
[PMID: 24640583]

CHAPTER 5

Complement Blocking Therapeutic Strategies: A Prospective Approach for the Treatment of Cardiovascular Diseases

Yaw Asare[1], **Santosh Vijayan**[2], **Gansuvd Shagdarsuren**[3] and **Erdenechimeg Shagdarsuren**[4,*]

[1] *Institute for Stroke and Dementia Research, Klinikum der Universität München, Ludwig-Maximilians University, Munich, Germany*

[2] *Institute for Translational Immunology, University Hospital, Johannes Gutenberg-University Mainz, Germany*

[3] *Department of Internal Medicine, School of Medicine, Mongolian National University of Medical Sciences, Ulaanbaatar, Mongolia*

[4] *Institute for Molecular Cardiovascular Research (IMCAR), University Hospital, RWTH Aachen, Germany*

Abstract: Despite huge improvements in clinical diagnosis as well as numerous options in patient care and treatment, the incidence of cardiovascular disease (CVD) has been on the rise in the last decade potentially due to hitherto deteriorating lifestyle. As a chronic inflammatory response of the arterial vessel wall, atherosclerosis and its clinical sequelae such as coronary heart disease, cerebrovascular disease and peripheral artery disease continue to be the leading causes of morbidity and mortality worldwide. This makes it necessary to explore novel therapeutic strategies to control and manipulate the mediators of atherosclerosis and cardiac repair processes in order to help combat cardiovascular events. The complement system, an important part of the innate immune response, constitutes a complex network of plasma proteins and membrane cofactors which act in concert with other immunological systems of the body for a rapid defense against foreign intrusions and infections. Activation of the complement cascade in CVD is well established. Numerous well-conducted studies on

* **Corresponding author Erdenechimeg Shagdarsuren:** Institute for Molecular Cardiovascular Research (IMCAR), University Hospital, RWTH Aachen, Germany, Pauwelsstraße 30, 52074 Aachen, Germany; Tel: +49-241-8036584; Fax: +49-241-8082703; Email: eguenther@ukaachen.de.

Atta-ur-Rahman and M. Iqbal Choudhary (Eds.)

targeting specific components of the complement cascade in CVD have opened avenues for targeted pharmacological inhibition of the complement system at different levels of complement activation. The use of gene targeting and neutralizing antibodies as well as small molecule inhibitors in animal models of human CVD has provided a clear beneficial role for blocking complement C5, C5a, C5a receptor (C5aR1, CD88) and the soluble complement receptor 1 (sCR1) and different regulators at C3 convertase level. Moreover, the discovery of the second receptor for C5a, the C5aR2 (C5L2, C5a receptor-like 2) and recent studies on the functional role in atherosclerosis has raised the intriguing possibility of the use of this receptor as a novel anti-inflammatory strategy. Though work is still in progress to determine whether there is a global effect of this receptor in pathogenesis of cardiovascular disease, there is no doubt that complement blocking strategies is an emerging field in medical pharmacology.

Keywords: Atherosclerosis, Cardiac and vascular remodelling, Cardiovascular disease, Complement inhibitors, Complement system and activation, Myocardial infarction.

Cardiovascular disease (CVD) is the leading cause of death worldwide and the underlying pathological condition has been primarily attributed to atherosclerosis. It is well established that atherosclerosis is a chronic inflammatory process of the arterial vessel wall orchestrated by variety of mediators of innate and adaptive immunity [1, 2]. As a major and crucial component of both innate and adaptive immune system, the complement system maybe envisioned to have a pivotal role in the pathomechanisms of CVD. Indeed, substantial evidence supports complement-mediated pathogenesis of CVD through pleiotropic effects on multiple cell types strongly implicated in CVD [3, 4]. Several components of the complement system have been strongly associated with the outcome of cardiovascular events in patients [5 - 8]. Employing *in vitro* mechanistic studies and diverse *in vivo* models that mimic human CVD, the functional role of complement components in CVD has been established. In line with its well characterized pro-inflammatory effects, function in immune complexes and debris as well as apoptotic cells removal, the activation of the complement system has both beneficial and detrimental effects. Several studies using gene targeting, neutralizing antibodies and small molecule inhibitors have helped in identifying specific complement components harboring therapeutic potential. In this chapter, we discuss both established and emerging paradigms in complement-mediated mechanisms underlying CVD. We summarize naturally occurring complement inhibitors and regulators, at various levels of complement activation, which could be harnessed for the treatment of CVD.

1. COMPLEMENT ACTIVATION CASCADE AND PATHWAYS

Complement system was first reported in 1896 by Jules Bordet, who found that antibodies present in fresh serum assisted in bacterial killing, but serum heated at 56°C or higher lost this property [9, 10]. The complement system, part of the innate and adaptive immune system, is usually regarded as the primary host-defense mechanism against pathogenic infections [11, 12]. This system is considered to be part of the primitive defense mechanism coordinating innate and adaptive immune systems [11, 13]. The mammalian complement system consists of more than 50 circulatory and membrane bound proteins. These proteins aid in differentiating between host and pathogen. Once a foreign body is detected by these proteins, they interact with one another and form immune complexes thereby aiding in pathogen clearance [14, 15]. The complement cascade can be activated by at least three major pathways - 1) Classical pathway 2) Lectin pathway and 3) Alternate pathway [16, 17]. The simplified version of the three pathways is depicted in Fig. (**1**). Additionally, the proteolytic enzymes in the newly described extrinsic protease pathway cleave C3 and C5 independent of conventional convertases. Furthermore, a new activation pathway exists for generation of C5a, especially in the absence of C3, with thrombin acting as a potent C5 convertase [16].

1.1. Classical Pathway of Complement Activation

The classical pathway of complement activation has always been regarded as the primary responder (major effector) to various stimulants such as Fc portion of immunoglobulin (Ig) in antigen-antibody complexes, enzymes like trypsin and numerous endotoxins, cell membranes, viruses and a string of other external stimulants [18]. It is the only complement pathway with functions in the adaptive immune system [19]. The classical pathway is activated when antibodies from pathogens are recognized and bound to multiple sites on the cell surface, specifically to IgG and IgM proteins [20].

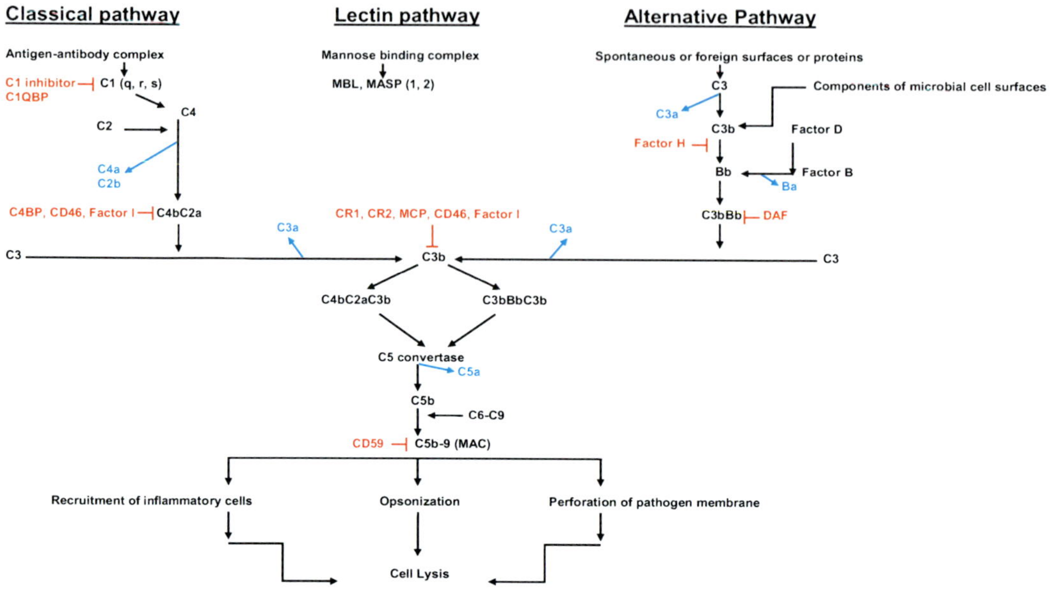

Fig. (1). Three classical pathways of complement activation.

Complement C1 complex is a derivative of three proteins C1q, C1r (2 components) and C1s (2 components). C1q aids in recognizing and binding to Fc region of the antibody. Free antibodies present in the stream are unable to bind to C1q because of the presence of C1-inhibitor. IgM (Immunoglobulin-M) is the most efficient isotype that is capable of activating the system [21]. IgM has five Fc regions, each of which can present a binding site to C1q and thereby leads to stable interactions. In addition, Immunoglobulin-G (IgG 1, 2, 3) is also capable of activating the complement system, though they have only one Fc region and hence attain more feeble interactions with C1q. Inactive serine proteases C1r and C1s, are activated when C1q binds to the Fc receptors. One molecule of C1r cleaves, activates itself and then cleaves the remaining C1r and C1s molecules [22]. Upon activation, C1s further induces the activity of the serine proteases C4 and C2. Activated C1s binds to the alpha chain of C4, degrades it and releases a smaller component C4a and a larger fragment C4b. C1s also binds to C2 and cleaves it to a larger C2b and a smaller C2a fragment. C4b and C2b form a complex called C3 convertase, which aids in cleaving C3 component [23].

Cleavage of C3 results in C3a and C3b fragments, with the former inducing inflammatory response. C3b further forms a complex with C4b and C2b called C5 convertase. Similar to C3 convertase, C5 convertase plays a role in the cleavage of C5 component to C5a and C5b. C5a is involved in inflammatory processes whiles C5b initiates the formation of membrane attack complex (MAC; C5b-9) Small transmembrane channels are formed from a complex involving C5b, C6, C7 and C8. C9 penetrates the transmembranes and binds to C5b-8 complex, initiates the process of oligomerization and forms the MAC. MAC then creates a transmembrane pore leading to lysis of foreign cells [24].

1.2. Mannose-Binding Lectin (MBL) Pathway

The Lectin Pathway also known as MBL activates the complement system in antibody-independent manner. MBL is an oligomeric subunit of identical polypeptide chains containing a cysteine, collagen and a carbohydrate recognition domain. This pathway is initiated when MBL Protein-1 binds to the carbohydrate chains (mannose, glucose or other sugar chains) on the surface of pathogens in a calcium-dependent manner leading to the activation of MBL-associated serine proteases [25]. These serine proteases form a proenzyme complex with MBL. In *Homo sapiens,* 3 kinds of Mannose-binding lectin-Associated Serine Protease (MASP) are present; namely MASP-1, MASP-2, and MASP-3. Activated MASP-1 cleaves complement protein C3 and C2, whiles MASP-2 cleaves C4 and C2 [26]. MASP-2 cleaves C4 complement protein to C4b and C4a. C4b binds to microbial surface whereas C4a triggers the stimulation of inflammation and other inflammatory molecules. MASP-2 also aids in cleaving C2 complement protein to C2a and C2b. C2b and C4b bind together to form C3 convertase as in the case of classical pathway. C3 convertase further cleaves C3 protein to C3b and C3a. C3b either binds to the surface of microbes or assist in the recognition of phagocytes and other inflammatory host molecules [26]. C3b may also associate with C4b-C2b complex to form C5 convertase that cleaves C5 into C5b and C5a. C5a drives inflammatory responses whiles C5b form a complex with C6, C7 and C8 giving rise to small transmembrane channels. C9 penetrates the transmembranes and binds with C5b-8 complex initiating the process of oligomerization and forming MAC, which creates a transmembrane pore leading to lysis of foreign cells [20, 24].

1.3. Alternative Pathway of Complement Activation

This is the humoral arm of the complement system and serves as a defense mechanism against infections without the involvement of antibodies. It may be presumed that this is the permanently active pathway in our system [23]. The proteins C3, complement factors B, D, H, P and I are responsible for initiation, recognition and amplification, of the alternative complement pathway, resulting in the formation of C3/C5 convertase [20]. This arm of the complement system is activated upon spontaneous conversion of C3 to active proteases. C3 is spontaneously broken down to generate C3(H_2O). Once complement factor B associates with C3(H_2O), factor B itself changes conformation and can then be cleaved by the factor D, generating Ba and away Bb. C3 convertase formed as a result of spontaneous activation is influenced by Factor P. Factor P aids in binding to cell bound C3b and thereby playing a role in stabilizing C3/C5 convertase. Complement factor Ba is released and C3b Factor Bb complex remains. This complex is homologous to classical C3 convertase in structure as well as function and hence is considered as alternative C3 convertase [27]. The presence of freely available C3b in close proximity in the medium boosts C3 convertase and thereby act as C5 convertase and binds to Factor P. At this point, the alternate pathway follows the ways of classical and MBL pathways. Thus, recruiting additional complement proteins (C6, C7, C8 and C9) and forming the MAC complex that initiates transmembrane pore and protein lysis [24].

Of importance, the three different ways of complement activation converge on precursor protein C3, giving rise to cleavage products C3a, C3b, C5a, C5b that drive inflammation or triggers the formation of MAC. complex (away). These pathways help in eliminating the pathogen from the host system [18].

1.4. Complement Anaphylatoxins

Complement anaphylatoxins are number of cleaved bioactive products released into the host as a result of complement activation [28]. The well-described ones are C3a and C5a. C4a is another one of these anaphylatoxins present in rare diseases such as Lyme disease and acquired immunodeficiency syndrome in human beings. It is also found to be present in lower vertebrates like guinea pigs in extremely high proportions [29, 30]. These complement peptides (anaphylatoxins) are conserved regions in the animal kingdom that are produced as a result of proteolysis of C3, C4 and C5 protein complexes [30 - 33]. C3a and C5a are generated in classical or alternative pathways, and sometimes released by mast cells and lung macrophages [34 - 36]. C4a on the other hand is released only in the classical pathway [36]. The relative potency of anaphylatoxins is in the following order: C5a>C3a>C4a [37].

C4a is a 77 amino acid peptide with characteristics close to C3a and C5a [38]. However, C4a enhances vascular permeability to a lesser extent than either C5a or C3a [39, 40]. C4a is composed of α, β and γ chains linked by inter- and intra-chain disulphide bonds [41] and notably affects phagocytes. C3a is a 77 residue peptide that forms a knot of six conserved cysteine residues and encompasses a basic charge [42]. C3a is a common bioactive product released upon activation of all three complement pathways and acts *via* C3aR present on leukocytes and epithelial cells. Serum carboxypeptidases act on C3a and cleave it to C3a desArg. C3a desArg is an adipocyte derived protein and can bind to C5aR2 receptor (C5L2 - C5a receptor-like 2, GPR77) thereby affecting the functional role of C5a [43, 44]. Unlike C4a and C3a, which have 77 amino residues, C5a is a 74 amino acid peptide that is pro-inflammatory in nature with a strong chemoattractant property towards all myeloid cells and induces vascular permeability [45, 46]. It is the only known complement protein that promotes chemotaxis of granulocytes [47]. C5a is released either by the cleavage of C5 by C5 convertase or proteolytic enzymes like thrombin and kallikrien [48]. Serum carboxypedtidases act on C5a and cleave it to C5a desArg, which is not as potent as C5a and hence acts as a weak chemoattractant [49, 50]. Nevertheless, both C5a and C5a desArg are present at sites of inflammation where they attract leukocytes and other inflammatory molecules. C5a interacts primarily with its two receptors C5aR1 and C5aR2. Both receptors consist of seven transmembrane proteins and belong to a rhodopsin like family. There are important differences between these two receptors even though they share structural similarities [51].

Notably, C3a and C5a peptides have pro-inflammatory property. Both activate eosinophils, mast cells and basophils, however, only C5a has direct effect on neutrophils [52]. C3a and C5a consist of α and β chains composed of disulphide bridges [41]. Whiles C5a is a post-translationally modified single carbohydrate complex chain bound to asparagine residue, the other peptides C3a and C4a bear no such carbohydrate modifications [41]. C3a and C5a act *via* the receptors C3aR and C5aR1/C5aR2 respectively. On the other hand no receptor for C4a has been reported, however it has been suggested to signal *via* either C3aR or C5aR1 [23].

1.5. Complement Anaphylatoxin Receptors

The three known complement anaphylatoxins receptors C3aR, C5aR1 and C5aR2 belong to the seven-transmembrane domain G-protein coupled receptor protein family [53, 54]. They comprise an extracellular N-terminus and seven helical transmembrane domains connected by intra and extracellular loops [55, 56]. C3aR, also known as complement component 3a receptor 1 (C3aR1), is a canonical C3a receptor [57]. It contains a small N-terminal domain and a greatly enlarged second extracellular domain that appears to be conserved across all species [55, 58, 59]. C3aR is known to undergo post-translational modifications like glycosylation, tyrosine sulfation, phosphorylation and acylation [55]. The receptor is capable of binding to the anaphylatoxins C3a and C4a [60]. C3aR is ubiquitously expressed in all tissues with varying levels of expression [58, 61]. It is known to be expressed on myeloid cells such as macrophages, dendritic cells, neutrophils and on non-myeloid cells like endothelial cells, smooth muscle cells and astrocytes [33, 62]. With its presence on neuronal cells, it may have a role in development and inflammation process in the nervous system [63, 64].

The main core of C5a interacts with acidic residues in the N-terminus whereas the transmembrane region interacts with the C-terminus of C5aR1 [65, 66]. C5a receptors are known to be expressed in numerous tissues such as those in the circulatory system, connective tissues and various organs as reviewed elsewhere [51]. Signalling occurs *via* mitogen activated protein kinases leading to nuclear factor kappa light chains with increased production of chemokines and intracellular calcium [45, 67]. C5aR1 is also known to undergo post-translational modifications like glycosylation, tyrosine sulfation and phosphorylation [55]. After binding and translational modifications, the receptor is internalised into clathrin-coated pits where it can be dephosphorylated or recycled to the plasma membrane or degraded in lysosomes [68]. As second receptor for C5a, C5aR2

(GPR77), is also expressed on both immune and non-immune cells and exhibits higher affinity to C5a desArg than C5aR1 does [51]. C5aR2 has a similar pattern of tyrosine and acidic N-terminal residues as C5aR1. A major feature of extracellular binding of C5a to its receptors is the presence of these tyrosine and acidic N-terminal residues [51]. Although most tissues co-express both receptors for C5a, the expression of C5aR2 is known to vary with the degree of pro- or anti-inflammatory response [69].

The CRs and their functions are in itself a bigger topic to be reviewed [51, 55] and hence detailed description is omitted here as it is out of the scope of this chapter.

2. NATURALLY OCCURRING COMPLEMENT INHIBITORS AND REGULATORS

Complement activation presents a potential threat to host cells and inappropriate activation may contribute to tissue damage and provides an important role in pathogenesis of many diseases. Complement is ubiquitously expressed and regularly activated; however, human cells express a variety of complement regulators to protect themselves from complement attack. They are membrane-bound or soluble proteins and control every step of the complement cascade (Tables **1-4**). These include the main important complement inhibitors among others: C1-esterase inhibitor (C1-INH), decay-accelerating factor (DAF; CD55), membrane cofactor protein (MCP; CD46) and complement receptor 1 (CR1; CD35), which act on the early as well as central stages of the pathway and CD59, which acts on the terminal lytic stage. The detailed molecular mechanisms of activation and regulation of the complement system has been nicely reviewed [23]. Tables **1-4** summarize the naturally occurring regulators at different levels of complement activation cascade and the drugs and inhibitors developed based on their functions.

2.1. Natural Regulators at the Early level of Complement Activation

C1-Esterase Inhibitor

The classical and lectin pathway is modulated by intrinsic **C1-esterase inhibitor** (C1-INH) (see below). In the classical pathway, a C4b-binding protein inhibits the action of the classical and the lectin pathways, more specifically C4 and also has ability to bind C3b [70]. C1-INH shuts down the proteolytic activity of C1r and C1s restricting again the time window allowed for cleaving C4 and C2. When not inhibited, however, the C3 convertases continue to act on C3 to generate C3a and C3b; in extreme cases C3 depletion will occur.

Table 1. Regulators at the initiation of the activation cascade.

Targets	Naturally occurring inhibitors/regulators	Existing form and expression	Function	Ref.	Drugs/Agents
Classical pathway	C1-INH	soluble	Binds C1r and C1s, inhibits C1qrs complex	[94]	C1-INH (Berinert-P, CSL Behring, Marburg, Germany) [94, 221]
	C1qR	membrane-bound, monocytes and B cells	Binds C1q, inhibits phagocytosis and cell adhesion	[266]	
Classical and lectin pathway	Carboxypeptidase N	soluble	Binds C3a, C4a and C5a, inactivation of anaphylatoxins	[267]	Synthetic Carboxypeptidase N Inhibitor [268]
	C1-INH	soluble	Restricts cleavage of C4 and C2	[94]	
Alternative pathway	Properdin	soluble	Stabilizes C3bBb complex, binds to apoptotic surfaces	[269]	Anti-properdin Ab (TSR 5/6) [270]
	Factor H (fH)	membrane-bound	Cofactor for factor I and limit formation of C3bBb complex	[271]	
	FHL-1/reconectin	soluble	Binds C3b, Cofactor for factor I and acceleration of C3 convertase decay	[272]	
			Inhibits alternative and lectin pathway, plasma Bb, C3a, sMAC	[273]	Anti-human Factor D mAb (Genetech, San Francisco, CA) [274]
			prevents formation of the C3bBb complex		Anti-Factor B mAb (Taligen Therapeutics) [274]

Factor H (fH) is a plasma protein that also regulates the alternative pathway and the amplification loop at the C3 convertase step. The carboxy terminus of this protein binds surface deposited C3b and surface-expressed polyanionic glycosaminoglycans (GAG). After they are bound, the N-terminal domains of fH exhibit decay accelerating and cofactor activities. Also, it serves as a cofactor for C3b inactivation by Factor I and induces C3bBb complex dissociation [71]. fH restrains complement activation on host surfaces that do not express other complement regulators including exposed basement membranes in the glomerulus (which express glycosaminoglycans), explaining in part the association between mutations in fH or Factor I and various C3 associated nephropathies [72]. Table **1** describes the naturally occuring regulators and drugs based on their function at the initiation of the complement activation cascade.

2.2. Natural Regulators at the C3-Convertase Level

Regulation of C3 convertase activity is accomplished by multiple molecules with overlapping but discrete functions. Nearly all naturally occurring complement regulators directly or indirectly inhibit and retain the C3 convertase activity [73]. The very short half-life of C3b due to rapid binding by red cells results in a limited period of time where it can bind factor B; one of these mechanisms that limit C3 convertase activity [74]. fH, a cofactor for factor I, further limits the reaction by displacing factor B from the C3 convertase which interrupts the positive feedback loop and limits formation of C3bBb, and by facilitating the natural property of factor I, which degrades C3b within the convertase [71].

Decay accelerating factor (DAF; CD55) is a glycophosphatidylinositol (GPI)-anchored, membrane-bound intrinsic regulator that inhibits the formation of C3 convertases and accelerates the decay of cell surface-assembled classical and alternative pathway C3 and C5 convertases. DAF inhibits the alternative C3 convertase by binding Bb, allows the disassociation of Bb from C3bBb and C2b from C4b thereby preventing amplification, downstream cleavage events, and formation of the MAC [75]. This decay accelerating activity functions only on the cell surface on which DAF is expressed. Most cell types of both vascular and non-vascular origin including red blood cells, epithelial cells and endothelial cells express GPI anchor. DAF expression is reduced in persons with mutations that reduce GPI levels such as those with paroxysmal nocturnal hemoglobinuria; in that disorder, red blood cells with very low levels of DAF and CD59 undergo complement-mediated hemolysis [76].

Membrane Cofactor Protein (MCP; CD46) and its murine homolog Crry (complement receptor type-1 related gene Y) are surface-expressed regulators with cofactor activity. MCP and Crry are expressed in all cells except red blood cells and function as cofactors for serine protease factor I that cleaves C3b to iC3b thereby irreversibly preventing reassembly of the C3 convertase [77]. The cleavage product iC3b is an opsonin and it can further be broken down to C3c. Its presence may indicate recent complement activation in tissues and C3dg. C3dg interacts further with CR2 on B cells to facilitate B-cell activation [78].

Complement Receptors (CRs)

Opsonized products by C3 cleavage fragments can be recognized by CR (CR1, CR2, CR3, CR4 and CRIg). CR1 and CR2 contain CCP modules, CR3 and CR4 belong to integrin family and CRIg belongs to immunoglobulin superfamily members [79]. CR1 is expressed on monocytes/macrophages, neutrophils and erythrocytes and renal podocytes [80]. CR2 (CD21) is found on B cells interacting with C3d and iC3b on the surface antigens forming a co-receptor complex with CD19 and CD81 [81]. Integrin family CR3 (CD11b/CD18 or Mac-1) and CR4 (CD11c/CD18) are expressed by macrophages/monocytes, dendritic cells, neutrophils, natural killer cells and bind multiple ligands participating in phagocytosis, cell adhesion, leukocyte trafficking and co-stimulation [79]. Both receptors bind to iC3b, however, CR3 binds to C3d, while CR4 recognizes C3c [79]. CRIg is expressed on macrophages as well as Kupffer cells in the liver and binds to C3b as well as iC3b and mediates the phagocytosis of opsonized particles [82] (Table **2**).

Table 2. Regulators at the C3 convertase level.

Targets	**Naturally occurring inhibitors/regulators**	**Existing form and expression**	**Function**	**Ref.**	**Drugs/Agents**	**Ref.**
C3 convertase	CD46 (membrane cofactor protein)	membrane-bound, all cells except erythrocytes	Binds C3b and C4b, degrades C3, cofactor for factor I and factor H	[77]		

(Table 2) contd.....

Targets	Naturally occurring inhibitors/regulators	Existing form and expression	Function	Ref.	Drugs/Agents	Ref.
C3 convertase	CD55 (decay-accelerating protein)	membrane-bound, most cell types, including erythrocytes, epithelial and ECs	Binds C4b2b and C3bBb, retains both DAF and MCP activities and blocks both C3 and C5 convertases	[75]	CAB-2, recombinant soluble fusion protein of sDAF and sMCP) XOMA Ltd. and Millennium Pharmaceuticals	[275]
	CR1 (CD35)	Membrane-bound, nucleated cells, erythrocytes, B cells, monocytes	Blocks the common pathway by binding C3b and C4b, limits half-life of C3b, participates in immune complex clearance, enhances phagocytosis	[80]	sCR1 (TP10) (Avant Immunotherapeutics), and CDX 1135 (Celldex Therapeutics)	[98]
	CR2 (CD21)	membrane-bound, B- and T-lymphocytes, follicular DC	Binds C3dg, C3d and iC3b, retains C3d, regulates B cell function	[75, 79]	sCrry, the rodent analog of human CR1/CR2	[77]
			CR2 domain of TT30 recognizes and binds to tissue bound C3bi and C3dg, delivers the regulatory domain of fH specifically to sites where complement regulation is required		TT30 (Taligen Therapeutics, Cambridge, MA)	[100]

(Table 2) contd.....

Targets	Naturally occurring inhibitors/regulators	Existing form and expression	Function	Ref.	Drugs/Agents	Ref.
	CR3 (Mac1, integrin)	membrane-bound, monocytes, macrophages, natural killer cells, neutrophils, T cells	Binds iC3b and factor H, enhances opsonisation, drives phagocytosis	[276]		
	CR4 (integrin)	Membrane-bound, monocytes and macrophages	Binds iC3b, enhances phagocytosis	[79]		
			Binds to C3 and inhibits the cleavage of C3 to C3b and C3a		Compstatin (cyclic tridecapeptide, POT-4, Potentia Pharmaceuticals, Louisville, KY)	[95]

2.3. Natural Regulators at the C5-Convertase Level

CD59 (Protectin) is GPI-anchored membrane protein, which blocks membrane perforation by C5b-8 as well as C5b-9 (MAC) and is expressed on most nucleated cell types as well as in red blood cells. CD59 does not bind free C8 and C9. The free C8, in the absence of a cell membrane, binds to C5b-7 and induces conformation changes that result in a loss of ability to form pores causing it to act as a MAC inhibitor [23, 83]. Moreover, the fluid phase soluble end products (sC5b-7 - sC5b-9) are scavenged by **clusterin** and **vitronectin** [84, 85]. (Table **3**).

Table 3. Regulators at the C5 convertase level and terminal pathway.

Targets	Naturally occurring inhibitors/regulators	Existing form and expression	Function	Ref.	Drugs/Agents	Ref.
Terminal pathway	Clusterin (SP-40)	soluble	Forms complex with C5b9 to generate inactive sC5b9, transports cholesterol, HDL, ApoA1 and lipids	[277]		

(Table 3) contd.....

Targets	Naturally occurring inhibitors/regulators	Existing form and expression	Function	Ref.	Drugs/Agents	Ref.
Terminal pathway	Vitronectin (Protein S)	soluble	Binds and blocks C5b-7 and MAC, adhesion protein	[85]		
	CFHR1 (complement factor H–related 1)	soluble	Inhibition of C5 convertase and MAC assembly	[278]		
	CD59 (Protectin)	Membrane-bound, erythrocyte and most nucleated cells	Inhibits formation of MAC by blocking C9 coupling on C5b-8 and MAC and the binding of C5b-7 to membrane targets	[83]		
			Prevents formation of C5a and C5b and formation of MAC		Anti-C5 mAb; Pexelizumab and Eculizumab (Alexion Pharmaceuticals, USA, humanized mAb)	[106, 108]

3. COMPLEMENT INHIBITORS/REGULATORS AS THERAPEUTICS

Molecular and structural basis of naturally occurring complement regulators as well as inhibitors and progress on the in-depth understanding of their mechanisms of action have opened many possibilities for the development and rational design of complement inhibitors for treatment of diseases. Here, we discuss some examples of complement-based drugs, which may be relevant for treatment of CVD.

3.1. C1-esterase Inhibitor (C1-INH)

The early stage of classical pathway is modulated by intrinsic C1-IHN, which binds to C1r and C1s and thereby completely inhibits the proteolytic activity of the C1qrs complex [86, 87]. It inactivates MASP-1, and MASP-2, restrict the time window allowed for cleaving C2 and C4 and thereby limiting MBL pathway activation. Moreover, C1-INH regulates the kallikrein-kinin system where it prevents the formation of bradykinin [86, 87]. Human C1-INH away is available in clinical practice for substitution therapy of hereditary angioedema (C1-INH deficiency, a rare disorder that maybe genetic or less commonly acquired angioedema). It manifests with episodic attacks of bradykinin-mediated, life-threatening localized recurrent subcutaneous/submucosal and or gastro-intestinal or oropharynx swellings [88]. In the past years, it has become apparent that C1-INH has additional anti-inflammatory functions independent of protease inhibition [89]. Cai *et al.* have reported that C1-INH can bind to both E- and P-selectin *via* a Sialyl-Lewis^x tetrasaccharide presented on its *N*-linked glycan and can thus interfere with leukocyte-endothelial cell interactions *in vitro* and *in vivo* and in turn results in suppression of transmigration of leukocytes across the endothelium [90]. In addition, C1-INH suppresses gram negative sepsis and endotoxin shock partly *via* direct interaction with endotoxin that interferes with its interaction with macrophages thereby suppressing TNF-α (tumor necrosis factor-alpha) and other inflammatory mediators. C1-INH treatment is beneficial in a number of disease models including sepsis, malaria, ischemia-reperfusion injury (intestinal, hepatic, muscle, cardiac, brain), hyper-acute transplant rejection, and other inflammatory disease models [91 - 93]. This effectiveness may be a result of mechanisms that do not require protease inhibition in addition to both complement and contact system activation [94] (Table **1**).

3.2. Inhibitors at the C3 Convertase Level

As listed in Table **1**, several drugs have been developed as synthetic mimics of naturally occurring complement inhibitors.

Compstatin is a cyclic tridecapeptide whose derivative POT-4, developed by Potentia Pharmaceuticals, binds to C3 and inhibit the cleavage of C3 to C3b and C3a. This substance is now been developed for local therapy of AMD (age-related macular degeneration) [95, 96]. Because of its species specificity, which is active only in humans and primates, it has been difficult to use in well-established animal models of CVD. Moreover, considering the central role of C3 in complement activation cascade and the fact that individuals deficient in C3 have a high incidence of bacterial infections, targeting C3 may results in the loss of immune protection conferred by complement activation [97].

Soluble CR1 was first developed as TP10 (Avant Immunotherapeutics) and showed beneficial effects in several animal studies [98]. CR1 is an endogenous membrane-bound C3 inhibitor and it has both decay accelerating and cofactor activity. It limits the half-life of C3b, thereby decreasing the levels of C3b and broadly inhibiting the generation of all effectors [79]. The now designated CDX1135 is being considered for a clinical trial in antibody-mediated organ rejection. In patients with deficiency in C3 nephritic factor or fH deficiency such as aHUS (atypical hemolytic uremic syndrome) and membranoproliferative glomerulonephritis, sCR1 would be expected to block the excessive activation of complement and thereby could be therapeutically beneficial [99].

CR2-fH and mAb 1379

A novel promising drug as a directed regulator to injured cell and tissue sites, TT30 (CR2-fH) is being developed by Taligan Therapeutics. TT30 is designed to deliver the complement regulatory domain of fH (second and third short consensus repeat (SCR) domain of fH) specifically to tissues with injury and activated complements by linking it to the ligand-binding domain of CR2 (CD21) [100]. When reached tissues by systemic administration, the CR2 domain of TT30 selectively bind to tissues/cells decorated with C3bi and C3dg, thereby blocking local complement activation and control inflammation [100]. This is a potent and specific inhibitor of the alternative pathway of complement activation, leaving the classical and lectin pathway relatively intact. The beneficial effects of TT30 have been shown in animal models of intestinal ischemia, retinal neovascularization and arthritis [101 - 103]. TT30 is at the end of preclinical trials for treatment of AMD, aHUS and autoimmune diseases [99].

mAb 1379 (TA106), is novel inhibitor developed by Taligen Therapeutics. It is a fusion protein comprised of the SCR domains of mouse factor B linked to a mouse IgG1 Fc domain and inhibits the alternative pathway activation by preventing formation of the C3bBb complex. This mAb is in preclinical studies and the effectiveness of this substance has been tested in mouse models of airway hyper-responsiveness and antiphospholipid antibody-induced pregnancy loss [104, 105] (Table **2**).

3.3. Inhibitors at the C5 Convertase Level and Formation of MAC

Pexelizumab and Eculizumab

They are humanized monoclonal antibodies binding to human C5 preventing its cleavage to C5a and C5b and specifically inhibits the terminal pathway. At the same time, it spares the generation of C3a and C3b, maintaining the functions of opsonizing pathogenic microorganisms and immune complexes, and can thereby preserve the host-defense mechanisms against infection. This drug has proven to be effective and safe in Paroxysmal nocturnal hemoglobinuria (PNH) and atypical aHUS. PNH and aHUS are 2 diseases with distinctly different underlying molecular mechanisms [106 - 108]. However, critical to the development of both diseases is the activation of the terminal complement pathway. Small molecules and compounds may have more advantages due to high potency and fewer adverse effects. A short aptamer directed against C5 (ARC1905) has been developed and is now in a phase 1 study to treat wet AMD [109] (Table **3**).

4. COMPLEMENT SYSTEM IN ATHEROSCLEROSIS-RELEVANT CELL TYPES

Atherogenic cells do not only secrete complement components but also represent potential targets of active products of the activated complement cascade. Therefore, understanding the interplay between the complement system and atherogenic cells may be beneficial in the design of complement-targeted therapeutics. Herein, we focus on vascular endothelial cells (ECs), smooth muscle cells (VSMCs), macrophages and platelets.

4.1. Complement Activation in Vascular Endothelial Cells

Endothelial cells (ECs) can participate directly in the initiation of inflammation by releasing or activating factors that influence not only the growth but also death and migration of vascular cells. This induces changes in the composition of the extracellular matrix leading to the recruitment of inflammatory cells to sites of injury. ECs express receptors for C1q, a subunit of the first component of the classical complement pathway. Ligand binding of C1q stimulates ECs to express E-selectin, the adhesion molecules intercellular adhesion molecule-1 (ICAM-1] and vascular cell adhesion molecule-1 (VCAM-1) and to release the chemotactic factors interleukin (IL)-8, IL-6 and chemokine (C-C motif) ligand-2 (CCL-2)(MCP-1, monocyte chemotactic protein-1) (reviewed in [110]). gC1qR can also interact with components of the coagulation and kinin system, and thus may play a crucial role not only in the initiation of local inflammatory processes but also in thrombotic complications related to atherosclerosis [111]. Vice versa, the activation of ECs by pro-inflammatory cytokines such as interferon (IFN)-γ, TNF-α and LPS is associated with a significant up-regulation of gC1qR in ECs [110]. Circulating leukocytes including neutrophils, monocyte/macrophages and T-cells recognize C1q, thus binding and deposition of C1q on ECs at sites of inflammation may also promote interactions between ECs and circulating leukocytes. This in turn contributes to the release of inflammatory mediators. The up-regulation of C1q on activated ECs may thus be part of a pro-inflammatory amplification loop sustaining EC activation as well as leukocyte recruitment and contribute to thrombosis, which might be relevant to the pathogenesis of chronic inflammatory conditions such as autoimmune diseases, ischemia/reperfusion injury or transplant rejection [112]. However, a protective role for the classical pathway has been suggested [113], which might possibly be due to effects in the clearance of apoptotic cells and immune complexes. This was demonstrated in atherosclerotic hypercholesterolemic mice deficient in C1q, which resulted in an accumulation of apoptotic cells within atherosclerotic lesions leading to an increase in lesion size and complexity of early lesions [114]. Moreover, vascular ECs also express receptors for C5a and C3a [110]. C3a can upregulate IL-1β and the chemokines IL-8 and Regulated on Activation, Normal T Cell Expressed and Secreted (RANTES) in ECs [115]. An enhanced surface and mRNA expression of C5aR was detected in microvascular ECs after exposure to LPS, IFN-γ, IL-6, and TNF-α concomitant with an upregulation of macrophage-inflammatory protein-2 and MCP-1 [116]. Vice versa, the stimulation of ECs with C5a in turn leads to an increase in EC gene expression of E-selectin, ICAM-1, VCAM-1, cytokines/

chemokines and related receptors, for example, vascular endothelial growth factor receptor-C, IL-6, IL- 18R [110]. In addition, C5a can also mediate EC chemotaxis as well as cell retraction and actin polymerization [117]. The immediate effects of purified C5b-9 (MAC) in EC cultures are the retraction of the plasma membrane with the exposure of underlying extracellular matrix and the translocation of P-selectin and von Willebrand factor (vWF) from Weibel–Palade storage granules to the plasma membrane (reviewed in [118]). In addition to releasing preformed mediators, MAC-activated ECs synthesize IL-8, MCP-1, P-selectin, tissue factor (TF), platelet-derived growth factor (PDGF) and basic fibroblast growth factor (bFGF) [110]. This process is crucially regulated by CD59. When CD59 is inactivated by glycation, as may occur in diabetes, ECs increase their production of PDGF and bFGF [118]. Furthermore, ECs have been shown to produce C1s and C4, C3 and factor B and appear to be the major producers of circulating C7, previously shown to be primarily synthesized at extrahepatic sites based on the analysis of C7 allotypes in liver transplant recipients [110]. In ECs, however, the direct exposure to hemodynamic shear stress can also abrogate the complement-induced pro-inflammatory response by the upregulation of the complement-inhibitory protein clusterin [119]. C5 has also been implicated in fibrocyte dedifferentiation and fibroblast proliferation, and thus may also contribute to fibrosis during remodeling. In a model of chronic bleomycin-induced pulmonary fibrosis, in complement C5-sufficient mice, the deleterious C5 activity was associated with increased expression of matrix metalloproteinase-3 (MMP-3) and transforming growth factor-β1 [120]. In addition, small molecule inhibitors of C5a decreased collagen production and hepatic fibrosis in genetically susceptible mice [121]. In patients with advanced atherosclerosis, elevated serum C5a levels strongly associated with increased risk of cardiovascular events [7] whereas C5a and sMAC were independently associated with plasma markers of endothelial dysfunction [122]. Taken together, complement activation products play crucial roles in the initiation of inflammation by ECs, and EC-derived complement products promote vascular inflammation (Fig. **2**).

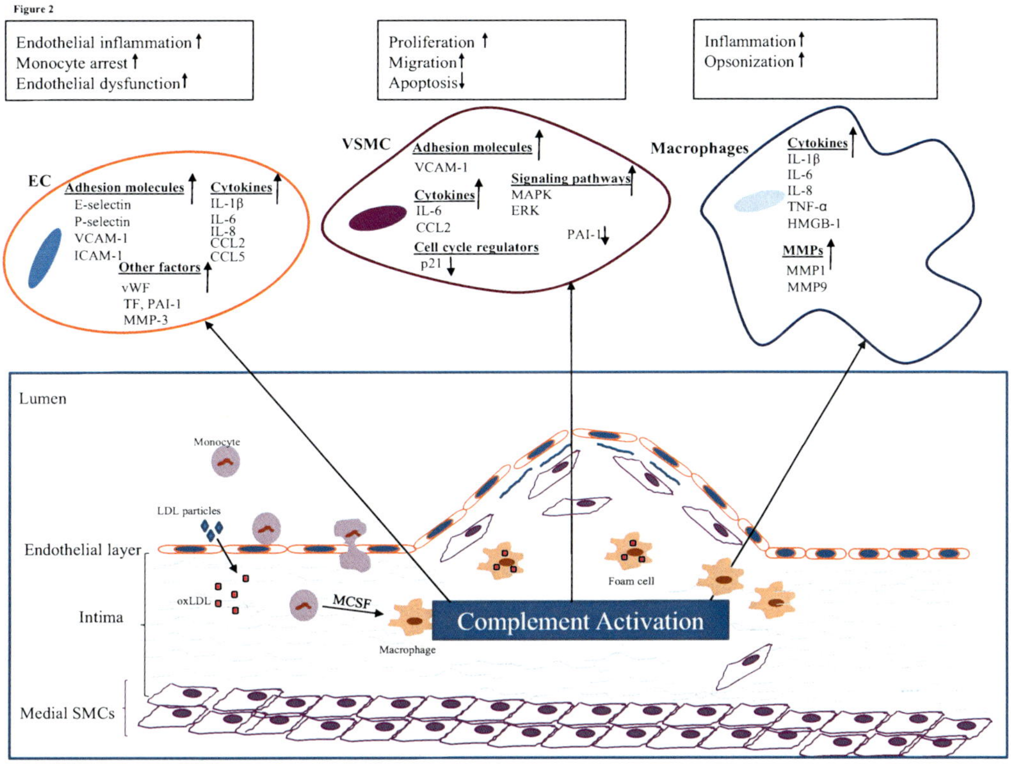

Fig. (2). Consequences of complement activation within the atherosclerotic plaque: vascular cells do not only secrete complement components but also represent potential targets of active products of the activated complement cascade.

4.2. Vascular Smooth Muscle Cells and the Complement Activation

Vascular smooth muscles cells (VSMCs) exhibit the ability to increase their rate of proliferation, migration and synthetic capacity in response to different vascular changes, *e.g.* after vascular injury and hypertension and play a critical role in vascular remodeling [123]. Indeed, neointimal SMCs differ from medial SMCs in regard to morphology, proliferative potential and gene expression, and exhibit a phenotype resembling fetal SMCs. In contrast to medial SMCs, neointimal SMCs exhibit a constitutively enhanced expression of P-selectin, CC and CXC chemokines. Having the capacity to permanently replace ECs after injury, neointimal SMCs exposed to circulating blood are important in amplifying leukocyte recruitment, as shown for monocyte and T-cell arrest under flow conditions [124]. VSMCs are initially targeted by the MAC complement attack within lesions, supported by the observation that MAC co-localizes with VSMCs during early atherogenesis. Furthermore, sublytic concentrations of MAC might contribute to SMC-mediated leukocyte recruitment by increasing the expression of MCP-1 and IL-6 [125, 126]. Several complement components, such as C1q, C3, C3c and MAC, have been detected in VSMCs in a model of angiotensin-I--induced renal vasculopathy [127]. Human aortic VSMCs themselves were shown to produce C3 and C4 in response to TNF-α and IFN-γ [128]. Similarly, CRP and TNF-α enhanced C3 expression in rat VSMCs both *in vitro* and *in vivo* [127]. In addition to modifying leukocyte recruitment, sublytic concentrations of MAC might also contribute to vascular remodeling by increasing the proliferation of human VSMCs concomitant with an activation of the MAPK and extracellular signal-regulated kinase (ERK). Importantly, inhibition of 3-hydroxy-3-methylglutaryl coenzyme A (HMG-CoA) reductase, with cerivastatin, reduced MAC-induced ERK1/2 activation, the proliferation of VSMCs and the synthesis of the pro-inflammatory IL-6 independent of lowering plasma cholesterol [129]. Additionally, complement activation may alter VSMC phenotype as reported by Lin and colleagues who showed that exogenous C3 induces a shift towards a synthetic VSMC phenotype [93]. In line with this, VSMCs isolated from angiotensin II and hypertensive rats showed a higher proliferation rate and pro-inflammatory gene expression profile in contrast to the more contractile phenotype in normotensive vessels [93, 127]. Interestingly, sublytic MAC concentrations have been shown to stimulate the proliferation of SMCs by reducing the cell cycle inhibitor p21 [130]. MAC can also amplify mitogenic signals from other growth factors such as PDGF adding a further level of complexity. MAC can also inhibit SMC apoptosis by activating an autocrine insulin-like growth factor-1 (IGF-1) loop [131] (Fig. **2**). While apoptosis of vascular cells is a prominent feature of vascular remodeling, antiapoptotic effects of MAC might protect VSMCs in early lesions [132]. Ruptured plaques also contain higher numbers of apoptotic VSMCs than do stable lesions, suggesting that VSMC apoptosis may promote plaque rupture. This is supported by the detection of higher expression of surface Fas on human plaque-derived SMCs and macrophages can also induce apoptosis in these cells [133], but a role of complement on this process has not yet been investigated. Complement activation may thus significantly contribute to the imbalance between cell death and proliferation observed during atherogenesis [130]. Physiologically, the proliferative response may be important in tissue repair during the resolution of inflammation. We previously reported the expression of C5aR1 in VSMCs. Human and mouse VSMCs express C5aR1 at mRNA and protein levels, which are markedly increased upon TNF-α stimulation. In the context of arterial neointima formation, we identified a specific role of C5aR1 in the regulation of VCAM-1 and PAI-1 in VSMCs [134]. The capacity of C5a to elicit migration of VSMCs or their progenitors and C5a-C5aR1-mediated regulation of vasoactive substances or their intracellular signal transduction in VSMCs still remains to be elucidated.

4.3. Macrophages and Complement Activation

In more advanced atherosclerotic lesions, MAC is colocalized with macrophages [130], and is very likely associated with apoptosis and necrosis of lipid-laden macrophages, and important for the clearance of apoptotic and necrotic material. Of note, macrophages can synthesize all components of complement system allowing for the local production and activation of complement at sites of inflammation. Macrophage production of C3 and C5 is increased by stimulation through both Fc and C1q receptor [135], further amplifying the local production of complement within vessel wall. Moreover, macrophages express receptors for C1q, C3b, iC3b, C3a, C5a and Fc. Complement C3a and C5a trigger the chemotaxis and activation of macrophages through C3aR and C5aR1, and the expression as well as synthesis of C3 in arterial tissue after vascular injury coincides with increasing infiltrates of macrophages [136]. In acute intestinal injury, C3a/C3aR axis is engaged in neutrophil mobilization [137] indicating a broader role of anaphylatoxins in leukocyte recruitment. The activation of monocytes through C5aR1 causes not only the upregulation of complement receptor (CR) 1 and CR3 but also the production of pro-inflammatory cytokines IL-1, IL-6, IL-8 and TNF-α [138] (Fig. **2**). The larger split product C3b and its subsequent cleavage product iC3b can bind covalently to cell membranes, serving as accessory adhesion molecules that strengthen the contact to macrophages that express CR1 and CR3. CR3 and C5a were in addition shown to mediate the secretion of MMP-9 from bovine and human neutrophils as well as human eosinophils [139, 140], which is a crucial proteinase utilized to transmigrate through extracellular basement membranes. Thus, the activation of the complement cascade not only contributes to leukocyte recruitment, but also enhances inflammation and cell activation within lesion. A study demonstrated that locally produced complement fragments C3a and C5a interacting with their receptors (C3aR and C5aR1) on T cells provide both costimulatory and survival signals to T cells [141]. The second alternative receptor for C5a, the C5aR2 is expressed in macrophages within human and mouse atherosclerotic plaques and have a contributory role for recruitment of inflammatory cells and expression of proinflammatory cytokines IL-1β and TNF-α [142].

4.4. Interplay between Platelets and the Complement Cascade

The complement system is involved in platelet-associated immune processes: (i) CRs on platelets contribute to the sensing of various pathogens and of infectious and non-infectious inflammatory reactions; (ii) the complement system can induce or support platelet activation, which triggers antimicrobial attack; and (iii) platelets can modulate the activity of the complement system, and *vice versa*. Furthermore, the interaction of platelets with other immune elements can involve complement molecules [143]. Intravascular aggregation of P-selectin- and vWF-expressing platelets is a prominent feature in experimental models of antibody-mediated vascular graft rejection that is decreased in the absence of MAC deposition [144]. By contributing to the recruitment of leukocytes which in turn secrete cytokines and pro-coagulatory tissue factor (TF), platelet-monocyte interactions provide an atherogenic milieu at the vascular wall that supports plaque formation. The finding that P-selectin on activated platelets can bind C3b and thus propagate the complement cascade suggests that platelets are active players in the complement system. C1q, MBL and CRP enter the equation when phospholipids are exposed to the plasma membrane of activated platelets. Furthermore, it was recently demonstrated that platelet microparticles, which are released from platelets upon activation, express complement components and inhibitors [145]. Thus, a carpet of activated platelets and platelet microparticles would enrich and extend the area available for complement interactions. Importantly, C5a upregulates plasminogen activator inhibitor-1 (PAI-1) in human plaque-derived macrophages *via* the activation of transcriptional factor nuclear factor kappa B (NF-κB) and thus may also contribute to thrombotic complications at the lesion site. However, on the contrary, this may act as a defense mechanism against plaque destabilization and rupture [146]. Likewise, C5a can upregulate PAI-1 in human mast cells and basophils that could be inhibited by the treatment with plasmin [147]. Considering the suggested role for mast cells and components of the complement system in the development of cardiovascular diseases, it could be hypothesized that mast cells by producing t-PA in a resting state and by expressing PAI-1 when activated by C5a, might participate in the modulation of the balance between proteases and protease inhibitors regulating tissue injury and repair mechanisms that follow. Together, increasing evidence indicates that the complement system plays a pivotal role in multiple cell types implicated in atherosclerosis, the underlying cause of cardiovascular diseases.

4.5. Lipids and Complement

Lipid-lowering drug therapy is frequently used for primary prevention of CVD, an evidence of LDL-cholesterol as established risk factor and a major player in atherosclerotic plaque formation [148]. The deposition of LDL in subendothelial space, during the initiation of atherogenesis, triggers expression of chemokines and adhesion molecules but also activates the complement system. This was demonstrated by the binding of enzymatically modified LDL to CRP inducing complement activation in early human atherosclerotic lesions [149]. Of note, C3, C4, C1s, and C1q levels were upregulated in plasma and aorta of hypercholesterolemic Apoe$^{-/-}$ mice as well as in plasma of familial hyper-cholesterolemia (FH) patients [150]. Importantly, C3-enriched FH plasma potentiated mitogenic activity in macrophages, an effect that was significantly reduced by anti-C3 neutralizing antibody [150]. C1q and MBL bind to modified lipoproteins as oxLDL and enhance their uptake by macrophages [151]. Also, an increased efflux of cholesterol to ATP-binding cassette transporters mediated by C1q and MBL has been reported [5]. Notably, accumulated cholesterol in macrophages induces the expression of C3 [152] but also several genes implicated in complement activation [153]. A cleavage product of C3, ASP or C3 adesArg, promotes fatty acid uptake in adipose tissue, an effect mediated by C5aR2 [154]. Indeed, *C5ar2*-deficient mice have reduced ability to synthesize triglyceride and increased potential to oxidize fatty acid in adipose tissue [155]. There is, therefore, increasingly interesting data on lipids and complement that deserves attention in understanding complement-mediated mechanisms underlying CVD.

5. COMPLEMENT SYSTEM IN ATHEROSCLEROSIS

5.1. Atherosclerosis and Complement-mediated Effects in the Vasculature

Atherosclerosis, the major cause of cardiovascular diseases, is a progressive chronic inflammatory disease characterized by the thickening of the arterial vessel wall and the clinical evidence is thrombus formation following plaque rupture [156]. It is orchestrated by interactions between modified lipids, immune and vascular cells as well as a variety of mediators of both innate and adaptive immunity that ultimately leads to the formation of lesion that protrude into the arterial lumen [1, 157]. The initiation of atherosclerotic plaque formation is triggered by hyperlipidemia and turbulent blood flow at arterial branching points resulting in endothelial cell (EC) dysfunction and activation. Low-density lipoprotein (LDL) particles leak into subendothelial space, are modified by enzymes such as myeloperoxidases, lipoxygenases as well as reactive oxygen species like hypochlorous (HOCl) and phenol radical intermediates and are retained [156, 158]. Modified LDL further triggers EC activation leading to the secretion of chemokines such as CCL2 and macrophage migration inhibitory factor (MIF), and the expression of adhesion molecules such as ICAM-1, VCAM-1 and P-selectin to recruit inflammatory cells like monocytes, granulocytes and T cells into the intima [159, 160]. In the intima, monocytes differentiate into macrophages that accumulate lipids leading to expression of wide array of cytokines that maintain plaque inflammatory milieu and also results in fatty streaks formation. Matrix components are deposited and smooth muscle cells (SMCs) are recruited giving rise to the fibroproliferative progression of the plaque. In the advanced stages, death of lipid-laden cells results in necrotic core formation and SMCs migrate to the subendothelial space to form fibrous cap. In addition, neovascularization may occur within the plaque and from the adventitia, and leakage of fragile vessels could lead to plaque hemorrhage. In unstable plaques, the rupture of fibrous cap exposes thrombogenic material leading to platelet aggregation and thrombus formation which is a major risk for myocardial infarction and stroke.

The atherosclerotic lesion is rich in triggers for the activation of the complement system and evidence for complement activation within the atherosclerotic plaque is enormous [3]. The complement anaphylatoxin C5a is a potent and multifunctional pro-inflammatory mediator of the innate immune system promoting the recruitment and subsequent activation of monocytes and neutrophils [46]. The initial report implicating C5a in atherosclerosis dates back in the early 80s when high levels of activated C5a in plasma of a patient with severe ulcerating atherosclerosis and the cholesterol embolization syndrome was observed. This led to the hypothesis that crystalline cholesterol might activate C5a to exacerbate ischemic injury in atherosclerotic states. Indeed crystalline cholesterol-triggered activation of C5a was able to induce the aggregation of PMNs and provoked them to damage cultured ECs *in vitro* [161]. The authors described this as a possible mechanism underlying ischemic manifestations in atherosclerosis. As a chronic inflammatory disease, atherosclerosis is marked by inflammatory mechanisms from initiation and progression to the point of clinical manifestation [2]. The complement anaphylatoxin C5a was, few years later, demonstrated to potently trigger the secretion of pro-inflammatory mediators as TNF and IL-1 from human mononuclear cells *in vitro* [162]. Employing human umbilical vein endothelial cells, Foreman and colleagues could show a C5a-induced expression of P-selectin in time and dose-dependent manner [163]. The pro-inflammatory nature of the atherosclerotic lesion is characterized and sustained by enhanced expression of chemokines such as CCL2 and MIF as well as adhesion molecules like ICAM-1, VCAM-1, E-selectin and P-selectin that work in concert to recruit inflammatory cells into the intima [1, 160, 164]. Of significance, C5a is able to induce the expression of not only pro-inflammatory mediators as TNF, IL-1 and IL-6 but also classical cell adhesion molecules as VCAM-1, ICAM-1 and E-selectin [162, 165]. Therefore, C5a is pivotal in inflammatory cell recruitment by either directly or indirectly triggering the expression of the molecules required initiating cell recruitment. Indeed, adhesion of neutrophils to C5a-activated endothelium has been described [163]. Interestingly, C5a is extremely potent chemotactic factor that directly guide monocytes, mast cells and T-lymphocytes to the site of inflammation [166, 167]. Injection of C5a into blood-perfused hind limb of normal and atherosclerotic monkeys resulted in significant reduction in leukocyte count in venous blood drainage from the hind limb. C5a-activated leukocytes induced a marked constriction of large arteries in atherosclerotic monkeys, an effect which was abolished by thromboxane A2 receptor antagonist. This may indicate that C5a-driven vascular responses are mediated partly by release of thromboxane A2 [168].

Evidence for a possible functional role of anaphylatoxin in atherosclerosis was further corroborated by identification of C5a and C3a receptors in human atherosclerotic coronary artery plaques. These anaphylatoxin receptors were expressed in multiple cell types including macrophages, T cells, mast cells, endothelial and smooth muscle cells present in the atherosclerotic plaque. However, the principal cell type expressing both C3aR and C5aR1 were macrophages whereas T cells expressed mainly C5aR1 and a small fraction expressed C3aR. Plaque endothelial and smooth muscle cells also expressed both C3aR and C5aR1 whereas mast cells expressed only C5aR1 [169]. Recently, anaphylatoxin receptors were found to be expressed on platelets from coronary heart disease patients [170]. This extends the repertoire of complement anaphylatoxin expression in the vasculature. However, whether anaphylatoxins modulate atherosclerotic plaque formation through effects in multiple atherogenic cell types is poorly explored.

In addition to anaphylatoxins, complement components like C1q [171], CD59 [172] and several others are expressed in human atherosclerotic lesion. This warrants the targeting of the complement system in atherosclerotic plaque formation.

5.2. Targeting Complement System in Experimental Atherosclerosis

Gene targeting and neutralizing antibodies have been very useful in the study of the functional role of the complement system in atherosclerosis. Employing C1q-deficient mice (*C1qa*$^{-/-}$) with low-density lipoprotein receptor knockout (*Ldlr*$^{-/-}$) background, a role for the classic complement pathway in atherosclerotic plaque formation was demonstrated. *C1q* deficiency exacerbates atherosclerotic lesion formation but with a rather complex plaque cellular composition including accumulation of apoptotic cells suggesting the need for effective apoptotic cell clearance for containing the size and complexity of early lesions [173]. C1q synergizes with IgM to opsonize apoptotic cells which facilitates their clearance by macrophages [174]. Intuitively, the absence of IgM would augment atherosclerotic lesion and exhibit features of defective clearance of cellular debris. Indeed, IgM was shown to be protective against atherosclerotic lesion formation in *Ldlr*$^{-/-}$ mice. This was however independent of C1q-induced complement activation and the underlying mechanisms may not involve apoptotic cell clearance [175].

Several other components of the complement pathway have been studied in atherogenesis. Genetic ablation of CD55 enhances leukocyte accumulation as well as neointima thickening and protects against atherosclerotic lesion formation *via* lowering of serum lipid profile [176, 177]. CD59, a key regulator of complement membrane attack complex (MAC) assembly protects against atherosclerosis by restricting the formation of complement membrane attack complex. Blockade of C5, with neutralizing antibody, or treatment with CR2-Crry, a small molecule inhibitor targeting C3 activation, in *mCd59ab*$^{-/-}$/*Apoe*$^{-/-}$ mice attenuated lesion formation [178, 179]. Paradoxically, C5-deficient and control *Apoe*$^{-/-}$ mice have comparable lesion size [180] and may indicate cooperation between C5 and CD59 that requires dual inhibition for atheroprotection. In contrast to the ambivalent role of C5 in atherosclerosis, C3, a central molecule in both classical and alternate pathway, has somewhat direct role. C3 deficiency exacerbates atherosclerotic lesion formation and induces features of vulnerable plaque phenotype [181]. In rabbits, C6 deficiency has atheroprotective effect on diet-induced atherosclerosis. The contrasting roles, *i.e.* atheroprotecting *vs.* atheropromoting, of the complement components described above warrants their specific manipulation that may serve as therapeutic strategy in the treatment of atherosclerosis.

A key biological outcome of complement activation is the generation of complement anaphylatoxins. The presence of anaphylatoxin receptors in human coronary artery plaque was a hint that they may have functional role in atherosclerotic lesion formation *in vivo* [169]. However, descriptive observations frequently cannot predict exacerbating *versus* inhibitory effects in a disease situation *in vivo* or exclude a bystander role. Thus *in vivo* models of vascular inflammation were needed to decipher the functional role of anaphylatoxin receptors in the development of atherosclerosis. In view of this, the first functional data on the role of C5aR1 in acute and accelerated atherosclerotic plaque formation *in vivo* after vascular injury was reported. Employing small molecule antagonist JPE1375 and blocking monoclonal antibody targeting C5aR1, we unequivocally demonstrated that in a wire-induced endothelial denudation of the carotid artery, mimicking injury to the endothelium during vascular interventions, in apolipoprotein E-deficient mice, C5aR1 targeting limited neointima formation. Mechanistically, this was attributed to reduced *Vcam-1* expression and a concomitant decreased in neutrophil and monocyte influx. In addition, C5aR1 inhibition resulted in a decreased PAI-1 expression and may explain the increased smooth muscle cell content likely *via* enhanced migration [134]. The candidacy of C5aR1 as a therapeutic target in vascular inflammation was thus confirmed. This was further corroborated by the use of a second antagonist of C5aR1, PMX53, which showed a decrease in atherosclerotic lesion formation in *Apoe*$^{-/-}$ mice [154]. C5a and its receptor C5aR1-mediated mechanisms underlying atherosclerotic plaque formation may include the induction of MMPs in human macrophages. C5a induces the expression but also the activity of MMP1 and MMP9, effects that could be blocked by C5aR1 neutralizing antibody. Importantly, C5a and C3a are present in high levels in human coronary lesions and this is associated with late lumen loss of drug eluting stents [182, 183].

The discovery of the second receptor for C5a, C5aR2, provided avenue to expand and pursue the cellular and molecular mechanisms underlying C5a and its receptor-driven initiation and progression of inflammatory diseases. In accord with their adjacent location on the genome, C5aR2 and C5aR1 are expressed in similar tissue and cellular locations [51]. Intuitively, in spite of the lack of G-protein coupled receptor signaling, C5aR2 would have similar effects as C5aR1. Indeed, like C5aR1, C5aR2 has been implicated in many inflammatory diseases as sepsis and atherosclerosis [184, 185]. In the vasculature, C5aR2 is highly expressed in advanced human carotid artery atherosclerotic plaques. This upregulation of C5aR2 upon atheroprogression correlates with high expression of pro-inflammatory cytokines. C5aR2 is mainly expressed in human atherosclerotic plaques by macrophages, neutrophils and endothelial cells. To determine the relevance of C5aR2 in vascular inflammation, *C5ar2*-deficient macrophages exposed to either C5a or oxidized LDL alone or both led to reduced pro-inflammatory cytokine production compared to control wild type (WT) [142]. This confirmed the pro-inflammatory role of C5aR2 reported to be mandatorily required for the production of the pro-inflammatory molecule HMGB1 and critical for the development of sepsis [184]. C5aR2 promotes mononuclear cell arrest on TNF-α-activated ECs by enhancing integrin expression and thus indicate a pro-atherosclerotic role of C5aR2 [142]. As descriptive and *in vitro* studies frequently do not predict the functional role in disease situation *in vivo*, *C5ar2*-deficient mice with hyperlipidemic background have been employed to address the functional role of C5aR2 in atherosclerotic plaque formation. *C5ar2* deficiency attenuates atherosclerotic as well as neointimal plaque formation after vascular injury and induces features of stable plaque phenotype. The atherosclerotic phenotype of *C5ar2*-deficient mice is attributed partly to reduced expression of *Vcam-1*, *Tnf-α* and *C5ar1*, all well described for their pro-inflammatory and pro-atherosclerotic roles [185]. Dual blockade of C5a receptors has been shown to be beneficial in "high-grade" sepsis [184] suggesting that C5aR1 and C5aR2 work in concert to regulate inflammatory conditions. Therefore, the combined blockade of C5a receptors may be more beneficial in the treatment of inflammatory diseases. Indeed, blocking C5ar1 with the small molecule antagonist JPE1375 in *C5ar2*-deficient mice resulted in further reduction of neointimal plaque size [185]. Whether blocking of C5ar2 in *C5ar1*-deficient mice would also lead to further reduction in plaque size is still unresolved partly due to the absence of good C5aR2 neutralizing antibodies and inhibitors. Nevertheless targeting anaphylatoxins particularly C5a and its receptors provides new therapeutic option for the treatment of atherosclerosis. Of note, the recent reports on the crosstalk between C5a and cholesterol crystals in the induction of cytokine production and inflammasome/caspase-1 activation provides another interesting mechanistic insights in complement activation in atherosclerosis that needs to be harnessed for the treatment of atherosclerosis [186, 187]. Together, data from both gene targeting and neutralizing antibody demonstrate the therapeutic potential of targeted complement inhibition.

5.3. Intervening Human Atherosclerosis *via* Complement Blocking Strategies

Epidemiological studies have been very useful in determining the association between the complement system and the development of human atherosclerosis [188]. Serum C3 and C4 levels have been closely linked to an increased risk of cardiovascular diseases [189]. Indeed, gene targeting and neutralizing antibodies have corroborated the critical role of the complement system in experimental atherosclerosis. Though mice are not humans, knowledge gained from various atherosclerosis models represents an important step in understanding the cellular and molecular mechanisms underlying the disease. Thus, may help in the design of therapeutic strategies to treat the disease. The candidacy of C5 as a potential therapeutic target was shown by the ability of C5-inhibitors to attenuate atherosclerosis in experimental models [134, 190]. In line with this, a precursor of the recombinant anti-C5 antibody eculizumab, pexelizumab, reduced mortality rate in patients undergoing coronary artery bypass grafting [191, 192]. Though complement inhibition in human atherosclerosis hitherto has not been fully explored, increasing evidence indicates the therapeutic potential of complement targeting in atherosclerosis and therefore warrants its exploration in clinical trials.

5.4. Complement As Circulating Biomarkers

In assessing risk of CVD, markers with strong predictive potential are critical in clinical decision making and the therapeutic strategy that follows. Prospective clinical studies have demonstrated that a substantial number of complement components are associated with risk of major cardiovascular events [3]. Serum C3 levels, from cohorts of 444 men and 416 women with mean age of 53.9 years without prior ischemic events and hence classified as healthy individuals, were associated with risk of MI [6]. Thus it is not surprising that atherosclerotic patients have high levels of C3 [193, 194] but also C4 [195]. In advanced stage of atherosclerosis, serum levels of anaphylatoxin C5a predicted risk of major cardiovascular events independent of markers as CRP, serum amyloid A and fibrinogen [7]. Additionally, C5a predicted risk of restenosis after superficial femoral artery balloon angioplasty and this was again independent of CRP [196]. High levels of MBL had a protective effect on MI in diabetic and hyper-cholesterolemic patients [197] whereas in healthy individuals MBL was a risk factor for coronary artery disease [198]. Recently, the potential of C3a and C3 to predict carotid intima-media thickness, ankle-arm blood pressure index and CVD was studied in a large cohort. High C3a, but not C3, levels associated with carotid intima-media thickness and ankle-arm blood pressure index. However, in heavy smokers, both C3a and C3 were independently associated with CVD [199]. Taken together, it appears circulating levels of specific components of the complement system may serve as useful predictors of major cardiovascular events.

6. COMPLEMENT AND MYOCARDIAL INFARCTION

6.1. Complement System is Activated in Myocardial Infarction

Myocardial infarction (MI) is a prominent cardiovascular event with high morbidity and mortality rates. Most common reason for MI is the buildup of atherosclerotic plaques and compromised blood flow to the myocardium deprives these muscles of oxygen. This impaired perfusion of the myocardium or myocardial necrosis results in not only systemic, but also a local inflammatory response that comprises a complicated interaction between ischemic myocardial and inflammatory cells, cytokines, complement factors, and acute-phase proteins. The activation of the complement system is an essential part of the innate immune response which is triggered after MI [200], where all components of the classical and alternative pathway are up-regulated [201]. The presence of complement activity in infarcted heart was detected as early as 1971 [138]. This has been verified by numerous studies that followed [130, 202, 204]. Immune complexes, autoantibodies against heart tissues, mitochondrial proteins and phospholipids released by ischemia and reperfusion as well as elevated CRP are mediators for direct activation of complement cascade in infarct heart; they directly bind C1q or the MBL. Following MI, complement components C3, C4, C5, and MAC have been reported to be expressed in the infarcted tissue. These components are found bound to mitochondria, plasma membrane and nuclei of cardiac myocytes [204]. Humans tend to have reduced levels of C1, C3 and C4 components in the plasma after MI and increase in circulatory levels of MAC, suggesting the activation of complement system [205, 206]. There have been studies which show that C3 predicts cardiovascular related risks in both genders [6, 207]. Likewise the early reference of complement and MI was reported in baboon model, where it is shown that C3, C4 and C5 are deposited in infarcted myocardial tissues and inactivating the complement system showed a significant reduction in myocardial damage [204, 208, 209]. Plasma levels of iC3b, C3d, C3a, C4d, Ba, Bb is shown to be significantly increased in patients with MI [210, 211]. C5a is known to alter the function of myocardium and is also known to reduce coronary blood flow in MI [212]. Once complement is activated, it recruits neutrophils and monocytes and thereby promotes the inflammatory process [213].

With respect to the complement system after MI, it is activated in the plasma and hence induces changes in vascular flow, promisingly increasing vascular permeability, leukocyte extravasation and chemotaxis (as primary response). The components C3a, C4a and C5a act as regulatory or inflammatory mediators and help by associating themselves by binding directly to the injured myocardium [214]. Though how complement is activated in MI is still unclear, the fact that all complement pathways play crucial roles in MI is well-established [215]. There have been reports of the lectin pathway being prominent contributor in MI or repair after MI but no clear-cut evidence suggests that other pathways do not contribute in cardiac repair [117]. Post MI, usually left ventricular (LV) remodeling begins and progresses with the course of time and the underlying factors like treatment or recurring MI contribute to the cause [118, 119, 216]. Due to this the heart could alter in various ways: thinning of ventricular wall, cardiomyocyte lengthening, infarct expansion, inflammation and reabsorption, scar formation, dilation and reshaping of LV, myocyte loss and accumulation of collagen [111]. A number of underlying mechanisms have been proposed. Briefly, the healthy myocytes stretch to replace the injured ones that stimulate expression of various proteins and release excessive angiotensin, hence contributing to myocyte hypertrophy. This lowers the cardiac output and performance, which further releases a stream of invading cytokines. Collagen synthesis is promoted resulting in scar tissue formation thereby remodeling the heart. Either way the complement components are found deposited on the surface near the infarcted heart. The fibroblast/endothelium layer express adhesion molecules as a result of complement deposition and the usual complement components of C3b, C5b act as ligands for integrins. Leukocytes infiltrate and accumulate in the vascular compartment. Finally, the MAC is formed causing selectins to be released [120, 121]. The terminal complex, as mentioned previously, triggers the release of IL8 and other cytokines thereby changing the vascular microenvironment. Also, the release of complement anaphylatoxins stimulates similar effect. Therefore, there is a crosstalk between different components of the immune system in cardiac remodeling and hence no single pathway is hitherto considered as the most effective one. Combating the inflammatory infiltrate, in a timely manner, and optimal positive repair mechanism is essential for cardiac remodeling and hence the role of immune system should be probed further for therapeutic options. In addition, vascular occlusion process occurring in acute myocardial infarction is potentiated by local complement activation enhanced neutrophil infiltration [217].

The complement system, as discussed above, is elevated during MI and cardiac repair, hence, various complement based strategies and drugs are being developed to control MI.

6.2. Complement Inhibition with C1-INH by MI and Myocardial IR-Injury

The blockade of complement system by C1-INH, a serine protease inhibitor, which inhibits the classical or the lectin pathways, has been shown to reduce the necrotic myocardium by 65%, attenuate plasma CK activity and improved cardiac function in animal models [123, 125]. Mechanistically, the endothelial function is preserved by inhibiting neutrophil endothelium interaction and hence increasing the contractile function of the heart [93, 133]. The exact mode of action is not known but it is speculated that C1-INH attenuate the anaphylatoxins directly or play major role in regulating the influx of leukocytes particularly neutrophils to the infarct site [123]. They may as well limit endothelial leukocyte interaction by inhibiting the expression of selectins [133]. The beneficial effects of this inhibitor are observed in human studies [126, 128, 129]. In randomised double-blinded study, C1-INH inhibition in patients with ST-elevation MI (STEMI), who underwent surgical reperfusion resulted in reduced serum cardiac troponin I (cTnI) levels with improved cardiac parameters [129, 218].

The effect of intravenous C1-INH has been studied following reperfusion therapy in 22 patients with acute myocardial infarction, at least 6 hours after onset of acute MI, in order to prevent interference with thrombolytic therapy. A loading dose of C1-INH was followed by a continuous infusion for 48 hours using three escalating dosage schemes. The loading doses of 50 U/kg and 100 U/kg increased plasma C1-INH activity. In this study, C1-INH was well tolerated and drug-related adverse events were not observed. In 13 patients who received early thrombolytic therapy, the release of troponin T and creatine kinase-MB mass was reduced by 36% and 57% and the 18 control patients [128]. Moreover, the investigation of pharmacokinetic behavior of C1-INH in patients with acute myocardial infarction to calculate the amount of C1-INH required for optimal efficacy. Higher dosage of C1-INH were required in patients in MI that differ from those found in healthy subjects, indicating the continuous and enhanced consumption of C1-INH by target proteases in patients with MI [219]. The drawback of the use of C1-INH in a clinical practice is the thrombogenic complications that follow treatment. In doses ranging from 20 U/kg - 60 U/kg, it was deemed cardio-protective and contrastingly, in higher doses above 100 IU/kg all the cardioprotective affects vanish due to the thrombogenic complications as reported in animal studies [131, 132]. Even though the treatment with C1-INH humans has been demonstrated to be safe for many years [220, 221], there have been recent reports suggesting increased risk of thromboembolic complications associated with the use of C1-INH [222, 223], particularly beyond the approved clinical indications and doses. The need of high dose of C1-INH for the treatment of MI compromised the thromboembolic complication of C1-INH at recommended or off-label, high doses. These adverse events were believed to be at least partly associated with C1-INH treatment due to its inhibitory effects on the fibrinolytic system [224, 225]. To support the safety of a recombinant C1-INH product, Relan *et al.* recently evaluated the effects of C1-INH treatment on coagulation and fibrinolysis in a randomised clinical trial in symptomatic HAE patients and observed no thromboembolic events in HAE patients following recombinant C1-INH treatment at doses up to 100 IU/kg [225]. Recent study evaluated the potential prothrombotic risk of C1-INH treatment in high doses using a preclinical rabbit model. Following intravenous infusion of C1-INH at doses up to 800 IU/kg, the exposure and the pharmacodynamic efficacy of C1-INH were confirmed by activity measurements of C1-esterase, and coagulation factors XIa and XIIa, respectively. Potential prothrombotic effects were assessed following induction of venous and arterial thrombosis using *in vivo* models of venous and arterial stasis, complemented by various *in vitro* assays of coagulation markers. Interestingly, high-dose C1-INH administration to rabbits did not potentiate venous thrombosis, and interestingly inhibited arterial thrombosis.

Moreover, decreased thrombin generation and platelet aggregation, as well as prolonged activated partial thromboplastin time, clotting time, and clot formation time were observed upon high dose administration of C1-INH [225]. This study was conducted in healthy rabbits and future investigations of the prothrombotic risk of C1-INH in various disease models, reflecting the potentially complex influences of underlying disease, are warranted.

6.3. Complement Inhibition at C3 Convertase Level in MI

C3 holds a convergence point in the complement activation pathways and hence blocking C3 may be a therapeutic option in interfering with complement-mediated pathologies [135]. Antibodies against C3b or factor B, which prevent the formation of the pro-convertase have been tested. TA106 developed by Taligen Therapeutics, which block the conversion to the active convertase is yet to be tested in models of MI. In addition, C3 may also be depleted *via* cleavage by cobra venom factor (CVF) or anti-C3 proteases [135]. CVF is a complement activating protein in cobra venom, which functionally resembles C3b, and has been used for decades for decomplementation of serum to investigate the role of complement in many model systems of disease. However, the use of CVF for clinical practice is considered impractical because of immunogenicity issues. The humanization of CVF was recently demonstrated to yield a potent CVF-like molecule. Mice treated with recombinant humanized CVF (HC3-1496) are protected from myocardial ischemia-reperfusion (MI/R) injuries with resultant preservation of cardiac function, indicating the potential of clinical use [226]. C3 inhibitors of the compstatin family that protect native C3 by preventing its binding to and cleavage by C3 convertases are most promising drug candidates [97]. Compstatin is a cyclic tridecapeptide that binds to C3 and inhibits C3 cleavage. It is found to be specific to human C3 without affecting other plasma proteins [139, 140, 227]; neither did it moderate leukocyte influx or show any adverse effect on the heart [140, 227]. In clinical conditions in which excessive C3 activation is a major driver, such as I/R injury in the context of transplantation or in C3 glomerulopathies, compstatin promise as alternative therapeutics [97]. Due to the species specifity of compstatin, which is active only in humans and primates, it has been difficult to test in other well-defined animal models [139]. Another disadvantage of this approach is that by centrally inhibiting all of the complement pathways, the risk of losing the immune protective effects offered by complement activation increases. A recent animal study reveal an additional indication that C3 is necessary to preserve myocardium and myocardial function in chronic MI [228], indicating that the usage of C3 inhibitors in MI is limited.

Targeting CR1 may represent a potential option for treatment of MI, since low levels of plasma soluble CR1 has been detected in patients receiving thrombolytic therapy for acute myocardial infarction and elevation of plasma sCR1 might limit complement-mediated injury in this setting [229]. The sCR1 bivalently bound dimeric forms of its ligands, C3b and methylamine-treated C4, and promoted their inactivation by factor I. The sCR1 had complement inhibitory and anti-inflammatory activities in a rat model of reperfusion injury of ischemic myocardium, reducing myocardial infarction size by 44% [230]. TP-10 is a recombinant sCR1 which block the common pathways formed by the C3 and C5 convertases by binding C3b and C4b. AVANT Immunotherapeutics is developing TP-10 for the potential treatment of reperfusion injury (following surgery, ischemic disease and organ transplantation), organ rejection, acute inflammatory injury to the lungs and autoimmune diseases [231]. As reported by Rioux *et al.*, TP-10 has also shown immense potential by influencing various complement-mediated interactions in animal studies as well as phase I Trials in patients at risk for adult respiratory distress syndrome (ARDS), adult patients with first-time MI (heart attack), and pediatric patients undergoing cardiac surgery [231]. Safety and efficacy of TP10 in adult women undergoing cardiopulmonary Bypass Surgery further went into phase II clinical study, however, the study was completed without any comments (ClinicalTrials.gov).

6.4. Complement Inhibition at C5 level with Anti-C5 Antibodies (Eculizumab) in MI

In the past few years, therapeutic strategies to block the formation of MAC in ischemic heart disease have received increased attention. Pexelizumab is a humanized monoclonal antibody consisting of a single-chain fragment against C5. It binds with high affinity and prevents cleavage products C5a and C5b, thus preventing the formation of MAC [232, 233]. Animal model of MI/R injury have been employed to show the protective role of blocking C5 in reducing infarct size and apoptosis [234]. In MI, inhibition of complement system by targeting antibodies against C5 significantly reduced necrosis, apoptosis and neutrophil infiltration in a rat model of MI/R injury. Though there are ample C3 deposits available, the mechanism by which it reduces or initiates the reduction is unclear [234]. Pexelizumab was further evaluated in several clinical studies and initial studies demonstrated clinical benefits in phase II study - the COMMA trial and phase III study - the PRIMO-CABG trial. In the COMMA trial, pexelizumab resulted in a statistically significant reduction in mortality but not in reduction of infarct size as assessed by creatine kinase MB (CK-MB) [233]. In the PRIMO-CABG trial, pexelizumab significantly reduced the amount of myocardial damage [235]. However, negative results of pexelizumab were observed in the COMPLY trial [232] and the APEX-AMI trial. In the APEX-AMI trial, the effectiveness of pexelizumab has conceived to be prominent in high-risk patients [236]. Similarly, an exploratory analysis of the combined PRIMO-CABG I and II data set using an established predictive risk model demonstrated a mortality benefit for high-risk surgical patients [237]. A systematic review and meta-analysis on 15,196 patients including seven trials (7019 patients with STEMI addition, insight from a sub study of theand 8177 undergoing coronary bypass surgery) reported no benefit of adding pexelizumab as seen in overall analysis of major adverse events, death, MI, stroke, heart failure, nor in the settings of patients with ST elevation MI treated with mechanical or pharmacologic reperfusion therapy. However, pexelizumab was associated with 26% reduction of the risk of death in setting of coronary artery bypass [238]. This lack of benefit of pexelizumab in setting of patients with STEMI contrasts with the apparent benefit observed in patients undergoing CABG. The authors discussed that the delivery of pexelizumab before surgery may reduce the "generalized" inflammatory process accompanying cardiopulmonary bypass. On the other hand, once microvascular damage and myocardial death owing to necrosis, "local" inflammation, and apoptosis have become irreversible in the setting of STEMI, complement activation is likely to have progressed to MAC formation, nullifying any benefit derived from the administration of pexelizumab. However, despite some similarities, the different effect of pexelizumab might reflect the presence of different activation pathways and/or magnitudes of activation of the complement cascade. In this regard, Lin *et al.* commented that pexelizumab may be hazardous to patients with ST-segment elevation myocardial infarction undergoing primary percutaneous coronary intervention without using adequate anti-thrombotic agents (glycoprotein IIb-IIIa antiplatelet inhibitors, clopidogrel and haparin non-responders) and they established a mathematical model to explain their observation related to estimation of the relative risks [237, 239]. Therein, Lin *et al.* proposed a mediational model to account for the effectiveness of pexelizumab [237]. In addition, insight from a sub study of the assessment of Pexelizumab in Acute Myocardial Infarction (APEX-AMI) trial showed that pexelizumab fails to inhibit assembly of the terminal complement complex in patients with ST-elevation myocardial infarction undergoing primary percutaneous coronary intervention [240, 241].

Another drug eculizumab which is a terminal complement C5 blocker, binds to C5 and prevents its entry into the C5 convertase, thus blocking completely the generation of C5a and the formation of MAC [107, 242]. This therapeutic is approved for use in Paroxysmal Nocturnal Hemoglobinuria (PNH) and aHUS and gives excellent results [243 - 246]. Treating systemic thrombotic microangiopathy (TMA) patients with aHUS with the anti-C5 monoclonal antibody eculizumab showed reduced levels of all known complement biomarkers especially those pertaining to complement activation such as C5a and C5b, followed by reduction in plasma levels. Moreover inflammation and endothelial modifications were also showed to be reduced [242]. This drug is known to abrogate intravascular haemolysis and subsequently normalizes the risk of thrombosis [245 - 247]. Moreover, patients using eculizumab have been shown to be highly susceptible to serious meningococcal infections [248]. Therefore, anti-meningococcal vaccine is administered 2-3 weeks before using eculizumab. In children high risk of streptococcus infections are observed. There are other side-effects like nasal congestion, tachycardia, hypertension, diarrhea and cough reported [249]. The best frequency of eculizumab injections is by detecting the increase in MAC levels in patients with aHUS [250, 251]. At the present time, there are no known studies with eculizumab in myocardial infarction, excluding one case report in which a timely administration of a specific treatment for complement-mediated haemolysis (eculizumab) prevented from the occurrence of complications such as intracerebral haemorrhage in patients with acute MI. Coronary thrombosis was caused in this patient by a hypercoagulable state related to a haemolytic crisis of PNH and the patient was treated conservatively with antithrombotic agents [247]. Currently, clinical trials are ongoing for many different diseases, where complement system is overactivated. An scFv form of the antibody (Pexelizumab, Alexion) was evaluated for use in myocardial infarction and cardiopulmonary bypass surgery, among other models [238, 252], but appears to be discontinued after those studies did not meet expectations [192].

6.5. Inhibiting MBL-Pathway

MBL (mannan-binding lectin) is present in ischemic areas and relatively recent studies in animal models have reported the protective effect of MBL using MBL-KO mice or MBL-inhibition in myocardial infarction. Lectin pathway-specific carbohydrate recognition subcomponent MBL plays an essential role in the pathophysiology of thrombosis and ischemia/reperfusion injury [253]. Indeed, endogenous MBL-ficolin-associated protein-1 (MAP-1) that inhibits complement activation was able to preserve cardiac function by decreasing infarct size and C3 deposition as well as inhibiting MBL deposition. This prevented thrombogenesis and displaced MBL-associated serine proteases (MASP)-1, MASP-2 and MASP-3 from the MBL complex. MAP-1 at pharmacological doses represents a novel therapeutic approach for human diseases involving the lectin pathway and its associated MASPs [253]. Moreover, recent study reported that the use of human MBL inhibitor (Monoclonal antibody 3F8) prevented myocardial injury, preserved cardiac function and decreased infarct size, fibrin deposition and arterial thrombogenesis in an animal model [254]. These novel data demonstrate the therapeutic window for MBL2 inhibition for effective treatment of disease and its complications.

6.6. Complement Inhibition at Effector Levels using C5a Receptor 1 Inhibitors

One of the first selective peptidic antagonists of the C5a receptor (C5aR1, CD88), was developed through modification of hexapeptide agonists [255] and partial agonists based on C-terminus of C5a [256], and binds human CD88 with higher affinity. Numerous studies have reported a series of full antagonists based on the modification of CD88 and chemical stabilization [257]. This cyclic hexapeptide PMX53 and its modified form, a linear peptidomimetic antagonist JPE-1375 have shown therapeutic potential in numerous animal models of inflammatory diseases such as arthritis [258], renal fibrosis and in an accelerated model of atherosclerosis [134, 259]. Several studies have shown the protective effect of C5aR1-inhibition in cardiac I/R-injury and myocardial infarction in different animal models. C5aR1-blocking with antagonists limits MI size and improves cardiac function by reducing the microvascular obstruction and neutrophil recruitment into the infarcted area [260, 261]. Infarct size, leukocyte recruitment into infarctions and TNF-α expression were reduced in mice treated with the C5aR1-antagonist JPE1375. Genetic C5ar1 deficiency blunts the inflammatory response in murine MI/R resulting in reduced inflammatory cell recruitment, which is due to a C5ar1-dependent effect on leukocyte transmigration across inflamed endothelium into the ischemic myocardium. This effect could be related to MMP-9 and JAM-A expression in response to ischemia and reperfusion [262]. CGS 32359, a large molecule compound which display full antagonist activity on human CD88, has been shown to reduce infarct size after surgical coronary occlusion due to the attenuation of neutrophil activation in pigs [260]. Similarly, C5aR1-blockade with an antibody attenuated I/R-induced MI size and markedly decreased microvascular permeability in the ischemic area and leukocyte adherence to coronary artery endothelium; an effect associated with the inhibition of protein kinase C-delta activation in cardiomyocytes [263]. ADC-1004, a truncated 113-residue mutated recombinant form of chemotactic inhibitory protein of *S. aureus* (CHIPS), which selectively blocks CD88, has shown potency in a porcine model of myocardial infarction and reduces microvascular obstruction [261] (Table **4**).

All these studies focused on C5aR1-mediated pro-inflammatory effects in I/R-injury and MI, however, a little is known about the C5aR1-mediated effects in cardiac repair processes. Despite the success in animal models and some early clinical studies, potential limitations have restricted the therapeutic usage of C5aR1 inhibitors. Potential drawback to PMX53 and related compounds are off-target activities at other receptors including tachykinin NK2 receptors [264] and Mas-related gene 2 receptors [265]. The linear piptidomimetic antagonist JPE-

1375 is unlikely to display oral activity and the large size as well as immunogenicity of CGS 32359 limits its therapeutic usage. Moreover, molecular mechanisms underlying myocardial I/R injury is poorly understood and C5aR1-mediated effects on cardiac repair processes need to be further investigated. A better therapeutic approach maybe to locate the damaged heart tissue and redevelop host myocytes and improve protein release system that would aid the damaged heart. The myocytes should be reversed into their primitive state and thereby help the host damaged heart to replace the dead tissue.

Table 4. Inhibitors/regulators at the effector level.

Targets	Naturally occurring inhibitors/regulators	Existing form and expression	Function	Ref.	Drugs/Agents	Ref.
Receptors for complement effector proteins	C3aR	Express on most immune cells and non-immune cells (ECs and VSMCs) and in different tissues	Binds C3a, regulates inflammation and immune cell recruitment	[59]		
	C5aR1 (CD88)	Express on most immune cells and non-immune cells (ECs, VSMCs) and in different tissues	Binds C5a, regulates inflammation and immune cell recruitment	[33, 51]	C5aR peptides PMX53 (Arana Therapeutics, Sydney, Australia) JPE 1375, JPT; Berlin	[257, 264]
			Binds C5a, regulates inflammation and immune cell recruitment	[33, 51]	Neutrazumab, anti-C5aR1 blocking antibody (G2 therapies); TNX 558 (Tanox)	[279]
	C5aR2 (C5L2, GPR77)	Macrophages, neutrophils, immune cells, ECs	Binds C5a and $C5a_{desarg}$, acts as a decoy receptor with anti- and pro-inflammatory property	[33, 51]	Competitive antagonist of C5a and $C5a_{desArg}$ on C5aR1 and C5aR2	[280, 281]

7. FUTURE OF COMPLEMENT INHIBITING THERAPEUTIC STRATEGIES

The first complement-directed drug is in therapeutic use. The purified or recombinant C1-INH and the anti-C5 antibody Eculizumab (Alexion) are two drugs that have been approved in humans. Fueled by the discovery of new functional roles, immune crosstalk mechanisms, and an increasing number of disease associations, complement has emerged as focal point of interest in immunomodulatory and anti-inflammatory strategies. A potential therapeutic option would be the targeted pharmacological inhibition of the complement system at different levels of complement activation depending on the pathogenic role of the individual complement components in the disease settings. In disorders with known initiator, the upstream inhibition of a single pathway may be preferred. In many aspects, tipping the balance between excessive and effective complement response may be an essential and highly promising strategy for restoring immune homeostasis and resolution of inflammation. The ideal level of intervention will be different for each disease and may even vary within groups of affected patients. This would prevent complement activation in the target tissues without affecting systemic complement activation and immunological functions essential for maintaining an effective immune defense such as the ability to kill intruding pathogens and cancer cells. Ongoing research efforts have produced a plethora of innovative and diverse drug candidates that demonstrate great promise in many clinical conditions. CR2-fH and mAb379, novel drugs designed as directed regulators to injured cell and tissue sites are being developed by Taligan Therapeutics. The safety and efficacy of this drug is currently being tested. As a major mediator of immune responses, C5a signaling can be an attractive target to tame inflammation without affecting opsonization or lytic property of the complement system. In some diseases, it may be more important to disrupt the amplification cycle to avoid perpetual opsonization and immune cell recognition. Furthermore, the expression and functional characterization of the second receptor for C5a, the C5aR2, in cardiovascular diseases like atherosclerosis or in other inflammatory diseases such as sepsis would help to develop novel therapeutic options. Therefore, the development of selective C5aR2 inhibitors is extremely necessary. An alternative approach may be the use of endogenous complement inhibitors such as C1-INH that exert their effects through a variety of mechanisms including protease inhibition. Restoration of local endothelial function should be a strategy by which vascular remodeling could be stimulated without the destabilization of local plaque. This may thus provide a multimodal approach for the treatment of arterial disease and remodeling. There is no doubt that harnessing the complement system is an emerging field in medical pharmacology.

CONFLICT OF INTEREST

The authors confirm that they have no conflict of interest to declare for this publication.

ACKNOWLEDGEMENTS

This work was supported by the FöFoLe program of the Ludwig-Maximilians University Munich to YA and by the Deutsche Forschungsgemeinschaft (DFG) grants GU1223/3-1 to ES.

REFERENCES

[1] Weber C, Noels H. Atherosclerosis: current pathogenesis and therapeutic options. Nat Med 2011; 17(11): 1410-22. [eng.].
[PMID: 22064431]

[2] Libby P. Inflammation in atherosclerosis. Nature 2002; 420(6917): 868-74. [eng.].
[PMID: 12490960]

[3] Speidl WS, Kastl SP, Huber K, Wojta J. Complement in atherosclerosis: friend or foe? J Thromb Haemost 2011; 9(3): 428-40. [eng.].
[PMID: 21155967]

[4] Carter AM. Complement activation: an emerging player in the pathogenesis of cardiovascular disease Scientifica (Cairo) 2012; 2012: 402783. Pubmed Central PMCID: 3820556. Epub 2012/01/01. eng.
[PMID: 24278688]

[5] Hovland A, Jonasson L, Garred P, *et al.* The complement system and toll-like receptors as integrated players in the pathophysiology of atherosclerosis. Atherosclerosis 2015; 241(2): 480-94. [eng.].
[PMID: 26086357]

[6] Muscari A, Bozzoli C, Puddu GM, *et al.* Association of serum C3 levels with the risk of myocardial infarction. Am J Med 1995; 98(4): 357-64. [eng.].
[PMID: 7709948]

[7] Speidl WS, Exner M, Amighi J, *et al.* Complement component C5a predicts future cardiovascular events in patients with advanced atherosclerosis. Eur Heart J 2005; 26(21): 2294-9. [eng.].
[PMID: 15917276]

[8] Hertle E, Arts IC, van der Kallen CJ, *et al.* The alternative complement pathway is longitudinally associated with adverse cardiovascular outcomes. The CODAM study. Thromb Haemost 2016; 115(2): 446-57.
[PMID: 26446431]

[9] Zhang S, Cui P. Complement system in zebrafish. Dev Comp Immunol 2014; 46(1): 3-10. [eng.].
[PMID: 24462834]

[10] Abadesso C, Almeida HI, Virella D, Carreiro MH, Machado MC. Use of palivizumab to control an outbreak of syncytial respiratory virus in a neonatal intensive care unit. J Hosp Infect 2004; 58(1): 38-41. [eng.].
[PMID: 15350712]

[11] Fujita T, Endo Y, Nonaka M. Primitive complement system--recognition and activation. Mol Immunol 2004; 41(2-3): 103-11. [eng.].
[PMID: 15159055]

[12] Medzhitov R, Janeway C Jr. Innate immune recognition: mechanisms and pathways. Immunol Rev 2000; 173: 89-97. [eng.].
[PMID: 10719670]

[13] Dzik JM. The ancestry and cumulative evolution of immune reactions. Acta Biochim Pol 2010; 57(4): 443-66. [eng.].
[PMID: 21046016]

[14] Niculescu F, Rus H. The role of complement activation in atherosclerosis. Immunol Res 2004; 30(1): 73-80. [eng.].
[PMID: 15258311]

[15] Gros P, Milder FJ, Janssen BJ. Complement driven by conformational changes. Nat Rev Immunol 2008; 8(1): 48-58. [eng.].
[PMID: 18064050]

[16] Huber-Lang M, Sarma JV, Zetoune FS, *et al.* Generation of C5a in the absence of C3: a new complement activation pathway. Nat Med 2006; 12(6): 682-7. [eng.].
[PMID: 16715088]

[17] Lepow IH, Rosen FS. Pathways to the complement system. N Engl J Med 1972; 286(17): 942-3. [eng.].
[PMID: 5013978]

[18] Sarma JV, Ward PA. The complement system. Cell Tissue Res 2011; 343(1): 227-35. [eng.].
[PMID: 20838815]

[19] Nonaka M. Evolution of the complement system. Subcell Biochem 2014; 80: 31-43. [eng.].
[PMID: 24798006]

[20] Ricklin D, Hajishengallis G, Yang K, Lambris JD. Complement: a key system for immune surveillance and homeostasis. Nat Immunol 2010; 11(9): 785-97. [eng.].
[PMID: 20720586]

[21] Li L, Li Y, Ijaz M, Shahbaz M, Lian Q, Wang F. Review on complement analysis method and the roles of glycosaminoglycans in the complement system. Carbohydr Polym 2015; 134: 590-7. [eng.].

[PMID: 26428162]

[22] Ratnoff OD, Pensky J, Ogston D, Naff GB. The inhibition of plasmin, plasma kallikrein, plasma permeability factor, and the C'1r subcomponent of the first component of complement by serum C'1 esterase inhibitor. J Exp Med 1969; 129(2): 315-31. [eng.].
[PMID: 4178758]

[23] Merle NS, Church SE, Fremeaux-Bacchi V, Roumenina LT. Complement System Part I - Molecular Mechanisms of Activation and Regulation. Front Immunol 2015; 6: 262. [eng.].
[PMID: 26082779]

[24] Janeway CA. Jr TP, Walport M Immunobiology: The Immune system in Health and Disease. 5th ed., New York: Garland Science 2001.

[25] Genster N, Takahashi M, Sekine H, Endo Y, Garred P, Fujita T. Lessons learned from mice deficient in lectin complement pathway molecules. Mol Immunol 2014; 61(2): 59-68. [eng.].
[PMID: 25060538]

[26] Matsushita M, Endo Y, Fujita T. Structural and functional overview of the lectin complement pathway: its molecular basis and physiological implication. Arch Immunol Ther Exp (Warsz) 2013; 61(4): 273-83. [eng.].
[PMID: 23563865]

[27] Kulkarni AP, Ghebremariam YT, Kotwal GJ. Curcumin inhibits the classical and the alternate pathways of complement activation. Ann N Y Acad Sci 2005; 1056: 100-12. [eng.].
[PMID: 16387680]

[28] Massey WA, Hubbard WC, Liu MC, Kagey-Sobotka A, Cooper P, Lichtenstein LM. Profile of prostanoid release following antigen challenge *in vivo* in the skin of man. Br J Dermatol 1991; 125(6): 529-34. [eng.].
[PMID: 1760357]

[29] Lienenklaus S, Ames RS, Tornetta MA, *et al.* Human anaphylatoxin C4a is a potent agonist of the guinea pig but not the human C3a receptor. J Immunol 1998; 161(5): 2089-93. [eng.].
[PMID: 9725198]

[30] Stricker RB, Savely VR, Motanya NC, Giclas PC. Complement split products c3a and c4a in chronic lyme disease. Scand J Immunol 2009; 69(1): 64-9. [eng.].
[PMID: 19140878]

[31] Peng Q, Li K, Sacks SH, Zhou W. The role of anaphylatoxins C3a and C5a in regulating innate and adaptive immune responses. Inflamm Allergy Drug Targets 2009; 8(3): 236-46. [eng.].
[PMID: 19601884]

[32] Morris CA, Carey JC. Three diagnostic signs in Williams syndrome. Am J Med Genet Suppl 1990; 6: 100-1. [eng.].
[PMID: 2118769]

[33] Klos A, Tenner AJ, Johswich KO, Ager RR, Reis ES, Köhl J. The role of the anaphylatoxins in health and disease. Mol Immunol 2009; 46(14): 2753-66. [eng.].
[PMID: 19477527]

[34] Schwartz LB, Kawahara MS, Hugli TE, Vik D, Fearon DT, Austen KF. Generation of C3a

anaphylatoxin from human C3 by human mast cell tryptase. J Immunol 1983; 130(4): 1891-5. [eng.]. [PMID: 6339618]

[35] Mulligan MS, Schmid E, Beck-Schimmer B, *et al.* Requirement and role of C5a in acute lung inflammatory injury in rats. J Clin Invest 1996; 98(2): 503-12. [eng.]. [PMID: 8755663]

[36] Marc MM, Korosec P, Kosnik M, *et al.* Complement factors c3a, c4a, and c5a in chronic obstructive pulmonary disease and asthma. Am J Respir Cell Mol Biol 2004; 31(2): 216-9. [eng.]. [PMID: 15039137]

[37] Hugli TE. Structure and function of C3a anaphylatoxin. Curr Top Microbiol Immunol 1990; 153: 181-208. [eng.]. [PMID: 2404694]

[38] Gorski JP, Hugli TE, Müller-Eberhard HJ. Characterization of human C4a anaphylatoxin. J Biol Chem 1981; 256(6): 2707-11. [eng.]. [PMID: 6970745]

[39] Tsuruta T, Yamamoto T, Matsubara S, *et al.* Novel function of C4a anaphylatoxin. Release from monocytes of protein which inhibits monocyte chemotaxis. Am J Pathol 1993; 142(6): 1848-57. [eng.]. [PMID: 8506953]

[40] Goldstein IM, Perez HD. Biologically active peptides derived from the fifth component of complement. Prog Hemost Thromb 1980; 5: 41-79. [eng.]. [PMID: 6999532]

[41] Barnum SR. C4a: An Anaphylatoxin in Name Only. J Innate Immun 2015; 7(4): 333-9. [eng.]. [PMID: 25659340]

[42] Pasupuleti M, Walse B, Nordahl EA, Mörgelin M, Malmsten M, Schmidtchen A. Preservation of antimicrobial properties of complement peptide C3a, from invertebrates to humans. J Biol Chem 2007; 282(4): 2520-8. [eng.]. [PMID: 17132627]

[43] Chen NJ, Mirtsos C, Suh D, *et al.* C5L2 is critical for the biological activities of the anaphylatoxins C5a and C3a. Nature 2007; 446(7132): 203-7. [eng.]. [PMID: 17322907]

[44] Coulthard LG, Woodruff TM. Is the complement activation product C3a a proinflammatory molecule? Re-evaluating the evidence and the myth. J Immunol 2015; 194(8): 3542-8. [eng.]. [PMID: 25848071]

[45] Ward PA. Role of C5 activation products in sepsis. Sci World J 2010; 10: 2395-402. [eng.]. [PMID: 21170490]

[46] Gerard C, Gerard NP. C5A anaphylatoxin and its seven transmembrane-segment receptor. Annu Rev Immunol 1994; 12: 775-808. [eng.]. [PMID: 8011297]

[47] Schreiber RD. The chemistry and biology of complement receptors. Springer Semin Immunopathol 1984; 7(2-3): 221-49. [eng.]. [PMID: 6238434]

[48] Walport MJ. Complement. First of two parts. N Engl J Med 2001; 344(14): 1058-66. [eng.].
[PMID: 11287977]

[49] Crass T, Bautsch W, Cain SA, Pease JE, Monk PN. Receptor activation by human C5a desArg74 but not intact C5a is dependent on an interaction between Glu199 of the receptor and Lys68 of the ligand. Biochemistry 1999; 38(30): 9712-7. [eng.].
[PMID: 10423250]

[50] Oppermann M, Götze O. Plasma clearance of the human C5a anaphylatoxin by binding to leucocyte C5a receptors. Immunology 1994; 82(4): 516-21. [eng.].
[PMID: 7835913]

[51] Monk PN, Scola AM, Madala P, Fairlie DP. Function, structure and therapeutic potential of complement C5a receptors. Br J Pharmacol 2007; 152(4): 429-48. [eng.].
[PMID: 17603557]

[52] Ehrengruber MU, Geiser T, Deranleau DA. Activation of human neutrophils by C3a and C5A. Comparison of the effects on shape changes, chemotaxis, secretion, and respiratory burst. FEBS Lett 1994; 346(2-3): 181-4. [eng.].
[PMID: 8013630]

[53] Sim RB, Laich A. Serine proteases of the complement system. Biochem Soc Trans 2000; 28(5): 545-50. [eng.].
[PMID: 11044372]

[54] Möhle R, Drost AC. G protein-coupled receptor crosstalk and signaling in hematopoietic stem and progenitor cells. Ann N Y Acad Sci 2012; 1266: 63-7. [eng.].
[PMID: 22901257]

[55] Klos A, Wende E, Wareham KJ, Monk PN. International union of basic and clinical pharmacology. [corrected]. LXXXVII. Complement peptide C5a, C4a, and C3a receptors. Pharmacol Rev 2013; 65(1): 500-43.
[PMID: 23383423]

[56] Findlay JB, Pappin DJ. The opsin family of proteins. Biochem J 1986; 238(3): 625-42. [eng.].
[PMID: 2948499]

[57] Shinjyo N, de Pablo Y, Pekny M, Pekna M. Complement peptide C3a promotes astrocyte survival in response to ischemic stress. Mol Neurobiol 2015. Epub 2015/05/15. Eng.
[PMID: 25972241]

[58] Ames RS, Li Y, Sarau HM, *et al.* Molecular cloning and characterization of the human anaphylatoxin C3a receptor. J Biol Chem 1996; 271(34): 20231-4. [eng.].
[PMID: 8702752]

[59] Melillo D, Sfyroera G, De Santis R, *et al.* First identification of a chemotactic receptor in an invertebrate species: structural and functional characterization of Ciona intestinalis C3a receptor. J Immunol 2006; 177(6): 4132-40. [eng.].
[PMID: 16951378]

[60] Sacks SH. Complement fragments C3a and C5a: the salt and pepper of the immune response. Eur J Immunol 2010; 40(3): 668-70. [eng.].

[PMID: 20186746]

[61] Tornetta MA, Foley JJ, Sarau HM, Ames RS. The mouse anaphylatoxin C3a receptor: molecular cloning, genomic organization, and functional expression. J Immunol 1997; 158(11): 5277-82. [eng.]. [PMID: 9164946]

[62] Martin U, Bock D, Arseniev L, *et al.* The human C3a receptor is expressed on neutrophils and monocytes, but not on B or T lymphocytes. J Exp Med 1997; 186(2): 199-207. [eng.]. [PMID: 9221749]

[63] Yanamadala V, Friedlander RM. Complement in neuroprotection and neurodegeneration. Trends Mol Med 2010; 16(2): 69-76. [eng.]. [PMID: 20116331]

[64] Bénard M, Raoult E, Vaudry D, *et al.* Role of complement anaphylatoxin receptors (C3aR, C5aR) in the development of the rat cerebellum. Mol Immunol 2008; 45(14): 3767-74. [eng.]. [PMID: 18635264]

[65] Siciliano SJ, Rollins TE, DeMartino J, Konteatis Z, Malkowitz L, Van Riper G, *et al.* Two-site binding of C5a by its receptor: an alternative binding paradigm for G protein-coupled receptors. Proc Natl Acad Sci U S A 1994; 91(4): 1214-8. Pubmed Central PMCID: 43127. Epub 1994/02/15. eng. [PMID: 8108389]

[66] Méry PF, Pavoine C, Belhassen L, Pecker F, Fischmeister R. Nitric oxide regulates cardiac Ca2+ current. Involvement of cGMP-inhibited and cGMP-stimulated phosphodiesterases through guanylyl cyclase activation. J Biol Chem 1993; 268(35): 26286-95. [eng.]. [PMID: 7902837]

[67] Ward PA. Functions of C5a receptors. J Mol Med 2009; 87(4): 375-8. [eng.]. [PMID: 19189071]

[68] Scott MG, Benmerah A, Muntaner O, Marullo S. Recruitment of activated G protein-coupled receptors to pre-existing clathrin-coated pits in living cells. J Biol Chem 2002; 277(5): 3552-9. [eng.]. [PMID: 11602587]

[69] Johswich K, Martin M, Thalmann J, Rheinheimer C, Monk PN, Klos A. Ligand specificity of the anaphylatoxin C5L2 receptor and its regulation on myeloid and epithelial cell lines. J Biol Chem 2006; 281(51): 39088-95. [eng.]. [PMID: 17068344]

[70] Blom AM, Villoutreix BO, Dahlbäck B. Complement inhibitor C4b-binding protein-friend or foe in the innate immune system? Mol Immunol 2004; 40(18): 1333-46. [PMID: 15072852]

[71] Pouw RB, Vredevoogd DW, Kuijpers TW, Wouters D. Of mice and men: The factor H protein family and complement regulation. Mol Immunol 2015; 67(1): 12-20. [PMID: 25824240]

[72] Hofer J, Giner T, Józsi M. Complement factor H-antibody-associated hemolytic uremic syndrome: pathogenesis, clinical presentation, and treatment. Semin Thromb Hemost 2014; 40(4): 431-43. [PMID: 24799303]

[73] Ricklin D. Manipulating the mediator: modulation of the alternative complement pathway C3

convertase in health, disease and therapy. Immunobiology 2012; 217(11): 1057-66.
[PMID: 22964231]

[74] Ramadass M, Ghebrehiwet B, Smith RJ, Kew RR. Generation of multiple fluid-phase C3b:plasma protein complexes during complement activation: possible implications in C3 glomerulopathies. J Immunol 2014; 192(3): 1220-30.
[PMID: 24367026]

[75] Kim DD, Song WC. Membrane complement regulatory proteins. Clin Immunol 2006; 118(2-3): 127-36.
[PMID: 16338172]

[76] Parker C, Omine M, Richards S, *et al.* International PNH Interest Group. Diagnosis and management of paroxysmal nocturnal hemoglobinuria. Blood 2005; 106(12): 3699-709. [eng.].
[PMID: 16051736]

[77] Miwa T, Song WC. Membrane complement regulatory proteins: insight from animal studies and relevance to human diseases. Int Immunopharmacol 2001; 1(3): 445-59.
[PMID: 11367529]

[78] Agarwal V, Talens S, Grandits AM, Blom AM. A Novel Interaction between Complement Inhibitor C4b-binding Protein and Plasminogen That Enhances Plasminogen Activation. J Biol Chem 2015; 290(30): 18333-42. [eng.].
[PMID: 26067271]

[79] van Lookeren Campagne M, Wiesmann C, Brown EJ. Macrophage complement receptors and pathogen clearance. Cell Microbiol 2007; 9(9): 2095-102.
[PMID: 17590164]

[80] Khera R, Das N. Complement Receptor 1: disease associations and therapeutic implications. Mol Immunol 2009; 46(5): 761-72.
[PMID: 19004497]

[81] Matsumoto AK, Martin DR, Carter RH, Klickstein LB, Ahearn JM, Fearon DT. Functional dissection of the CD21/CD19/TAPA-1/Leu-13 complex of B lymphocytes. J Exp Med 1993; 178(4): 1407-17.
[PMID: 7690834]

[82] Helmy KY, Katschke KJ Jr, Gorgani NN, *et al.* CRIg: a macrophage complement receptor required for phagocytosis of circulating pathogens. Cell 2006; 124(5): 915-27.
[PMID: 16530040]

[83] Wickham SE, Hotze EM, Farrand AJ, *et al.* Mapping the intermedilysin-human CD59 receptor interface reveals a deep correspondence with the binding site on CD59 for complement binding proteins C8alpha and C9. J Biol Chem 2011; 286(23): 20952-62.
[PMID: 21507937]

[84] Preissner KP, Podack ER, Müller-Eberhard HJ. SC5b-7, SC5b-8 and SC5b-9 complexes of complement: ultrastructure and localization of the S-protein (vitronectin) within the macromolecules. Eur J Immunol 1989; 19(1): 69-75.
[PMID: 2465906]

[85] Preissner KT. The role of vitronectin as multifunctional regulator in the hemostatic and immune

systems. Blut 1989; 59(5): 419-31.
[PMID: 2479432]

[86] Aulak KS, Donaldson VH, Coutinho M, Davis AE III. C1-inhibitor: structure/function and biologic role. Behring Inst Mitt 1993; (93): 204-13.
[PMID: 8172569]

[87] Davis AE III, Whitehead AS, Harrison RA, *et al.* Human inhibitor of the first component of complement, C1: characterization of cDNA clones and localization of the gene to chromosome 11. Proc Natl Acad Sci USA 1986; 83(10): 3161-5.
[PMID: 3458172]

[88] Davis AE III. Hereditary and acquired deficiencies of C1 inhibitor. Immunodefic Rev 1989; 1(3): 207-26.
[PMID: 2698641]

[89] Davis AE III, Cai S, Liu D. C1 inhibitor: biologic activities that are independent of protease inhibition. Immunobiology 2007; 212(4-5): 313-23.
[PMID: 17544816]

[90] Cai S, Dole VS, Bergmeier W, *et al.* A direct role for C1 inhibitor in regulation of leukocyte adhesion. J Immunol 2005; 174(10): 6462-6.
[PMID: 15879149]

[91] Liu D, Lu F, Qin G, Fernandes SM, Li J, Davis AE III. C1 inhibitor-mediated protection from sepsis. J Immunol 2007; 179(6): 3966-72.
[PMID: 17785834]

[92] Lu F, Chauhan AK, Fernandes SM, Walsh MT, Wagner DD, Davis AE III. The effect of C1 inhibitor on intestinal ischemia and reperfusion injury. Am J Physiol Gastrointest Liver Physiol 2008; 295(5): G1042-9.
[PMID: 18787060]

[93] Lu F, Fernandes SM, Davis AE III. The effect of C1 inhibitor on myocardial ischemia and reperfusion injury. Cardiovasc Pathol 2013; 22(1): 75-80. [eng.].
[PMID: 22705194]

[94] Davis AE III, Mejia P, Lu F. Biological activities of C1 inhibitor. Mol Immunol 2008; 45(16): 4057-63.
[PMID: 18674818]

[95] Ricklin D, Lambris JD. Compstatin: a complement inhibitor on its way to clinical application. Adv Exp Med Biol 2008; 632: 273-92.
[PMID: 19025129]

[96] Chiu TL, Mulakala C, Lambris JD, Kaznessis YN. Development of a new pharmacophore model that discriminates active compstatin analogs. Chem Biol Drug Des 2008; 72(4): 249-56.
[PMID: 18844671]

[97] Mastellos DC, Yancopoulou D, Kokkinos P, *et al.* Compstatin: a C3-targeted complement inhibitor reaching its prime for bedside intervention. Eur J Clin Invest 2015; 45(4): 423-40. [eng.].
[PMID: 25678219]

[98] Lazar HL, Keilani T, Fitzgerald CA, *et al.* TP10 Cardiac Surgery Study Group. Beneficial effects of complement inhibition with soluble complement receptor 1 (TP10]during cardiac surgery: is there a gender difference? Circulation 2007; 116(11) (Suppl.): I83-8.
[PMID: 17846331]

[99] Emlen W, Li W, Kirschfink M. Therapeutic complement inhibition: new developments. Semin Thromb Hemost 2010; 36(6): 660-8.
[PMID: 20865643]

[100] Fridkis-Hareli M, Storek M, Mazsaroff I, *et al.* Design and development of TT30, a novel C3d-targeted C3/C5 convertase inhibitor for treatment of human complement alternative pathway-mediated diseases. Blood 2011; 118(17): 4705-13.
[PMID: 21860027]

[101] Huang Y, Qiao F, Atkinson C, Holers VM, Tomlinson S. A novel targeted inhibitor of the alternative pathway of complement and its therapeutic application in ischemia/reperfusion injury. J Immunol 2008; 181(11): 8068-76.
[PMID: 19017999]

[102] Song H, Qiao F, Atkinson C, Holers VM, Tomlinson S. A complement C3 inhibitor specifically targeted to sites of complement activation effectively ameliorates collagen-induced arthritis in DBA/1J mice. J Immunol 2007; 179(11): 7860-7.
[PMID: 18025232]

[103] Rohrer B, Long Q, Coughlin B, *et al.* A targeted inhibitor of the alternative complement pathway reduces angiogenesis in a mouse model of age-related macular degeneration. Invest Ophthalmol Vis Sci 2009; 50(7): 3056-64.
[PMID: 19264882]

[104] Taube C, Thurman JM, Takeda K, *et al.* Factor B of the alternative complement pathway regulates development of airway hyperresponsiveness and inflammation. Proc Natl Acad Sci USA 2006; 103(21): 8084-9. [eng.].
[PMID: 16702544]

[105] Thurman JM, Kraus DM, Girardi G, *et al.* A novel inhibitor of the alternative complement pathway prevents antiphospholipid antibody-induced pregnancy loss in mice. Mol Immunol 2005; 42(1): 87-97. [eng.].
[PMID: 15488947]

[106] Hillmen P, Muus P, Dührsen U, *et al.* Effect of the complement inhibitor eculizumab on thromboembolism in patients with paroxysmal nocturnal hemoglobinuria. Blood 2007; 110(12): 4123-8.
[PMID: 17702897]

[107] Dubois EA, Cohen AF. Eculizumab. Br J Clin Pharmacol 2009; 68(3): 318-9.
[PMID: 19740388]

[108] Whiss PA. Pexelizumab Alexion. Curr Opin Investig Drugs 2002; 3(6): 870-7.
[PMID: 12137406]

[109] Patel S. Combination therapy for age-related macular degeneration. Retina 2009; 29(6) (Suppl.): S45-

8. [eng.].
[PMID: 19553801]

[110] Dorn GW II, Robbins J, Sugden PH. Phenotyping hypertrophy: eschew obfuscation. Circ Res 2003; 92(11): 1171-5. [eng.].
[PMID: 12805233]

[111] Cohn JN, Ferrari R, Sharpe N. Cardiac remodeling--concepts and clinical implications: a consensus paper from an international forum on cardiac remodeling. Behalf of an International Forum on Cardiac Remodeling. J Am Coll Cardiol 2000; 35(3): 569-82. [eng.].
[PMID: 10716457]

[112] Olivetti G, Capasso JM, Sonnenblick EH, Anversa P. Side-to-side slippage of myocytes participates in ventricular wall remodeling acutely after myocardial infarction in rats. Circ Res 1990; 67(1): 23-34. [eng.].
[PMID: 2364493]

[113] Ilczuk T, Wasiutynski A, Wilczek E, Gornicka B. Possible role of complement factors and their inhibitors in the myocardial infarction: an immunohistochemical study. Cent Eur J Immunol 2014; 39(2): 253-9. [eng.].
[PMID: 26155132]

[114] Sun Y. Myocardial repair/remodelling following infarction: roles of local factors. Cardiovasc Res 2009; 81(3): 482-90. [eng.].
[PMID: 19050008]

[115] Frangogiannis NG. The immune system and cardiac repair. Pharmacol Res 2008; 58(2): 88-111. [eng.].
[PMID: 18620057]

[116] Danobeitia JS, Djamali A, Fernandez LA. The role of complement in the pathogenesis of renal ischemia-reperfusion injury and fibrosis. Fibrogenesis Tissue Repair 2014; 7: 16. [eng.].
[PMID: 25383094]

[117] Jordan JE, Montalto MC, Stahl GL. Inhibition of mannose-binding lectin reduces postischemic myocardial reperfusion injury. Circulation 2001; 104(12): 1413-8. [eng.].
[PMID: 11560858]

[118] Eaton LW, Bulkley BH. Expansion of acute myocardial infarction: its relationship to infarct morphology in a canine model. Circ Res 1981; 49(1): 80-8. [eng.].
[PMID: 7237703]

[119] Hochman JS, Bulkley BH. Expansion of acute myocardial infarction: an experimental study. Circulation 1982; 65(7): 1446-50. [eng.].
[PMID: 7074800]

[120] Markiewski MM, Lambris JD. The role of complement in inflammatory diseases from behind the scenes into the spotlight. Am J Pathol 2007; 171(3): 715-27. [eng.].
[PMID: 17640961]

[121] Markiewski MM, Nilsson B, Ekdahl KN, Mollnes TE, Lambris JD. Complement and coagulation: strangers or partners in crime? Trends Immunol 2007; 28(4): 184-92. [eng.].

[PMID: 17336159]

[122] Hertle E, Stehouwer CD, van Greevenbroek MM. The complement system in human cardiometabolic disease. Mol Immunol 2014; 61(2): 135-48. [eng.].
[PMID: 25017306]

[123] Buerke M, Murohara T, Lefer AM. Cardioprotective effects of a C1 esterase inhibitor in myocardial ischemia and reperfusion. Circulation 1995; 91(2): 393-402. [eng.].
[PMID: 7805243]

[124] Wouters D, Stephan F, Strengers P, *et al.* C1-esterase inhibitor concentrate rescues erythrocytes from complement-mediated destruction in autoimmune hemolytic anemia. Blood 2013; 121(7): 1242-4. [eng.].
[PMID: 23411737]

[125] Wouters D, Wagenaar-Bos I, van Ham M, Zeerleder S. C1 inhibitor: just a serine protease inhibitor? New and old considerations on therapeutic applications of C1 inhibitor. Expert Opin Biol Ther 2008; 8(8): 1225-40. [eng.].
[PMID: 18613773]

[126] Bauernschmitt R, Böhrer H, Hagl S. Rescue therapy with C1-esterase inhibitor concentrate after emergency coronary surgery for failed PTCA. Intensive Care Med 1998; 24(6): 635-8. [eng.].
[PMID: 9681790]

[127] Wąsek WC, Samul W, Ryczek R, Skrobowski A. Unique case of ST-segment-elevation myocardial infarction related to paradoxical embolization and simultaneous pulmonary embolization: clinical considerations on indications for patent foramen ovale closure in no-guidelines land. Circulation 2015; 131(13): 1214-23. [eng.].
[PMID: 25825398]

[128] de Zwaan C, Kleine AH, Diris JH, *et al.* Continuous 48-h C1-inhibitor treatment, following reperfusion therapy, in patients with acute myocardial infarction. Eur Heart J 2002; 23(21): 1670-7. [eng.].
[PMID: 12398824]

[129] Thielmann M, Marggraf G, Neuhäuser M, *et al.* Administration of C1-esterase inhibitor during emergency coronary artery bypass surgery in acute ST-elevation myocardial infarction. Eur J Cardiothorac Surg 2006; 30(2): 285-93. [eng.].
[PMID: 16829095]

[130] Entman ML, Michael L, Rossen RD, *et al.* Inflammation in the course of early myocardial ischemia. FASEB J 1991; 5(11): 2529-37. [eng.].
[PMID: 1868978]

[131] Horstick G, Berg O, Heimann A, *et al.* Application of C1-esterase inhibitor during reperfusion of ischemic myocardium: dose-related beneficial *versus* detrimental effects. Circulation 2001; 104(25): 3125-31. [eng.].
[PMID: 11748112]

[132] Horstick G, Heimann A, Götze O, *et al.* Intracoronary application of C1 esterase inhibitor improves cardiac function and reduces myocardial necrosis in an experimental model of ischemia and reperfusion. Circulation 1997; 95(3): 701-8. [eng.].

[PMID: 9024160]

[133] Cai S, Davis AE III. Complement regulatory protein C1 inhibitor binds to selectins and interferes with endothelial-leukocyte adhesion. J Immunol 2003; 171(9): 4786-91. [eng.].
[PMID: 14568956]

[134] Shagdarsuren E, Bidzhekov K, Mause SF, *et al.* C5a receptor targeting in neointima formation after arterial injury in atherosclerosis-prone mice. Circulation 2010; 122(10): 1026-36. [eng.].
[PMID: 20733098]

[135] Ricklin D, Lambris JD. Therapeutic control of complement activation at the level of the central component C3. Immunobiology 2015. Epub 2015/06/24. Eng.
[PMID: 26101137]

[136] Shagdarsuren E, Bidzhekov K, Djalali-Talab Y, *et al.* C1-esterase inhibitor protects against neointima formation after arterial injury in atherosclerosis-prone mice. Circulation 2008; 117(1): 70-8. [eng.].
[PMID: 18071075]

[137] Wu MC, Brennan FH, Lynch JP, *et al.* The receptor for complement component C3a mediates protection from intestinal ischemia-reperfusion injuries by inhibiting neutrophil mobilization. Proc Natl Acad Sci USA 2013; 110(23): 9439-44. [eng.].
[PMID: 23696668]

[138] Hill JH, Ward PA. The phlogistic role of C3 leukotactic fragments in myocardial infarcts of rats. J Exp Med 1971; 133(4): 885-900. [eng.].
[PMID: 4993831]

[139] Sahu A, Morikis D, Lambris JD. Compstatin, a peptide inhibitor of complement, exhibits species-specific binding to complement component C3. Mol Immunol 2003; 39(10): 557-66. [eng.].
[PMID: 12431389]

[140] Furlong ST, Dutta AS, Coath MM, *et al.* C3 activation is inhibited by analogs of compstatin but not by serine protease inhibitors or peptidyl alpha-ketoheterocycles. Immunopharmacology 2000; 48(2): 199-212. [eng.].
[PMID: 10936517]

[141] Strainic MG, Liu J, Huang D, *et al.* Locally produced complement fragments C5a and C3a provide both costimulatory and survival signals to naive CD4+ T cells. Immunity 2008; 28(3): 425-35.
[PMID: 18328742]

[142] Vijayan S, Asare Y, Grommes J, *et al.* High expression of C5L2 correlates with high proinflammatory cytokine expression in advanced human atherosclerotic plaques. Am J Pathol 2014; 184(7): 2123-33. [eng.].
[PMID: 24819959]

[143] Speth C, Rambach G, Würzner R, *et al.* Complement and platelets: Mutual interference in the immune network. Mol Immunol 2015; 67(1): 108-18.
[PMID: 25886718]

[144] Wehner J, Morrell CN, Reynolds T, Rodriguez ER, Baldwin WM III. Antibody and complement in transplant vasculopathy. Circ Res 2007; 100(2): 191-203.
[PMID: 17272820]

[145] Yin W, Ghebrehiwet B, Peerschke EI. Expression of complement components and inhibitors on platelet microparticles. Platelets 2008; 19(3): 225-33.
[PMID: 18432523]

[146] Kastl SP, Speidl WS, Kaun C, *et al.* The complement component C5a induces the expression of plasminogen activator inhibitor-1 in human macrophages *via* NF-kappaB activation. J Thromb Haemost 2006; 4(8): 1790-7.
[PMID: 16879222]

[147] Wojta J, Kaun C, Zorn G, *et al.* C5a stimulates production of plasminogen activator inhibitor-1 in human mast cells and basophils. Blood 2002; 100(2): 517-23.
[PMID: 12091343]

[148] Libby P, Ridker PM, Hansson GK. Progress and challenges in translating the biology of atherosclerosis. Nature 2011; 473(7347): 317-25. [eng.].
[PMID: 21593864]

[149] Bhakdi S, Torzewski M, Klouche M, Hemmes M. Complement and atherogenesis: binding of CRP to degraded, nonoxidized LDL enhances complement activation. Arterioscler Thromb Vasc Biol 1999; 19(10): 2348-54. [eng.].
[PMID: 10521363]

[150] Verdeguer F, Castro C, Kubicek M, *et al.* Complement regulation in murine and human hypercholesterolemia and role in the control of macrophage and smooth muscle cell proliferation. Cardiovasc Res 2007; 76(2): 340-50. [eng.].
[PMID: 17673191]

[151] Fraser DA, Tenner AJ. Innate immune proteins C1q and mannan-binding lectin enhance clearance of atherogenic lipoproteins by human monocytes and macrophages. J Immunol 2010; 185(7): 3932-9. [eng.].
[PMID: 20833838]

[152] Mogilenko DA, Kudriavtsev IV, Trulioff AS, *et al.* Modified low density lipoprotein stimulates complement C3 expression and secretion *via* liver X receptor and Toll-like receptor 4 activation in human macrophages. J Biol Chem 2012; 287(8): 5954-68. [eng.].
[PMID: 22194611]

[153] Suzuki M, Becker L, Pritchard DK, *et al.* Cholesterol accumulation regulates expression of macrophage proteins implicated in proteolysis and complement activation. Arterioscler Thromb Vasc Biol 2012; 32(12): 2910-8. [eng.].
[PMID: 23042816]

[154] Manthey HD, Thomas AC, Shiels IA, *et al.* Complement C5a inhibition reduces atherosclerosis in ApoE-/- mice. FASEB J 2011; 25(7): 2447-55. [eng.].
[PMID: 21490292]

[155] Paglialunga S, Schrauwen P, Roy C, *et al.* Reduced adipose tissue triglyceride synthesis and increased muscle fatty acid oxidation in C5L2 knockout mice. J Endocrinol 2007; 194(2): 293-304. [eng.].
[PMID: 17641279]

[156] Hansson GK, Hermansson A. The immune system in atherosclerosis. Nat Immunol 2011; 12(3): 204-

12. [eng.].
[PMID: 21321594]

[157] Hansson GK, Libby P. The immune response in atherosclerosis: a double-edged sword. Nat Rev Immunol 2006; 6(7): 508-19. [eng.].
[PMID: 16778830]

[158] Zhao L, Funk CD. Lipoxygenase pathways in atherogenesis. Trends Cardiovasc Med 2004; 14(5): 191-5. [eng.].
[PMID: 15261891]

[159] Zernecke A, Shagdarsuren E, Weber C. Chemokines in atherosclerosis: an update. Arterioscler Thromb Vasc Biol 2008; 28(11): 1897-908. [eng.].
[PMID: 18566299]

[160] Asare Y, Schmitt M, Bernhagen J. The vascular biology of macrophage migration inhibitory factor (MIF). Expression and effects in inflammation, atherogenesis and angiogenesis. Thromb Haemost 2013; 109(3): 391-8. [eng.].
[PMID: 23329140]

[161] Hammerschmidt DE, Greenberg CS, Yamada O, Craddock PR, Jacob HS. Cholesterol and atheroma lipids activate complement and stimulate granulocytes. A possible mechanism for amplification of ischemic injury in atherosclerotic states. J Lab Clin Med 1981; 98(1): 68-77. [eng.].
[PMID: 6265570]

[162] Okusawa S, Yancey KB, van der Meer JW, *et al.* C5a stimulates secretion of tumor necrosis factor from human mononuclear cells *in vitro*. Comparison with secretion of interleukin 1 beta and interleukin 1 alpha. J Exp Med 1988; 168(1): 443-8. [eng.].
[PMID: 3260938]

[163] Foreman KE, Vaporciyan AA, Bonish BK, *et al.* C5a-induced expression of P-selectin in endothelial cells. J Clin Invest 1994; 94(3): 1147-55. [eng.].
[PMID: 7521884]

[164] Bernhagen J, Krohn R, Lue H, *et al.* MIF is a noncognate ligand of CXC chemokine receptors in inflammatory and atherogenic cell recruitment. Nat Med 2007; 13(5): 587-96. [eng.].
[PMID: 17435771]

[165] Albrecht EA, Chinnaiyan AM, Varambally S, *et al.* C5a-induced gene expression in human umbilical vein endothelial cells. Am J Pathol 2004; 164(3): 849-59. [eng.].
[PMID: 14982839]

[166] Schulman ES, Post TJ, Henson PM, Giclas PC. Differential effects of the complement peptides, C5a and C5a desArg on human basophil and lung mast cell histamine release. J Clin Invest 1988; 81(3): 918-23. [eng.].
[PMID: 2449462]

[167] Nataf S, Davoust N, Ames RS, Barnum SR. Human T cells express the C5a receptor and are chemoattracted to C5a. J Immunol 1999; 162(7): 4018-23. [eng.].
[PMID: 10201923]

[168] Mügge A, Heistad DD, Densen P, *et al.* Activation of leukocytes with complement C5a is associated

with prostanoid-dependent constriction of large arteries in atherosclerotic monkeys *in vivo*. Atherosclerosis 1992; 95(2-3): 211-22. [eng.].
[PMID: 1418094]

[169] Oksjoki R, Laine P, Helske S, *et al.* Receptors for the anaphylatoxins C3a and C5a are expressed in human atherosclerotic coronary plaques. Atherosclerosis 2007; 195(1): 90-9. [eng.].
[PMID: 17234193]

[170] Patzelt J, Mueller KA, Breuning S, *et al.* Expression of anaphylatoxin receptors on platelets in patients with coronary heart disease. Atherosclerosis 2015; 238(2): 289-95. [eng.].
[PMID: 25544179]

[171] Peerschke EI, Minta JO, Zhou SZ, *et al.* Expression of gC1q-R/p33 and its major ligands in human atherosclerotic lesions. Mol Immunol 2004; 41(8): 759-66. [eng.].
[PMID: 15234555]

[172] Seifert PS, Roth I, Schmiedt W, *et al.* CD59 (homologous restriction factor 20], a plasma membrane protein that protects against complement C5b-9 attack, in human atherosclerotic lesions. Atherosclerosis 1992; 96(2-3): 135-45. [eng.].
[PMID: 1281630]

[173] Bhatia VK, Yun S, Leung V, *et al.* Complement C1q reduces early atherosclerosis in low-density lipoprotein receptor-deficient mice. Am J Pathol 2007; 170(1): 416-26. [eng.].
[PMID: 17200212]

[174] Quartier P, Potter PK, Ehrenstein MR, Walport MJ, Botto M. Predominant role of IgM-dependent activation of the classical pathway in the clearance of dying cells by murine bone marrow-derived macrophages *in vitro*. Eur J Immunol 2005; 35(1): 252-60. [eng.].
[PMID: 15597324]

[175] Lewis MJ, Malik TH, Ehrenstein MR, Boyle JJ, Botto M, Haskard DO. Immunoglobulin M is required for protection against atherosclerosis in low-density lipoprotein receptor-deficient mice. Circulation 2009; 120(5): 417-26. [eng.].
[PMID: 19620499]

[176] Sakuma M, Morooka T, Wang Y, *et al.* The intrinsic complement regulator decay-accelerating factor modulates the biological response to vascular injury. Arterioscler Thromb Vasc Biol 2010; 30(6): 1196-202. [eng.].
[PMID: 20299685]

[177] Lewis RD, Perry MJ, Guschina IA, Jackson CL, Morgan BP, Hughes TR. CD55 deficiency protects against atherosclerosis in ApoE-deficient mice *via* C3a modulation of lipid metabolism. Am J Pathol 2011; 179(4): 1601-7. [eng.].
[PMID: 21816131]

[178] Wu G, Hu W, Shahsafaei A, *et al.* Complement regulator CD59 protects against atherosclerosis by restricting the formation of complement membrane attack complex. Circ Res 2009; 104(4): 550-8. [eng.].
[PMID: 19131645]

[179] Liu F, Wu L, Wu G, *et al.* Targeted mouse complement inhibitor CR2-Crry protects against the development of atherosclerosis in mice. Atherosclerosis 2014; 234(1): 237-43. [eng.].

[PMID: 24685815]

[180] Patel S, Thelander EM, Hernandez M, *et al.* ApoE(-/-) mice develop atherosclerosis in the absence of complement component C5. Biochem Biophys Res Commun 2001; 286(1): 164-70. [eng.].
[PMID: 11485323]

[181] Buono C, Come CE, Witztum JL, *et al.* Influence of C3 deficiency on atherosclerosis. Circulation 2002; 105(25): 3025-31. [eng.].
[PMID: 12081998]

[182] Speidl WS, Kastl SP, Hutter R, *et al.* The complement component C5a is present in human coronary lesions *in vivo* and induces the expression of MMP-1 and MMP-9 in human macrophages *in vitro.* FASEB J 2011; 25(1): 35-44. [eng.].
[PMID: 20813982]

[183] Speidl WS, Katsaros KM, Kastl SP, *et al.* Coronary late lumen loss of drug eluting stents is associated with increased serum levels of the complement components C3a and C5a. Atherosclerosis 2010; 208(1): 285-9. [eng.].
[PMID: 19683238]

[184] Rittirsch D, Flierl MA, Nadeau BA, *et al.* Functional roles for C5a receptors in sepsis. Nat Med 2008; 14(5): 551-7. [eng.].
[PMID: 18454156]

[185] Selle J, Asare Y, Kohncke J, *et al.* Atheroprotective role of C5ar2 deficiency in apolipoprotein E-deficient mice. Thrombosis and haemostasis 2015; 114(4) Epub 2015/06/19. Eng.
[PMID: 26084965]

[186] Samstad EO, Niyonzima N, Nymo S, *et al.* Cholesterol crystals induce complement-dependent inflammasome activation and cytokine release. J Immunol 2014; 192(6): 2837-45. [eng.].
[PMID: 24554772]

[187] Niyonzima N, Samstad EO, Aune MH, *et al.* Reconstituted high-density lipoprotein attenuates cholesterol crystal-induced inflammatory responses by reducing complement activation. J Immunol 2015; 195(1): 257-64. [eng.].
[PMID: 26026058]

[188] Capuano V, D'Arminio T, La Sala G, Mazzotta G. The third component of the complement (C3]is a marker of the risk of atherogenesis. Eur J Cardiovasc Prev Rehabil 2006; 13(4): 658-60. [eng.].
[PMID: 16874160]

[189] Nilsson B, Hamad OA, Ahlström H, *et al.* C3 and C4 are strongly related to adipose tissue variables and cardiovascular risk factors. Eur J Clin Invest 2014; 44(6): 587-96. [eng.].
[PMID: 24754458]

[190] Lu X, Xia M, Endresz V, *et al.* Immunization with a combination of 2 peptides derived from the C5a receptor significantly reduces early atherosclerotic lesion in Ldlr(tm1Her) Apob(tm2Sgy) J mice. Arterioscler Thromb Vasc Biol 2012; 32(10): 2358-71. [eng.].
[PMID: 22837469]

[191] Shernan SK, Fitch JC, Nussmeier NA, *et al.* Pexelizumab Study Investigators. Impact of pexelizumab, an anti-C5 complement antibody, on total mortality and adverse cardiovascular outcomes in cardiac

surgical patients undergoing cardiopulmonary bypass. Ann Thorac Surg 2004; 77(3): 942-9. [eng.]. [PMID: 14992903]

[192] Verrier ED, Shernan SK, Taylor KM, *et al.* PRIMO-CABG Investigators. Terminal complement blockade with pexelizumab during coronary artery bypass graft surgery requiring cardiopulmonary bypass: a randomized trial. JAMA 2004; 291(19): 2319-27. [eng.]. [PMID: 15150203]

[193] Carter AM, Prasad UK, Grant PJ. Complement C3 and C-reactive protein in male survivors of myocardial infarction. Atherosclerosis 2009; 203(2): 538-43. [eng.]. [PMID: 18755462]

[194] Ajjan R, Grant PJ, Futers TS, *et al.* Complement C3 and C-reactive protein levels in patients with stable coronary artery disease. Thromb Haemost 2005; 94(5): 1048-53. [PMID: 16363249]

[195] Muscari A, Bozzoli C, Gerratana C, *et al.* Association of serum IgA and C4 with severe atherosclerosis. Atherosclerosis 1988; 74(1-2): 179-86. [eng.]. [PMID: 3214477]

[196] Speidl WS, Exner M, Amighi J, *et al.* Complement component C5a predicts restenosis after superficial femoral artery balloon angioplasty. Journal of endovascular therapy : an official journal of the international society of endovascular specialists 2007; 14(1): 62-9. Epub 2007/02/13. eng. [PMID: 17291149]

[197] Saevarsdottir S, Oskarsson OO, Aspelund T, *et al.* Mannan binding lectin as an adjunct to risk assessment for myocardial infarction in individuals with enhanced risk. J Exp Med 2005; 201(1): 117-25. [eng.]. [PMID: 15623574]

[198] Keller TT, van Leuven SI, Meuwese MC, *et al.* Serum levels of mannose-binding lectin and the risk of future coronary artery disease in apparently healthy men and women. Arterioscler Thromb Vasc Biol 2006; 26(10): 2345-50. [eng.]. [PMID: 16902159]

[199] Hertle E, van Greevenbroek MM, Arts IC, *et al.* Distinct associations of complement C3a and its precursor C3 with atherosclerosis and cardiovascular disease. The CODAM study. Thromb Haemost 2014; 111(6): 1102-11. [eng.]. [PMID: 24500020]

[200] Rossen RD, Michael LH, Kagiyama A, *et al.* Mechanism of complement activation after coronary artery occlusion: evidence that myocardial ischemia in dogs causes release of constituents of myocardial subcellular origin that complex with human C1q *in vivo.* Circ Res 1988; 62(3): 572-84. [PMID: 3257722]

[201] Yasojima K, Kilgore KS, Washington RA, Lucchesi BR, McGeer PL. Complement gene expression by rabbit heart: upregulation by ischemia and reperfusion. Circ Res 1998; 82(11): 1224-30. [PMID: 9633921]

[202] Kilgore KS, Friedrichs GS, Homeister JW, Lucchesi BR. The complement system in myocardial ischaemia/reperfusion injury. Cardiovasc Res 1994; 28(4): 437-44. [eng.]. [PMID: 8181029]

[203] Hugo F, Hamdoch T, Mathey D, Schäfer H, Bhakdi S. Quantitative measurement of SC5b-9 and C5b-9(m) in infarcted areas of human myocardium. Clin Exp Immunol 1990; 81(1): 132-6. [eng.].
[PMID: 2379317]

[204] McManus LM, Kolb WP, Crawford MH, O'Rourke RA, Grover FL, Pinckard RN. Complement localization in ischemic baboon myocardium. Lab Invest 1983; 48(4): 436-47. [eng.].
[PMID: 6339810]

[205] Pinckard RN, Olson MS, Giclas PC, Terry R, Boyer JT, O'Rourke RA. Consumption of classical complement components by heart subcellular membranes *in vitro* and in patients after acute myocardial infarction. J Clin Invest 1975; 56(3): 740-50.
[PMID: 808560]

[206] Langlois PF, Gawryl MS. Detection of the terminal complement complex in patient plasma following acute myocardial infarction. Atherosclerosis 1988; 70(1-2): 95-105.
[PMID: 3258520]

[207] Folsom AR, Aleksic N, Catellier D, Juneja HS, Wu KK. C-reactive protein and incident coronary heart disease in the Atherosclerosis Risk In Communities (ARIC) study. Am Heart J 2002; 144(2): 233-8. [eng.].
[PMID: 12177639]

[208] Pinckard RN, O'Rourke RA, Crawford MH, *et al.* Complement localization and mediation of ischemic injury in baboon myocardium. J Clin Invest 1980; 66(5): 1050-6. [eng.].
[PMID: 7000824]

[209] Maroko PR, Carpenter CB, Chiariello M, *et al.* Reduction by cobra venom factor of myocardial necrosis after coronary artery occlusion. J Clin Invest 1978; 61(3): 661-70. [eng.].
[PMID: 641147]

[210] Chumakova SP, Urazova OI, Novitskiĭ VV, *et al.* [Characteristic of the complement system in patients with ischemic heart disease with moderate and marked hemolysis after operations with cardiopulmonary bypass]. Kardiologiia 2013; 53(2): 4-9. [Characteristic of the complement system in patients with ischemic heart disease with moderate and marked hemolysis after operations with cardiopulmonary bypass]. [rus.].
[PMID: 23548384]

[211] Yasuda M, Takeuchi K, Hiruma M, *et al.* The complement system in ischemic heart disease. Circulation 1990; 81(1): 156-63. [eng.].
[PMID: 2297823]

[212] Martin SE, Chenoweth DE, Engler RL, Roth DM, Longhurst JC. C5a decreases regional coronary blood flow and myocardial function in pigs: implications for a granulocyte mechanism. Circ Res 1988; 63(2): 483-91. [eng.].
[PMID: 3396162]

[213] Frangogiannis NG, Smith CW, Entman ML. The inflammatory response in myocardial infarction. Cardiovasc Res 2002; 53(1): 31-47. [eng.].
[PMID: 11744011]

[214] Amsterdam EA, Stahl GL, Pan HL, Rendig SV, Fletcher MP, Longhurst JC. Limitation of reperfusion

injury by a monoclonal antibody to C5a during myocardial infarction in pigs. Am J Physiol 1995; 268(1 Pt 2): H448-57.
[PMID: 7840295]

[215] Shernan SK, Collard CD. Role of the complement system in ischaemic heart disease: potential for pharmacological intervention. BioDrugs : clinical immunotherapeutics, biopharmaceuticals and gene therapy 2001; 15(9): 595-607.
[PMID: 11580303]

[216] Chan W, Duffy SJ, White DA, *et al.* Acute left ventricular remodeling following myocardial infarction: coupling of regional healing with remote extracellular matrix expansion. JACC Cardiovasc Imaging 2012; 5(9): 884-93. [eng.].
[PMID: 22974800]

[217] Distelmaier K, Adlbrecht C, Jakowitsch J, *et al.* Local complement activation triggers neutrophil recruitment to the site of thrombus formation in acute myocardial infarction. Thromb Haemost 2009; 102(3): 564-72. [eng.].
[PMID: 19718478]

[218] Fattouch K, Bianco G, Speziale G, *et al.* Beneficial effects of C1 esterase inhibitor in ST-elevation myocardial infarction in patients who underwent surgical reperfusion: a randomised double-blind study. Eur J Cardiothorac Surg 2007; 32(2): 326-32. [eng.].
[PMID: 17576071]

[219] Diris JH, Hermens WT, Hemker PW, Lagrand WK, Hack CE, van Dieijen-Visser MP. Pharmacokinetics of C1-inhibitor protein in patients with acute myocardial infarction. Clin Pharmacol Ther 2002; 72(5): 498-504. [eng.].
[PMID: 12426513]

[220] Bork K, Gül D, Hardt J, Dewald G. Hereditary angioedema with normal C1 inhibitor: clinical symptoms and course. Am J Med 2007; 120(11): 987-92. [eng.].
[PMID: 17976427]

[221] Busse P, Bygum A, Edelman J, *et al.* Safety of C1-esterase inhibitor in acute and prophylactic therapy of hereditary angioedema: findings from the ongoing international Berinert patient registry. J Allergy Clin Immunol Pract 2015; 3(2): 213-9. [eng.].
[PMID: 25609333]

[222] Crowther M, Bauer KA, Kaplan AP. The thrombogenicity of C1 esterase inhibitor (human): review of the evidence. Allergy Asthma Proc 2014; 35(6): 444-53. [eng.].
[PMID: 25584911]

[223] Relan A, Bakhtiari K, van Amersfoort ES, Meijers JC, Hack CE. Recombinant C1-inhibitor: effects on coagulation and fibrinolysis in patients with hereditary angioedema. BioDrugs : clinical immunotherapeutics, biopharmaceuticals and gene therapy 2012; 26(1): 43-52. Epub 2011/12/17. eng.
[PMID: 22171564]

[224] Martinez-Saguer I, Cicardi M, Suffritti C, *et al.* Pharmacokinetics of plasma-derived C1-esterase inhibitor after subcutaneous *versus* intravenous administration in subjects with mild or moderate hereditary angioedema: the PASSION study. Transfusion 2014; 54(6): 1552-61. [eng.].
[PMID: 24266596]

[225] Schürmann D, Herzog E, Raquet E, *et al.* C1-esterase inhibitor treatment: preclinical safety aspects on the potential prothrombotic risk. Thromb Haemost 2014; 112(5): 960-71. [eng.].
[PMID: 25103795]

[226] Gorsuch WB, Guikema BJ, Fritzinger DC, Vogel CW, Stahl GL. Humanized cobra venom factor decreases myocardial ischemia-reperfusion injury. Mol Immunol 2009; 47(2-3): 506-10. [eng.].
[PMID: 19747734]

[227] Soulika AM, Khan MM, Hattori T, *et al.* Inhibition of heparin/protamine complex-induced complement activation by Compstatin in baboons. Clin Immunol 2000; 96(3): 212-21. [eng.].
[PMID: 10964539]

[228] Wysoczynski M, Solanki M, Borkowska S, *et al.* Complement component 3 is necessary to preserve myocardium and myocardial function in chronic myocardial infarction. Stem Cells 2014; 32(9): 2502-15. [eng.].
[PMID: 24806427]

[229] Karthikeyan G, Baalasubramanian S, Seth S, Das N. Low levels of plasma soluble complement receptor type 1 in patients receiving thrombolytic therapy for acute myocardial infarction. J Thromb Thrombolysis 2007; 23(2): 115-20. [eng.].
[PMID: 17131173]

[230] Weisman HF, Bartow T, Leppo MK, *et al.* Soluble human complement receptor type 1: *in vivo* inhibitor of complement suppressing post-ischemic myocardial inflammation and necrosis. Science 1990; 249(4965): 146-51. [eng.].
[PMID: 2371562]

[231] Rioux P. TP-10 (AVANT Immunotherapeutics). Curr Opin Investig Drugs 2001; 2(3): 364-71. [eng.].
[PMID: 11575706]

[232] Mahaffey KW, Granger CB, Nicolau JC, *et al.* COMPLY Investigators. Effect of pexelizumab, an anti-C5 complement antibody, as adjunctive therapy to fibrinolysis in acute myocardial infarction: the COMPlement inhibition in myocardial infarction treated with thromboLYtics (COMPLY) trial. Circulation 2003; 108(10): 1176-83. [eng.].
[PMID: 12925455]

[233] Granger CB, Mahaffey KW, Weaver WD, *et al.* COMMA Investigators. Pexelizumab, an anti-C5 complement antibody, as adjunctive therapy to primary percutaneous coronary intervention in acute myocardial infarction: the COMplement inhibition in Myocardial infarction treated with Angioplasty (COMMA) trial. Circulation 2003; 108(10): 1184-90. [eng.].
[PMID: 12925454]

[234] Vakeva AP, Agah A, Rollins SA, Matis LA, Li L, Stahl GL. Myocardial infarction and apoptosis after myocardial ischemia and reperfusion: role of the terminal complement components and inhibition by anti-C5 therapy. Circulation 1998; 97(22): 2259-67. [eng.].
[PMID: 9631876]

[235] Verrier ED, Shernan SK, Taylor KM, *et al.* PRIMO-CABG Investigators. Terminal complement blockade with pexelizumab during coronary artery bypass graft surgery requiring cardiopulmonary bypass: a randomized trial. JAMA 2004; 291(19): 2319-27. [eng.].
[PMID: 15150203]

[236] Armstrong PW, Granger CB. 1881; Pexelizumab and the APEX AMI trial. JAMA 2007; 297(17): 1881. author reply -2; Epub 2007/05/03. eng.
[PMID: 17473297]

[237] Lin GM. Pexelizumab, an Anti-C5 Complement Antibody for Primary Coronary Revascularization: A New Insight from Old Versions. Cardiovasc Hematol Disord Drug Targets 2011; 11(2): 97-101. [eng.].
[PMID: 22044037]

[238] Testa L, Van Gaal WJ, Bhindi R, *et al.* Pexelizumab in ischemic heart disease: a systematic review and meta-analysis on 15,196 patients. J Thorac Cardiovasc Surg 2008; 136(4): 884-93. [eng.].
[PMID: 18954626]

[239] Lin GM, Chu KM, Han CL. Pexelizumab may be hazardous to those with ST-segment elevation myocardial infarction undergoing primary percutaneous interventions without using glycoprotein IIb-IIIa inhibitors. Int J Cardiol 2011; 146(2): 280-2.
[PMID: 21109318]

[240] Martel C, Granger CB, Ghitescu M, *et al.* Pexelizumab fails to inhibit assembly of the terminal complement complex in patients with ST-elevation myocardial infarction undergoing primary percutaneous coronary intervention. Insight from a substudy of the Assessment of Pexelizumab in Acute Myocardial Infarction (APEX-AMI) trial. Am Heart J 2012; 164(1): 43-51. [eng.].
[PMID: 22795281]

[241] Lin GM, Li YH, Jaiteh LE, Han CL. Pexelizumab fails to inhibit assembly of the terminal complement complex in patients with ST-elevation myocardial infarction undergoing primary percutaneous coronary intervention. Insight from a substudy of the Assessment of Pexelizumab in Acute Myocardial Infarction (APEX-AMI) trial. Am Heart J 2012; 164(6): e19-author reply e21.
[PMID: 23194495]

[242] Cofiell R, Kukreja A, Bedard K, *et al.* Eculizumab reduces complement activation, inflammation, endothelial damage, thrombosis, and renal injury markers in aHUS. Blood 2015; 125(21): 3253-62. [eng.].
[PMID: 25833956]

[243] Hillmen P, Muus P, Röth A, *et al.* Long-term safety and efficacy of sustained eculizumab treatment in patients with paroxysmal nocturnal haemoglobinuria. Br J Haematol 2013; 162(1): 62-73.
[PMID: 23617322]

[244] Krishnan SK, Hill A, Hillmen P, *et al.* Improving cytopenia with splenic artery embolization in a patient with paroxysmal nocturnal hemoglobinuria on eculizumab. Int J Hematol 2013; 98(6): 716-8.
[PMID: 24318160]

[245] Wilson CH, Brown AL, White SA, Goodship TH, Sheerin NS, Manas DM. Successful treatment of de novo posttransplant thrombotic microangiopathy with eculizumab. Transplantation 2011; 92(8): e42-3. [eng.].
[PMID: 21989273]

[246] Chandran S, Baxter-Lowe L, Olson JL, Tomlanovich SJ, Webber A. Eculizumab for the treatment of de novo thrombotic microangiopathy post simultaneous pancreas-kidney transplantation--a case report. Transplant Proc 2011; 43(5): 2097-101. [eng.].
[PMID: 21693335]

[247] Gerber B, Kyburz T, Reinhart WH, Bonetti PO, Stussi G. Complement inhibition to treat myocardial infarction? BMJ Case Rep 2011; 2011 Pubmed Central PMCID: 3083014. Epub 2011/01/01. eng. [PMID: 22696664]

[248] Struijk GH, Bouts AH, Rijkers GT, Kuin EA, ten Berge IJ, Bemelman FJ. Meningococcal sepsis complicating eculizumab treatment despite prior vaccination 2013; Meningococcal sepsis complicating eculizumab treatment despite prior vaccination. American journal of transplantation : official journal of the American Society of Transplantation and the American Society of Transplant Surgeons 2013; 13(3): 819-20. Epub 2013/01/08. eng. [PMID: 23289494]

[249] Legendre CM, Licht C, Muus P, *et al.* Terminal complement inhibitor eculizumab in atypical hemolytic-uremic syndrome. N Engl J Med 2013; 368(23): 2169-81. [eng.]. [PMID: 23738544]

[250] Cugno M, Gualtierotti R, Possenti I, *et al.* Complement functional tests for monitoring eculizumab treatment in patients with atypical hemolytic uremic syndrome. J Thromb Haemost 2014; 12(9): 1440-8. [eng.]. [PMID: 24853860]

[251] Noris M, Galbusera M, Gastoldi S, *et al.* Dynamics of complement activation in aHUS and how to monitor eculizumab therapy. Blood 2014; 124(11): 1715-26. [eng.]. [PMID: 25037630]

[252] Smith PK, Shernan SK, Chen JC, *et al.* PRIMO-CABG II Investigators. Effects of C5 complement inhibitor pexelizumab on outcome in high-risk coronary artery bypass grafting: combined results from the PRIMO-CABG I and II trials. J Thorac Cardiovasc Surg 2011; 142(1): 89-98. [eng.]. [PMID: 20880552]

[253] Pavlov VI, Skjoedt MO, Siow Tan Y, Rosbjerg A, Garred P, Stahl GL. Endogenous and natural complement inhibitor attenuates myocardial injury and arterial thrombogenesis. Circulation 2012; 126(18): 2227-35. [eng.]. [PMID: 23032324]

[254] Pavlov VI, Tan YS, McClure EE, *et al.* Human mannose-binding lectin inhibitor prevents myocardial injury and arterial thrombogenesis in a novel animal model. Am J Pathol 2015; 185(2): 347-55. [eng.]. [PMID: 25482922]

[255] Konteatis ZD, Siciliano SJ, Van Riper G, *et al.* Development of C5a receptor antagonists. Differential loss of functional responses. J Immunol 1994; 153(9): 4200-5. [eng.]. [PMID: 7930622]

[256] Drapeau G, Brochu S, Godin D, Levesque L, Rioux F, Marceau F. Synthetic C5a receptor agonists. Pharmacology, metabolism and *in vivo* cardiovascular and hematologic effects. Biochem Pharmacol 1993; 45(6): 1289-99. [eng.]. [PMID: 8466549]

[257] Woodruff TM, Nandakumar KS, Tedesco F. Inhibiting the C5-C5a receptor axis. Mol Immunol 2011; 48(14): 1631-42. [eng.]. [PMID: 21549429]

[258] Woodruff TM, Strachan AJ, Dryburgh N, *et al.* Antiarthritic activity of an orally active C5a receptor antagonist against antigen-induced monarticular arthritis in the rat. Arthritis Rheum 2002; 46(9): 2476-85. [eng.].
[PMID: 12355496]

[259] Boor P, Konieczny A, Villa L, *et al.* Complement C5 mediates experimental tubulointerstitial fibrosis. J Am Soc Nephrol 2007; 18(5): 1508-15.
[PMID: 17389734]

[260] Riley RD, Sato H, Zhao ZQ, *et al.* Recombinant human complement C5a receptor antagonist reduces infarct size after surgical revascularization. J Thorac Cardiovasc Surg 2000; 120(2): 350-8.
[PMID: 10917953]

[261] van der Pals J, Koul S, Andersson P, *et al.* Treatment with the C5a receptor antagonist ADC-1004 reduces myocardial infarction in a porcine ischemia-reperfusion model. BMC Cardiovasc Disord 2010; 10: 45. [eng.].
[PMID: 20875134]

[262] Mueller M, Herzog C, Larmann J, *et al.* The receptor for activated complement factor 5 (C5aR) conveys myocardial ischemic damage by mediating neutrophil transmigration. Immunobiology 2013; 218(9): 1131-8. [eng.].
[PMID: 23642836]

[263] Zhang H, Qin G, Liang G, Li J, Barrington RA, Liu DX. C5aR-mediated myocardial ischemia/reperfusion injury. Biochem Biophys Res Commun 2007; 357(2): 446-52.
[PMID: 17416341]

[264] Schnatbaum K, Locardi E, Scharn D, *et al.* Peptidomimetic C5a receptor antagonists with hydrophobic substitutions at the C-terminus: increased receptor specificity and *in vivo* activity. Bioorg Med Chem Lett 2006; 16(19): 5088-92. [eng.].
[PMID: 16876401]

[265] Subramanian H, Kashem SW, Collington SJ, Qu H, Lambris JD, Ali H. PMX-53 as a dual CD88 antagonist and an agonist for Mas-related gene 2 (MrgX2]in human mast cells. Mol Pharmacol 2011; 79(6): 1005-13. [eng.].
[PMID: 21441599]

[266] Tarr J, Eggleton P. Immune function of C1q and its modulators CD91 and CD93. Crit Rev Immunol 2005; 25(4): 305-30.
[PMID: 16167883]

[267] Skidgel RA, Erdös EG. Structure and function of human plasma carboxypeptidase N, the anaphylatoxin inactivator. Int Immunopharmacol 2007; 7(14): 1888-99.
[PMID: 18039526]

[268] Fisher GH, Ryan JW, Chung A, Plumer TH Jr. Synthetic inhibitors of carboxypeptidase N. Adv Exp Med Biol 1986; 198(Pt A): 405-10.
[PMID: 3812090]

[269] Hourcade DE. Properdin and complement activation: a fresh perspective. Curr Drug Targets 2008; 9(2): 158-64.

[PMID: 18288967]

[270] Bertram P, Akk AM, Zhou HF, Mitchell LM, Pham CT, Hourcade DE. Anti-mouse properdin TSR 5/6 monoclonal antibodies block complement alternative pathway-dependent pathogenesis. Monoclon Antib Immunodiagn Immunother 2015; 34(1): 1-6.
[PMID: 25723276]

[271] Józsi M, Zipfel PF. Factor H family proteins and human diseases. Trends Immunol 2008; 29(8): 380-7.
[PMID: 18602340]

[272] Zipfel PF, Skerka C. FHL-1/reconectin: a human complement and immune regulator with cell-adhesive function. Immunol Today 1999; 20(3): 135-40.
[PMID: 10203705]

[273] Friese MA, Hellwage J, Jokiranta TS, *et al.* FHL-1/reconectin and factor H: two human complement regulators which are encoded by the same gene are differently expressed and regulated. Mol Immunol 1999; 36(13-14): 809-18.
[PMID: 10698334]

[274] Ricklin D, Lambris JD. Complement-targeted therapeutics. Nat Biotechnol 2007; 25(11): 1265-75.
[PMID: 17989689]

[275] Kroshus TJ, Salerno CT, Yeh CG, Higgins PJ, Bolman RM III, Dalmasso AP. A recombinant soluble chimeric complement inhibitor composed of human CD46 and CD55 reduces acute cardiac tissue injury in models of pig-to-human heart transplantation. Transplantation 2000; 69(11): 2282-9.
[PMID: 10868627]

[276] Zipfel PF, Skerka C. Complement regulators and inhibitory proteins. Nat Rev Immunol 2009; 9(10): 729-40.
[PMID: 19730437]

[277] Schwarz M, Spath L, Lux CA, *et al.* Potential protective role of apoprotein J (clusterin) in atherogenesis: binding to enzymatically modified low-density lipoprotein reduces fatty acid-mediated cytotoxicity. Thromb Haemost 2008; 100(1): 110-8.
[PMID: 18612545]

[278] Heinen S, Hartmann A, Lauer N, *et al.* Factor H-related protein 1 (CFHR-1]inhibits complement C5 convertase activity and terminal complex formation. Blood 2009; 114(12): 2439-47.
[PMID: 19528535]

[279] Sarma JV, Ward PA. New developments in C5a receptor signaling. Cell Health Cytoskelet 2012; 4: 73-82.
[PMID: 23576881]

[280] Otto M, Hawlisch H, Monk PN, *et al.* C5a mutants are potent antagonists of the C5a receptor (CD88] and of C5L2: position 69 is the locus that determines agonism or antagonism. J Biol Chem 2004; 279(1): 142-51.
[PMID: 14570896]

[281] Heller T, Hennecke M, Baumann U, *et al.* Selection of a C5a receptor antagonist from phage libraries attenuating the inflammatory response in immune complex disease and ischemia/reperfusion injury. J Immunol 1999; 163(2): 985-94.

CHAPTER 6

New Antiplatelet and Anticoagulant Agents: Towards Recognition and Reduction of Gastrointestinal Harm

Parth J. Parekh[1,*], **Edward C. Oldfield I.V.**[2] and **David A. Johnson**[3]

[1] *Department of Internal Medicine, Division of Gastroenterology and Hepatology, Tulane University, New Orleans, LA, USA*

[2] *Department of Internal Medicine, Eastern Virginia Medical School, Norfolk, VA, USA*

[3] *Department of Internal Medicine, Division of Gastroenterology and Hepatology, Eastern Virginia Medical School, Norfolk, VA, USA*

Abstract: The most important adverse effect of antiplatelet and anticoagulant therapy is the occurrence of bleeding. Gastroenterologists, cardiologists, and primary care physicians often find themselves balancing the benefits of antiplatelet and anticoagulant therapy with the risk of bleeding, namely gastrointestinal bleeding. While aspirin and warfarin have long been the mainstay of oral antiplatelet and anticoagulant therapy, respectively, recent discoveries of more precise targets for therapy have come to market in order to reduce the risk of cardiovascular events and overcome the well-known limitations that plague warfarin therapy (*e.g.* narrow therapeutic index, variable individual metabolic response, and numerous food and drug interactions). Despite the fact that these novel agents may increase the risk of gastrointestinal bleeding [1], their ease of use makes them more attractive than conventional agents. This review will provide an overview of the pharmacology of available antiplatelet agents and anticoagulants, outline risks that clinicians should be cognizant of when considering prophylactic therapy in order to reduce the risk of gastrointestinal toxicity, and provide up to date data on reversal agents that are currently available as well as those that are in the pipeline.

* **Corresponding author Parth J. Parekh:** Department of Internal Medicine, Division of Gastroenterology and Hepatology, Tulane University, New Orleans, LA, 70112, USA; Tel: (504)988-5606; Fax: (504)988-2188; E-mail: parthjparekh@gmail.com

Atta-ur-Rahman and M. Iqbal Choudhary (Eds.)

INTRODUCTION

Gastrointestinal bleeding (GIB) is a known adverse effect of antiplatelet agents [2]. and anticoagulants [1]. with significant morbidity and mortality in addition to an enormous burden on global health care resources [3]. The mean hospital cost for an episode of upper GIB, lower GIB, or small-bowel bleeding is upwards of $7,300 USD, $4,800 USD, and $40,000 USD, respectively [3]. Expanding indications and ease of use have made antithrombotic therapy robust, which in turn has increased the burden of GIB related to these agents [4]. Antiplatelet agents (*e.g.* aspirin and thienopyridines) cause ulcers and erosions by inhibiting cyclooxygenase (COX)-1 resulting in prostaglandin depletion, which plays a pivotal role in maintaining the gastric epithelium [5]. In addition, antiplatelet agents impair angiogenesis and these two mechanisms in concert are thought to result in GIB. Traditional anticoagulants and novel oral anticoagulants (nOACs) (*e.g.* direct thrombin inhibitors or factor Xa inhibitors) are thought to precipitate bleeding from pre-existing lesions [1]. The nOACs may even predispose susceptible patients to a higher rate of GIB than traditional anticoagulants. Both of the landmark trials (Randomized Evaluation of Long-Term Anticoagulation Therapy (RE-LY) [6] and Rivaroxaban *versus* Warfarin in Nonvalvular Atrial Fibrillation (ROCKET-AF) [7]) that established the relative efficacy/non-inferiority of dabigatran and rivaroxaban, respectively, compared with warfarin therapy in selected patients demonstrated there to be an increased risk of GIB with these agents compared to warfarin therapy. Here, we review the pharmacology of available antiplatelet and anticoagulants, both traditional and nOACs, outline risk factors that warrant prophylactic therapy in order to reduce the risk of gastrointestinal toxicity, and review the most up to date literature on reversal agents that are currently available as well as those that are in the pipeline.

PHARMACOLOGY OF AVAILABLE ANTIPLATELET AGENTS

Aspirin

Aspirin irreversibly inhibits both COX1 and COX2 *via* serine acetylation. Aspirin achieves its antiplatelet properties through its effects on COX1-mediated thromboxane A2, which is highly sensitive to aspirin [8]. Higher doses are required for aspirin to exhibit its anti-inflammatory *via* inhibition of COX-2 mediated prostaglandin I2 generation, thus larger daily doses at shorter dosing intervals are necessary in order to achieve its anti-inflammatory effects [8 - 10]. Fig. (**1**) depicts how differing doses of aspirin effect the COX pathway.

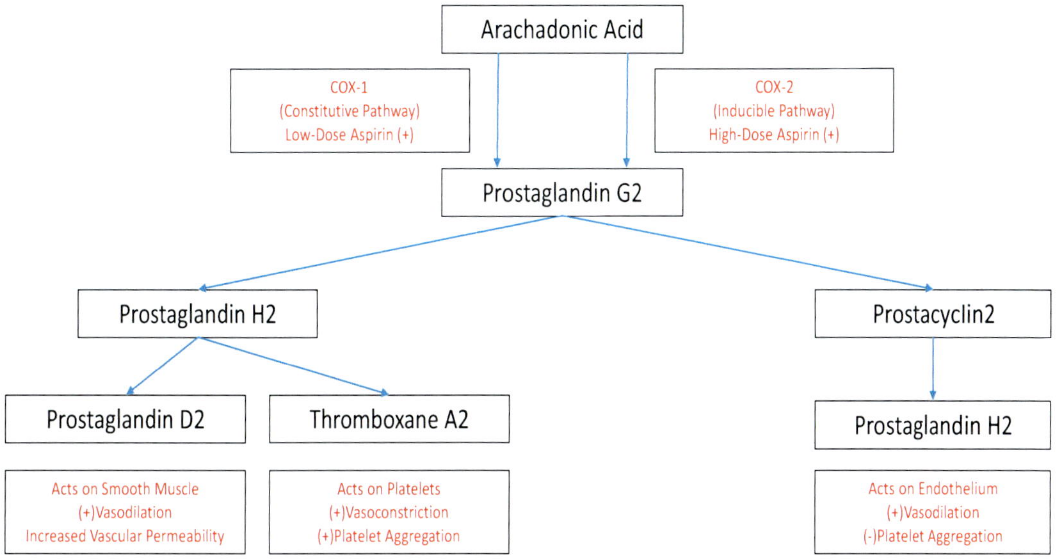

Fig. (1). Effect of differing doses of aspirin on the COX pathway.

Aspirin reaches its peak plasma concentrations within 40 minutes of ingestion, with notable platelet inhibition occurring within 1 hour [8]. Enteric-coated formulations have delayed onset, with peak plasma concentrations occurring within 4 hours after ingestion. Despite having a relatively short half-life of only 15 minutes, the effect of aspirin on platelets last for the entire lifespan of the platelet due to irreversible inhibition [8]. In addition, studies have also shown aspirin to effect COX1 on megakaryocytes (platelet precursors) thus affecting newly released platelets in addition to pre-existing ones [8, 10].

Thienopyridines– Clopidogrel, Prasugrel, and Ticagrelor

The thienopyridines and its derivatives are a group of antiplatelet agents that selectively bind to the $P2Y_{12}$ receptor on the platelet cell surface, thus inhibiting adenosine diphosphate (ADP) induced platelet aggregation [11]. Initially an inactive prodrug, clopidogrel undergoes a 2-step activation process in order to be biotransformed to its active state *via* various cytochrome (CYP) P450 enzymes, namely CYP2C19 and CYP3A4 [12]. Clopidogrel reaches its peak plasma concentration within 2 hours of ingestion [13], with notable platelet inhibition occurring within 4 hours after administering a 600 mg loading dose [14]. Prasugrel is similar to clopidogrel in that it is also a prodrug and irreversibly binds to $P2Y_{12}$ receptors, however it differs in that it only requires a single-step activation process *via* CYP3A4 and CYP2B6 in order to be biotransformed to its active state [15]. As a result the active metabolite of prasugrel is more readily available than that of clopidogrel allowing for a faster onset and more complete and consistent inhibition of ADP-induced platelet aggregation [15 - 17]. Prasugrel reaches its peak plasma concentration within 30 minutes of ingestion, with a half-life of 4 hours [8]. Ticagrelor is a thienopyridine derivative, classified as a cyclopentyltriazolopyrimidine, that does not require any active biotransformation [11]. In addition, it differs from clopidogrel and prasugrel in that it reversibly binds to $P2Y_{12}$ receptors thus exhibits linear kinetics in a dose-dependent fashion [18]. Prasugrel reaches its peak plasma concentration within 2 hours of ingestion, with a half-life of 7 hours [11].

BLEEDING RISK OF AVAILABLE ANTIPLATELET AGENTS

Anti-platelet agents are currently the cornerstone in the primary and secondary prevention of cardiovascular disease. Patients who have undergone percutaneous coronary intervention for acute coronary syndrome (ACS) or patients suffering from chronic stable angina may be subjected to a year or more of dual antiplatelet therapy in order to reduce the risk of subsequent cardiovascular events [19]. Aspirin therapy has long been associated with an increased risk of bleeding, and as studies have shown this appears to be a duration-related effect more so than a dose-related effect [20]. When a second antiplatelet agent is added to the regimen, the risk of overt GIB can be as high as 1.3% within the first 30 days of therapy [21].

Aspirin

Aspirin increases the risk of GIB, in particular upper GIB, through its impact on platelet aggregation as well as prostaglandin synthesis. Normally, prostaglandins generated *via* COX1 increase mucosal blood flow and stimulate mucous and bicarbonate secretion which acts to maintain epithelial integrity [22]. Aspirin, by way of COX1 inhibition resulting in a loss of alkali protectants, promotes an acidic environment which ultimately weakens the gastric mucosa and predisposes it to gastrointestinal injury [23].

Despite the overall increased risk for bleeding with aspirin use, the risk remains the lowest compared to all other antiplatelet agents [24]. A large population-based cohort study by De Berardis *et al.*, which totaled 372,850 individuals (n=186,425 individuals being treated with low-dose aspirin; n=186,425 individuals that were matched controlled without aspirin use), evaluated the incidence of gastro-intestinal bleeding [25]. The study totaled 1.6 million person-years with a median follow up of 5.7 years. They found that use of aspirin was associated with an excess risk of GIB (IRR 1.55; 95% CI – 1.46-1.65). A meta-analysis by Valkhoff *et al.*, which totaled 18 studies (10 case-control studies, 7 randomized control trials (RCTs, and 1 cohort study), evaluated the risk of upper GIB with use low-dose aspirin [26]. Pooled data from the observational studies found the risk of upper GIB associated with aspirin use was 3.1 (95% CI 2.5 -3.7, $p<0.0001$). The pooled odds ratio (OR) from subgroup analysis within the observational studies examining the risk of upper GIB with aspirin doses <100 mg daily, and for doses 300-325 mg daily was 2.6 (95% CI 1.9-3.7, $p<0.0001$) and 3.6 (95% CI 1.7-7.3, $p=0.001$), respectively. Pooled data from the RCTs found the OR of upper GIB with low dose aspirin use (75-325 mg daily) to be 1.5 (95% CI 1.2-1.8, $p<0.0001$).

Another meta-analysis by McQuaid *et al.*, which totaled 22 RCTs, evaluated the risk of clinically relevant adverse events with antiplatelet use, including aspirin [27]. They found aspirin use to increase the risk of major GIB (RR 2.07, 95% CI 1.61-2.66) when compared to placebo. In addition, this was not a dose-dependent phenomenon as there was no statistically significant difference between 75-162.5 mg daily and 162.5-325 mg daily. The absolute annual increase in major GIB attributable to aspirin was 0.12%. One study demonstrated an increased risk of major GIB with aspirin compared to clopidogrel (RR = 1.45, 95%CI – 1.00-2.10) with an absolute annual increase of 0.12% (95% CI 0.00-0.28). The authors found that applying this absolute increased risk of GIB with aspirin compared to clopidogrel would lead to a number needed to treat of 883 at a cost of greater than $1 million USD to prevent one major episode of GIB.

Thienopyridines– Clopidogrel, Prasugrel, and Ticagrelor

Thienopyridines increase the risk of GIB, in particular upper GIB, by impairing release of platelet-derived growth factors responsible for angiogenesis and mucosal healing, such as vascular endothelial growth factor and endostatin [28]. As a result, thienopyridines impair the background healing of ulcers, ultimately converting silent ulcers into bleeding ones [8, 29, 30]. A recent study by Lin *et al.* sought to clarify whether clopidogrel use is a risk factor for upper and lower GIB, and identify risk factors in users that further predispose them to GIB [31]. This nation-wide population based study included 3,238 clopidogrel users and 12,952 age- and sex-matched controls. Cox regression analysis demonstrated that clopidogrel use increased the risk of both upper (hazard ratio (HR) 3.66, 95% CI 2.96-4.51) and lower GIB (HR 3.52, CI 2.74-4.52). In addition, they found age, chronic kidney disease, history of peptic ulcer bleeding, and concomitant use of aspirin or other nonsteroidal anti-inflammatory drugs to be independent risk factors for upper GIB, and age, chronic kidney disease, history of peptic ulcer bleeding, and concomitant use of aspirin and selective serotonin reuptake inhibitors (SSRIs) to be independent risk factors for lower GIB.

Both of the landmark trials (Prasugrel *versus* Clopidogrel in Patients with Acute Coronary Syndromes (TRITON-TIMI) [32]. and Ticagrelor *versus* Clopidogrel in Patients with Acute Coronary Syndromes (PLATO) [33]) that established the relative efficacy/non-inferiority of prasugrel and ticagrelor, respectively, compared with clopidogrel therapy in patients with ACS demonstrated there to be an increased risk of GIB with these agents compared to clopidogrel therapy.

Current Strategies Towards Recognition and Reduction of Gastrointestinal Harm

It is important for clinicians to recognize risk factors for NSAID-related (*e.g.*

aspirin) gastrointestinal injury in order to risk stratify patients that warrant prophylactic therapy in order to reduce the risk of gastrointestinal toxicity. There have been many studies evaluating certain risk factors that may predispose patients to a higher risk of NSAID-related gastrointestinal injury [23, 34 - 42]. Table **1** provides a summary of the various risk factors that have been associated with an increased risk for NSAID-related gastrointestinal injury.

Chemoprophylaxis – Who to Treat? What Agents to Use? What is the Role of Helicobacter Pylori?

Expert consensus is also to use proton pump inhibitors (PPIs) for patient receiving dual antiplatelet therapy, have a history of upper GIB, or have risk factors as outlined in Table **1** [43].

Table 1. Summary of risk factors associated with an increased risk for NSAID-related gastrointestinal injury [8].

Risk Factor	Odds Ratio
History of complicated ulcer	13.5
Multiple concomitant NSAIDs (including aspirin)	9
High dose NSAID use	7
Concomitant use of anticoagulation	6.4
History of an uncomplicated ulcer	6.1
Age > 75 years old	5.8
Hemodialysis	3.3
Concomitant use of steroids	2.2

The role of empiric chemoprophylaxis with gastroprotective agents still remain a point of contention. Current consensus guidelines recommend the use of PPIs over any other gastroprotective agents [5]. A case-control study by Lanas*et al.* matched 2,777 consecutive patients with an upper GIB (confirmed endoscopically) with 5,532 controls in order to evaluate the effect of antisecretory drugs and nitrates on the risk of upper GIB associated with NSAIDs and antiplatelet agents [44]. They found that PPI use was associated with greater reductions in upper GIB as compared to H2-receptor antagonists (H2RAs) and nitrates amongst patients on traditional NSAIDs, low-dose aspirin, or clopidogrel. A cohort study by Ng *et al.*

evaluated the occurrence of upper GIB and the treatment effect of H2RAs and PPIs in 987 consecutive patients on dual antiplatelet therapy with aspirin and clopidogrel [45]. They found that upper GIB occurred in 4.0% (39/987) of patients. Patients were co-prescribed PPIs, H2RAs, and or control in 213, 287, and 487 patients, respectively. After adjustment for age, dose of aspirin, history of upper GIB and duration of treatment, the risk of upper GIB was significantly reduced by concomitant PPI use (OR = 0.04, 95% CI 0.002-0.21, p=0.002) and only marginally by H2RA (OR=0.43, 95% CI 0.18-0.91, p=0.04) as compared to control, which led the authors to conclude that for patients on dual antiplatelet therapy, co-prescription with PPI was associated with a lower risk of GIB.

For patients on dual antiplatelet therapy, concomitant use with PPI therapy does appear to result in a lesser incidence of GIB [44, 45]. Recently, despite some *in vitro* studies suggesting an interaction between PPIs (namely omeprazole and esomeprazole and clopidogre), there has been relatively little evidence of any clinically significant interaction between the two [46]. The COGENT Study (Clopidogrel with or without Omeprazole in Coronary Artery Disease) randomly assigned 3,873 patients (3,761 included in the analysis) with an indication for dual antiplatelet therapy to receive clopidogrel and aspirin in combination with either omeprazole or placebo with overt or occult GIB, symptomatic gastroduodenal ulcers or erosions, obstruction, or perforation being the primary gastrointestinal endpoint [47]. A total of 51 patients had a gastrointestinal event, with an event rate of 1.1% with omeprazole (HR 0.34, 95% CI 0.18-0.63, p<0.001) and 2.9% with placebo after 180 days. Notably, the rate of upper GIB reduced with omeprazole therapy when compared to placebo (HR 0.13, 95% CI 0.03-0.56, p=0.001). A total of 109 patients had a cardiovascular event, with event rates of 4.9% with omeprazole and 5.7% with placebo, without any significant heterogeneity seen in high-risk subgroups. It should be noted that the study was prematurely terminated due to funding and was underpowered for this outcome. As the CI approaches 1.44, an increase in cardiovascular rates up to 44% cannot be excluded. Thus, the authors concluded that among patients receiving dual antiplatelet therapy with aspirin and clopidogrel, concomitant use of a PPI reduced the rate of upper GIB without having any apparent cardiovascular interaction between clopidogrel and omeprazole. However, they could not definitely rule out any clinically meaningful difference in cardiovascular events due to use of a PPI, and as the drug-drug interaction between PPIs and clopidogrel does not appear to be a class-effect [48], clinicians exercising extreme caution, particularly when it comes to high-risk subjects, may want to consider co-prescribing a PPI other then omeprazole or esomeprazole in these patients.

Current estimates are that *Helicobacter pylori* (*H.pylori*) and NSAID use, or a combination of the two, account for approximately 95% of all gastric and duodenal ulcers [49]. *H.pylori* in the setting of concomitant NSAID use does appear to have synergistic effects on gastrointestinal injury. A meta-analysis by Huang *et al.*, which totaled 25 studies, evaluated the relationship between *H.pylori* infection and the use of NSAIDs in the pathogenesis of peptic ulcer disease [50]. They found the rates of uncomplicated peptic ulcer disease to be more common in patients positive for *H.pylori* than those negative (41.7% *vs* 25.9%, respectively). In addition, they found the presence of *H.pylori* infection and NSAID use to increase the risk of ulcer bleeding 1.79-fold and 4.85 fold, respectively, and if the two were present together the risk of ulcer bleeding increased by 6.13-fold. This led the authors to conclude that both *H.pylori* infection and NSAID use independently significantly increased the risk of peptic ulcer disease and ulcer bleeding, and that there appears to be synergism for ulcer development and ulcer bleeding between *H.pylori* and NSAID use.

Knowledge of the apparent synergism for ulcer development and ulcer bleeding between *H.pylori* and NSAID use begs the question as to whether or not *H.pylori* eradication prevents peptic ulcer formation in patients requiring long term NSAIDs. Pooled data from a meta-analysis by Tang *et al.* found the prevalence of peptic ulcer disease in NSAID users to be 31.2% and 17.9% in the presence or absence of *H.pylori* infection, respectively [51]. More notably, peptic ulcer development occurred in 6.4% and 11.8% of NSAID users who underwent or did not undergo *H.pylori* eradication therapy, respectively.

A meta-analysis by Vergara *et al.*, which totaled 5 studies and included 939 patients, evaluated whether *H.pylori* eradication prevented peptic ulcer formation in patients on chronic NSAIDs [52]. Patients who underwent *H.pylori* eradication were significantly less likely to develop a peptic ulcer compared to those who did not receive any treatment for their *H.pylori* (7.4% *vs.* 13.4%, respectively). Subgroup analysis further investigated the benefit of *H.pylori* treatment in NSAID-naïve patients *vs.* patients on chronic, long-term NSAID therapy. Patients in the naïve group were less likely to develop a peptic ulcer if they underwent *H.pylori* treatment prior to initiating NSAID therapy. This was not true of the NSAID-experienced group.

Given that the *H.pylori* and chronic NSAID use appear to have synergistic effects on gastrointestinal injury and that the greatest benefit of *H.pylori* eradication is derived prior to initiating NSAID therapy, current consensus recommendations are that patients should undergo *H. pylori* testing and treatment if positive prior to initiation of long-term NSAID therapy [53]. In addition, patients with bleeding peptic ulcers should undergo *H.pylori* testing and should be treated if positive [54]. The role of *H.pylori* testing in patients currently undergoing NSAID therapy, in the absence of ulcer bleeding, remains debatable as studies suggests that these patients may not benefit from *H.pylori* eradication [8].

PHARMACOLOGY OF TRADITIONAL AND NOVEL ANTI-COAGULANTS

Warfarin

It is important to first briefly review warfarin prior to discussing the nOACs since warfarin is the gold standard to which these new medications are compared. Warfarin is a vitamin K antagonist that produces an anticoagulant effect by inhibiting the vitamin K mediated γ-carboxylation of factors II, VII, IX, and X [55]. Warfarin is administered as a racemic mixture of two different active isomers and is rapidly absorbed with high bioavailability. Briefly, metabolism occurs by various pathways in the liver which can be affected by several factors (*e.g.* genetic polymorphisms of CYP isoenzymes, numerous food and drug interactions, other co-morbidities, and other environmental factors) [55]. As a result, pharma-cokinetics can be unpredictable and patients are subjected to frequent monitoring of their international normalized ratio (INR) and dose adjustments in order to combat the factors outlined above and achieve a therapeutic drug levels. As a result, patient compliance often becomes a major concern. Available data suggests that patients on warfarin may spend nearly 40% of the time outside the therapeutic window [56]. By comparison, the nOACs have a more rapid time to therapeutic effect, have a more predictable pharmacokinetics and pharmacodynamics, which allow them to be administered without the need for frequent laboratory measurements.

Direct Thrombin Inhibitors - Dabigatran

Dabigatran is a direct thrombin inhibitor that reversibly inhibits both free and fibrin-bound thrombin. This prevents the cleavage of fibrinogen to fibrin resulting in impaired thrombin-induced platelet aggregation [57]. Dabigatran also leads to decreased activation of factors V, VIII, XI, and XIII [57]. Fig. (**2**) depicts the mechanism of action of dabigatran.

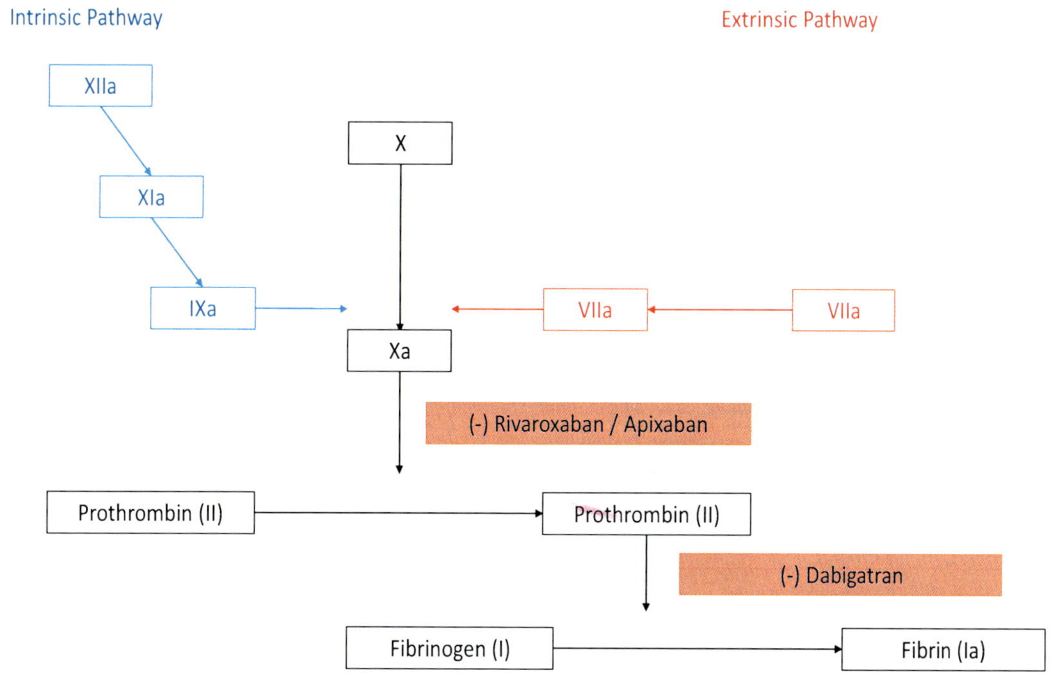

Fig. (2). Mechanism of action of the nOACs.

Dabigatran is administered as the prodrug, dabigatran etexilate, in order to improve bioavailability, as dabigatran by itself only has a bioavailability of 6-7% [58]. Once absorbed, dabigatran etexilate is rapidly hydrolyzed into dabigatran within the enterocytes, portal vein, and liver. Time to therapeutic effect ranges from 30 minutes to 2 hours [57]. Importantly, dabigatran is not a major substrate, inhibitor, or inducer of any CYP450 enzymes or other drug transporters [58, 59]. There are, however, two other factors that can potentially affect its absorption. First, it is important to discuss in detail with patients prior to prescribing dabigatran that the medication is packaged as drug pellets within a capsule shell. Removal of the pellets from this capsule shell be it by chewing, breaking, or emptying the contents of the capsule can result in increased exposure to the active metabolite [60]. Second, dabigatran etexilate has moderate affinity for the P-glycoprotein (P-gp) transporter and therefore P-gp inhibitors and inducers may alter drug absorption [58].

Dabigatran has a half-life of 12-17 hours and is predominately excreted in the urine, therefore in patients with renal insufficiency the half-life of dabigatran may be prolonged (18-27 hours). Renal dosing is suggested for patients with a creatinine clearance (CrCl) 15-30 mL/min when used for atrial fibrillation, but for other indications it is recommended to avoid dabigatran for CrCl less than 30mL/min [11]. There is little information available for patients with a CrCl less than 15 mL/min or for patients on dialysis [58].

Factor Xa Inhibitors - Rivaroxaban and Apixaban

Rivaroxaban and apixaban are both direct factor Xa inhibitors that reversibly inhibit factor Xa, which would otherwise normally form prothrombinase complexes [57]. This results in a reduction in thrombin formation, which ultimately decreases conversion of fibrinogen to fibrin [57]. Fig. (**2**) further illustrates this mechanism of action.

The bioavailability of rivaroxaban is dose dependent, ranging from 80-100% with the 10mg dose to 66% for the 20mg dose [58]. Time of onset ranges from anywhere between 1-4 hours [57]. Rivaroxaban is a substrate for both P-gp and CYP3A4, and consequently inhibitors of P-gp and CYP3A4 can lead to increased concentrations of rivaroxaban [58]. Rivaroxaban primarily undergoes renal excretion (66%) with a half life of 5-9 hours, thus dose reduction is recommended in patients with renal insufficiency (CrCl 15-50 mL/min) when used for the indication of stroke prevention in atrial fibrillation and not recommended for use whenCrCl<15 mL/min; the use of rivaroxaban for the treatment of deep vein thrombosis (DVT), pulmonary embolism (PE), or for the prevention of DVT following hip or knee replacement surgery is not recommended for patients with CrCl<30 mL/min [11, 58].

Apixaban has approximately 50% bioavailability with a time to onset of 3-4 hours [57]. Similar to rivaroxaban, apixaban is also a substrate for both P-gp and CYP3A4. In fact, current recommendations suggest a decreased dose of apixaban when co-administered with strong dual inhibitors of P-gp and CYP3A4 which include ketoconazole, itraconazole, ritonavir, and clarithromycin [11]. While apixaban primarily undergoes biliary excretion, approximately 25% is renally cleared and therefore dose reduction is should considered for atrial fibrillation patients with at least 2 of the following characteristics: greater than 80 years of age, weight less than 60 kilograms, or serum creatinine of greater than 1.5 mg/dL [58].

BLEEDING RISK OF TRADITIONAL AND NOVEL ANTICOAGULANTS

Warfarin therapy has long been the mainstay reducing cardiovascular and/or thromboembolic complications in patients with atrial fibrillation or patients that have recently suffered a myocardial infarction, and the prophylaxis and treatment of venous thrombosis and its extension, pulmonary embolism [11, 57]. As previously described there are many factors that plague warfarin therapy, making it extremely difficult for patients to achieve consistent therapeutic drug levels. As such, many nOACs were brought to market in order to overcome the limitations of warfarin. Unfortunately, warfarin and the nOACs carry a significant risk for GIB [61].

Warfarin

The overall risk of bleeding with warfarin has been estimated at 1.5-5.2% per year with a 13% mortality for major bleeding events [59]. When specifically looking at GIB, a recent systematic review found an OR of 3.21 (95% CI 1.32-7.82) for major GIB among warfarin users when compared to placebo [62]. Additionally, when warfarin was combined with aspirin there was an increased risk for major

GIB compared to warfarin therapy alone (OR 2.66, 95% CI 1.05-6.74) [62]. Subsequent studies have also found an increase risk for GIB with warfarin therapy (relative risk (RR) 1.8, 95% CI 1.3-2.4), with an even greater risk when combined with aspirin therapy (RR 5.3, 95% CI 2.9-9.5) [63].

Dabigatran, Rivaroxaban, and Apixaban

It has been proposed that the nOACs may cause an increased risk of GIB due prolonged exposure within the GI tract thereby precipitating bleeding from vulnerable lesions [64]. Where warfarin is virtually entirely absorbed (95%), the active metabolite of all three nOACs remain within the lumen of the GI tract thus exerting a local anticoagulant or topical caustic effect to preexisting vulnerable lesions [64].

An early focus was placed on the risk of GIB with the nOACs owing to an increased risk for GIB seen in the RE-LY and ROCKET-AF trials. In the RE-LY trial, dabigatran was associated with an increased risk for GIB compared to warfarin for both the 110mg dose (RR 1.10, 95% CI 0.86-1.41) and the 150mg dose (RR 1.50, 95% CI 1.19-1.89), however this was only significant in the 150mg group [6]. In the ROCKET-AF trial, rivaroxaban was associated with 224 major GIBs (3.2%) compared to 154 events in the warfarin group (2.2%) $p<0.001$ [7]. The results of these two trials contrast with those of ARISTOTLE trial (Apixaban *versus* Warfarin in Patients with Atrial Fibrillation) where apixaban was associated with a lower rate of GIB compared to warfarin (HR 0.89, 95% CI 0.70-1.15), albeit a non-significant finding [65]. This discrepancy in the risk between nOACs has become the target of recent studies aiming to further clarify the risk and various risk factors predisposing individuals to GIB with these medications [66 - 69].

In one of the most recent attempts to better characterize the risk for GIB among users of nOACs, Holster *et al.* performed a systematic review and meta-analysis of 43 RCTs comparing nOACs to the standard risk of bleeding, with 19 of 43 trials (44%) specifically reporting on GIB risk [1]. In total, there were 1,101 GIBs among 75,081 patients (1.5%), translating to an OR of 1.45 (95% CI, 1.07-1.97) that were included; however, there was also a significant amount of heterogeneity among these studies (I^2 61%). Overall, the combined number needed to harm (NNH) calculated from this study was 500 (95% -10,000 to 200), implying that one GIB would occur for every 500 patients treated with a nOAC. The overall risk of clinically relevant bleeding was also increased with nOACs compared to standard care (OR 1.16, 95% CI 1.00-1.34), however the data was again marked by significant heterogeneity (I^2 83%).

Interestingly, further analysis of the data showed some stratification of GIB risk among nOAC users by indication [1]. For instance, compared to controls, the GIB risk was highest among trials on ACS (5.3% *vs.* 1.0%), intermediate for both atrial fibrillation (2.1% *vs.* 1.6%) and deep vein thrombosis/pulmonary embolism (DVT/PE) (3.0% *vs.* 1.9%), and lowest for DVT prophylaxis following orthopedic surgery (0.1% *vs.* 0.2%). This variation in risk based on studied indication is important to note, as a large contribution for the overall increased risk of GIB was attributable to the 2 trials on ACS (pooled OR 5.2, 95% CI 2.58-10.53), which adjusts the NNH to 24, implying a much greater risk for GIB among users of nOACs with ACS. This is not a surprising finding, as standard care of ACS includes treatment with antithrombotic medications, which are well known to have a cumulative risk for GIB [8]. Importantly, it should also be noted that in these ACS trials the comparative drug is placebo *versus* other anticoagulants (warfarin or enoxaparin), thus the NNH will be lower by nature of study design. Further subgroup analysis by indication also showed that the studies on DVT/PE conferred a significantly increased risk of GIB (pooled OR 1.59, 95% CI 1.03-2.44), whereas atrial fibrillation (pooled OR 1.21, 95% CI 0.91-1.61) and DVT prophylaxis following orthopedic surgery (pooled OR 0.78, 95% CI 0.31-1.96) did not.[1]. When analyzed by agent, both dabigatran (OR 1.58, 95% CI 1.29-1.93) and rivaroxaban (OR 1.48, 95% CI 1.21-1.82) showed a significantly increased risk for GIB, whereas apixaban did not (OR 1.23, 95% CI 0.56-2.73). Among these subgroups, DVT/PE included only dabigatran and rivaroxaban, whereas atrial fibrillation included all three drugs; therefore, when taken in context with the findings for the individual drugs, it is possible that the non-significant effect in atrial fibrillation group may be related to the inclusion of apixaban compared to the other indications with only dabigatran and rivaroxaban.

Delving further into the risk for GIB with nOACs, Abraham *et al.* recently completed a retrospective, propensity matched cohort study comparing the risk of GIB between dabigatran, rivaroxaban, and warfarin [61]. Interestingly, this study demonstrated there to be an increased risk for GIB that was age-dependent for patients on dabigatran and rivaroxaban compared to warfarin. For patients under the age of 65, propensity score matched models showed failed to show an increased risk of GIB with nOACs compared to warfarin in both atrial fibrillation (dabigatran, HR 0.79 (95% CI, 0.61-1.03); rivaroxaban, HR 0.93 (95% CI, 0.69-1.25)) and non atrial fibrillation patients (dabigatran, HR 1.14 (95% CI, 0.54-2.39); rivaroxaban, HR 0.89 (95% CI, 0.60-1.32)) [2]; however, the risk for GIB from nOACs increased starting at age 65, eventually surpassing the risk of warfarin by age 75 for users of dabigatran with atrial fibrillation (HR 2.49, 95% CI 1.61-3.83) and users of rivaroxaban both with (HR 2.91, 95% CI 1.65-4.81) and without atrial fibrillation (HR 4.58, 95% CI 2.40-8.72).

Importantly, this increased risk of GIB seen among dabigatran users older than 75 years of age with atrial fibrillation was also seen in other studies. Graham *et al.* recently reviewed the safety of dabigatran *versus* warfarin among Medicare enrollees, finding an overall increased risk for major GIB among the dabigatran users (HR 1.28, 95% CI 1.14-1.44) [70]. Again, an important observation was that for both men and women under 75 years of age, there was no significant increase in the risk for GIB; however, the risk became significant for women >75 years old (HR 1.50, 95% CI 1.20-1.88) and men >85 years old (HR 1.55, 95% CI 1.04-2.32). Similar results were noted by Hernandez *et al.* in another retrospective cohort study using Medicare claims of dabigatran use in patients with atrial fibrillation [71]. Overall, the HR for the risk of GIB was 1.85 (95% CI 1.64-2.07), yet the risk was significant only for patients >75 years of age (HR 1.85, 95% CI 1.60-2.14), and not for those patients <75 years of age (HR 1.95, 95% CI 0.60-2.38). Also supporting the data demonstrating an increased risk for GIB among older patients, Miller *et al.* performed a meta-analysis using the results from the major trials of dabigatran (RE-LY) [6], rivaroxaban (ROCKET-AF) [7], and apixaban (ARISTOTLE) [64] to compare the efficacy and safety of these drugs compared to warfarin [72]. Their findings were notable for a decreased risk of all-cause stroke, systemic embolism, and all cause mortality, however, subgroup analysis to determine the risk of GIB demonstrated an increased, albeit inconclusive, risk (RR 1.25, 95% CI 0.91-1.72).

While there is evidence to suggest an increased risk of GIB with use of the nOACs, particularly in patients > 75 years of age, there are a number of studies that present evidence otherwise. Most recently, Chang *et al.* published results from a retrospective, population-based cohort study analyzing the risk of GIB among users of dabigatran, rivaroxaban and warfarin [73]. Overall, the authors found there to be no significant difference in risk of GIB between users of dabigatran and warfarin (adjusted HR 1.21, 95% CI 0.96-1.53) or rivaroxaban and warfarin (adjusted HR 0.98, 95% CI 0.36-2.69). When comparing the rate of GIB per 100 person years, the risk was greatest with dabigatran and lowest with rivaroxaban (the rate of GIB for dabigatran *versus* warfarin *versus* rivaroxaban was 9.01 *versus* 7.02 *versus* 3.41, respectively). Another important finding of this study was that age was not an independent risk factor for GIB for either dabigatran or rivaroxaban. Furthermore, another recent meta-analysis, which totaled 12 studies including 102,607 patients, also failed to find an increased risk of GIB among nOAC users when compared to warfarin users (RR 0.94, 95% CI .075-1.99, I^2 71%) [74]. In a subgroup analysis, however, there was a significant reduction in the risk of major GIB among patients being treated for venous thromboembolic disease (RR 0.64, 95% CI 0.41-0.99, I^2 = 16%), but not for patients treated for atrial fibrillation (RR 1.08, 95% CI 0.86-1.37, I^2 = 78%.

As demonstrated, the risk profiles appear to vary significantly between studies. Abraham *et al.* discussed potential several potential reasons for these conflicting results [61]. They noted that the average age of patients in the RELY trial [6] compared to their study was 71.5 years old *versus* 67.2 years old, respectively. In addition, they noted that the average age of patients in the ROCKET-AF [7] trial compared to their study was 73 years old *versus* 69 years old, respectively. Abraham *et al.* also noted a significant difference in the $CHADS_2$ score between the studies, with over 40% of the patients in their study scoring 0-1 compared to approximately 33% of patients in the RELY trial and 0% of patients in the ROCKET-AF scoring 0-1. It is important to consider these differences in study design, as they may explain some the variability in results between the various studies.

Finally, when attempting to analysis the risk of GIB among nOACs users, it is important to understand that none of these trials were specifically designed to assess this risk but rather, the information available is all the result of subgroup analyses from RCTs, population based cohort studies, or meta-analyses. As a result, many of the risk factors for GIB are not well-controlled or documented, including the use of over the counter antiplatelet, antithrombotic agents, or acid suppressing medications. This is certainly an important observation to consider, as the use of these agents is well documented to influence the risk of GIB [8]. Furthermore, patients enrolled in previous trials were thought to be at low risk for GIB complications, and not necessarily representative of the general patient population. In fact, it has been estimated that the risk of hemorrhage may be 3-15 times greater than estimated through trials, as 25-40% of future users may be high-risk patients [1, 75].

Overall, it is quite evident that regardless of the conflicting data, nOACs have the potential to increase the risk for GIB, especially in the elderly. As such, particular attention should to be paid to the use of nOACs in the elderly population. This includes dosing adjustments for age and other comorbidities. One important facet to discuss is that these studies were unable to account for differences in dosing. The RE-LY trial showed the risk for GIB was elevated in patients receiving 150mg daily (RR 1.49, 95% CI 1.21-1.84), but not in those receiving 110mg daily (RR 1.09, 95% CI 0.87-1.36) [76]. However, subgroup analysis from many of the other studies showing an elevated risk of GIB were not able to discern between varying doses, but rather they included only the pooled risk across all doses. As such, European consensus guidelines recommend the use of dabigatran 110mg among the elderly or for those at high risk for bleeding [77]. Unfortunately, the only doses of dabigatran approved for use in the United States are 75mg and 150mg. This complicates our understanding of the true risk of bleeding, as it precludes the extrapolation of findings from European studies to our population as demonstrated by Larsen *et al.* who demonstrated that the risk of GIB with dabigatran was lower than warfarin when the 110mg dose was used (adjusted HR 0.60, 95% CI 0.37-0.93) but not when 150mg dose was used (adjusted HR 1.12, 95% CI 0.67-1.83) [78]. This suggests that available data should be approached with some caution, as differences in dosing might mitigate some of the increased risk for GIB seen in these studies. Furthermore, the elderly population is also underrepresented in many of these clinical trials and therefore data may not accurately reflect the true bleeding risk [72]. This has proven true in the case with warfarin, where published rates of bleeding underestimate "real world" data [79].

Drug Monitoring (nOACs)

The nOACs have become a very attractive alternative to warfarin therapy for patients requiring anticoagulation. Their predictable pharmacology alleviates the need for patients to undergo routine laboratory monitoring. At the same time, this makes it difficult to test efficacy. Whereas the INR sets the foundation for optimizing warfarin therapy and guiding clinical management, nOACs do not have any single measure, nor do conventional laboratory measurements offer a precise estimation of anticoagulant function. There are, however, some laboratory measures that offer insight in the nOAC activity and new laboratory tests in development that may provide practitioners with tools for managing and optimizing nOACs.

Among the most common measures of anticoagulant function, activated partial thromboplastin time (aPTT) and thrombin time (TT) are both affected by dabigatran administration and offer varying levels of qualitative assessment [80]. Of these measures, the aPTT is the suggested measure on the package insert, however no therapeutic range is listed. Additionally, the aPTT does not have a linear dose relationship and also decreases in sensitivity more than 12 hours from last dosing [62, 81]. By comparison, the TT has actually been shown to be the most sensitive measure for dabigatran exposure, demonstrating a linear dose-response curve, albeit with increasing variability at supratherapeutic levels [57, 62]. The bottom line for use of these conventional measures would be that a normal aPTT or TT excludes therapeutic levels of dabigatran; similarly, an elevated TT suggests therapeutic effect and elevated aPTT suggests recent dabigatran ingestion [57, 82]. A number of other laboratory measure also exist for monitoring dabigatran activity, these include the dilute thrombin time (dTT), ecarin clotting time (ECT), and ecarin chromogenic assay (ECA), which all offer quantitate measures of dabigatran activity [62, 81]. However, in addition to not being FDA approved and of limited availability, but a prospective study comparing the efficacy of these tests showed that measured dabigatran levels varied in a statistically significant manner across a variety of different laboratories, even when the same methods were used [63]. Thus, for the time being, TT and aPTT are the best options for assessing drug effect until new techniques become FDA approved and are more widely accessible.

Similar to dabigatran, both apixaban and rivaroxaban do not require routine laboratory measurement. Unfortunately, there are no readily available measures to monitor the drug levels of these factor Xa inhibitors. While aPTT and TT showed some reliability in monitoring dabigatran activity, rivaroxaban and apixaban have no effect on TT and minimal effect on aPTT [57]. Instead, the PT appears to provide the most sensitive qualitative assessment of activity, in particular for rivaroxaban where it prolongs the PT in a linear dose-response over the therapeutic range; however, prolongation of the PT assay varies between institutions depending on the thromboplastin reagent used for rivaroxaban affecting the sensitivity of the test [57, 82, 83]. Apixaban has minimal effect on PT at therapeutic levels and is better assessed with quantitative measures using the chromogenic factor Xa assay, however, this must done with special care as it requires drug-specific calibration that may vary between institutions [84, 85]. Apixaban is also able to be assessed using a modified PT assay with diluted thromboplastin, however this too is of limited availability. Therefore, while there are measures for both apixaban and rivaroxaban, only rivaroxaban is widely able to be practically and reliably assessed using the PT until the chromogenic factor Xa assays become widely available [57].

Reversal Strategies and Clinical Management of nOACs

The clinical management and reversal of warfarin therapy in the setting of acute bleeding or supratherapeutic INR has been well established [8, 86]. Unfortunately, one of the main drawbacks to the use of nOACs is the lack of any widely accessible reversal agents. While there are specific reversal agents for each of these drugs, at present these are still investigational or just recently FDA approved and not widely available for clinical use. There are a number of methods for controlling and managing bleeding for patients on nOACs. Many of these approaches rely on an understanding of the pharmacokinetics, pharmacodynamics, and mechanism of action of the nOACs, as there are not clinical trials evaluating the efficacy of these techniques in patients with active bleeding. Included in these treatment options are activated charcoal, hemodialysis, prothrombin complex concentrate (PCC), factor eight inhibitor bypass activity (FEIBA) and recombinant Factor VIIa (rFVIIa) [11, 57, 82].

Idarucizumab is a humanized monoclonal antibody with high affinity for dabigatran that just recently received FDA approval on October 16th, 2015. Early animal studies and human trials with healthy volunteers demonstrated idarucizumab to reverse prolonged clotting times and had a safety adverse effects profile [87, 88]. Most recently, Pollack *et al.* completed a prospective trial on the safety and efficacy of idarucizumab for reversal of dabigatran in 90 patients with either serious bleeding or requiring an urgent procedure [89]. Overall, idarucizumab normalized test results within minutes in up to 98% of the patients, however fatal bleeding still occurred in 5 of the 90 patients. Among the patients requiring an urgent procedure, 92% had normal hemostasis with only mild to moderate impairment in the remaining 8% at a median time of 11.4 hours to achieve hemostasis. Importantly, idarucizumab now makes dabigatran the only nOAC with an FDA approved reversal agent. For many clinicians, however, idarucizumab may not be readily available for use so soon after its approval. Therefore, it is important to review other options for the clinical management of dabigatran induced bleeding.

Beginning with drug removal, two options exist for dabigatran: activated charcoal and dialysis. The role of activated charcoal is somewhat questionable, however, when taken in context with an appropriate patient history, activated charcoal seems appropriate when given within 1-2 hours of drug ingestion, particularly for life-threatening bleeding [62, 90, 91]. Since dabigatran has low protein binding, hemodialysis has been proven effective with nearly 57% of metabolite removed within 4 hours [8]. One recommendation for hemodialysis in these patients is to initiate dialysis in patients with life threatening bleeding or patients with a CrCl<30 mL/min, acute kidney injury, or if the last dose of dabigatran was between 2-12 hours prior to presentation [82].

Beyond drug removal, a number of other blood products are available for treating life-threatening bleeding in patients on dabigatran, however the results from available studies offer inconclusive evidence. The data from animal models with 4 factor PCC demonstrating reduction in hematoma size and even reduced mortality did not translate to healthy human volunteers (as there was no improvement in aPTT, ECT, or TT with 4 factor PCC administration); however, this does not rule out a potentially beneficial effect, as reversal of lab values may not be perfectly correlated with hemostasis [92 - 94]. Among the available case reports on life-threatening bleeding with dabigatran, the majority of studies point towards no clinical benefit for hemostasis with the use of fresh frozen plasma (FFP), rFVIIa, PCCs, fibrinogen, or platelets [82]. Overall, it appears among the available agents, 4 factor PCC is the best choice for reversing the anticoagulant effect of dabigatran, as such consideration of a single-dose of 25 units/kg (not to exceed 2500 units) is recommend. Furthermore, there appears to be consensus against reusing 4 factor PCC and also against the administration of rFVIIa or FEIBA within the same 24-hour period [57, 82].

The approach to reversal of the factor Xa inhibitors is quite similar to that of direct thrombin inhibitors with one major exception, namely there is no significant role for hemodialysis owing to their high protein binding [11]. Many of the other reversal techniques still apply, however. Activated charcoal within 1-2 hours may prevent the absorption of both rivaroxaban and apixaban. Even extending out to 6 hours, activated charcoal may reduce the concentration of apixaban, as the drug undergoes enterohepatic recirculation [57, 58]. Animal models concerning the reversal of bleeding associated with these agents show more benefit from the use of 4 factor PCC, FEIBA, and rFVIIa than compared to dabigatran [57, 82]. Unfortunately, there is not enough data from clinical trials to offer great insight into the efficacy of these therapeutic options in humans, although studies from healthy volunteers treated with rivaroxaban have shown significant improvement and even normalization of coagulation studies in patients given 4 factor PCC and rFVIIa [93, 95].

There is promise of a reversal agent in the future for reversal of bleeding in the setting of anticoagulation with factor Xa inhibitors. Andexanet alfa is a first in class, modified recombinant molecule that acts as a decoy molecule that has a higher affinity to the factor Xa inhibitor compared to host factor Xa and as a result binds to the drug (*e.g.* rivaroxaban or apixaban) rather than to factor Xa itself [96]. Recently, a phase III RCT study by Siegal *et al.* evaluated the efficacy of andexanet alfa in healthy older volunteers given 5 mg of apixaban twice daily or 20 mg of rivaroxaban daily [97]. Among patients treated with apixaban, anti-factor Xa activity was reduced by 94% who received andexanet alfa compared to 21% who received placebo ($p<0.001$). Among patients treated with rivaroxaban, anti-factor Xa activity was reduced by 92% who received andexanet alfa compared to 18% who received placebo ($p<0.001$). There were no serious adverse or thrombotic events reported, which led the authors to conclude that andexanet alfa safely reversed the anticoagulant activity of apixaban and rivaroxaban in older, healthy patients within minutes after administration and for the duration of infusion.

Table 2. Pharmacologic Properties of the nOACs [56, 57, 81, 85].

Drug	Dabigatran	Rivaroxaban	Apixaban
Dosing	75 or 150 mg; twice daily	10, 15, or 20 mg; daily	2.5 or 5mg; twice daily
Absorption	6.5% absolute	80%	50% absolute
Onset	30 minutes -2 hours	1-4 hours	3-4 hours
Half-life	12-17 hours	5-9 hours	6 hours (single dose); 12 hours (repeated dosing)
Protein binding	35%	>90%	87%
CYP Metabolism	None	Substrate 3A4, 2J2	Substrate 3A4
Excretion	80% renal, 20% feces	65% renal, 35% feces	27% renal, 70% feces
Potential monitoring	aPTT, PT, TT, dTT, ECA, ECT	PT, chromogenic factor Xa	PT, chromogenic factor Xa
Specific Reversal agents	Idarucizumab (Praxbind)	Andexanet-α (future)	Andexanet-α (future)
Potential drug removal options	Hemodialysis (49-57% removal in 4 hours) Activated charcoal	Activated charcoal	Activated charcoal
Potential reversal agents	Consider PCC, FEIBA, rFVIIa	Consider PCC, FEIBA, rFVIIa	Consider PCC, FEIBA, rFVIIa
Discontinue before surgery	CrCl > 50ml/min: 1-2 days CrCl < 50ml/min: 3-5 days	At least 24 hours	Moderate/high risk >48 hours Low risk >24 hours

Table **2** provides an overview of the pharmacology, potential monitoring laboratory studies, and potential reversal agents for patients on a nOAC.

CONCLUSION

The most common adverse event of antiplatelet, anticoagulant, or combination therapy is bleeding. Gastroenterologists, cardiologists, and primary care providers often find themselves walking a fine line balancing the benefits of antithrombotic therapy with the risk of bleeding, in particular GIB. Clinicians should be cognizant of the risk factors described in order to appropriately treat patients with chemoprophylactic therapy and ways to reduce the risk of gastrointestinal toxicity.

Additionally, ease of use without need for routine laboratory monitoring make nOACs an attractive alternative to warfarin therapy. Unfortunately, data suggests that patients may have a higher risk of GIB with nOACs compared to traditional therapy, which may even vary among the different agents. Further studies aimed to specifically address the risk of GIB in addition to identifying risk factors that that predispose patients to GIB are necessary. For now, clinicians should be aware of the reported increased risk of GIB that exists with these drugs. In order to mitigate the risk, clinicians should continue to work on risk factor modification and select the appropriate therapy for each drug based on their individual characteristics including, but not limited to: age, renal function, previous history of GIB, antiplatelet use, antithrombotic use, and acid suppressive therapy use. As a result, clinicians should be mindful of the potential risk of these drugs and continue to stay abreast on the most recent data to minimize the risk of harm as these drugs may pose in addition to reversal agents that are making their way through clinical trials. Certainly, an understanding of the variations in the pharmacology of the nOACs will further aid in the selection of an appropriate medication to maximize benefit while minimizing risk.

ABBREVIATIONS

aPTT = Activated partial thromboplastin time

CrCl = Creatinine clearance

CYP = Cytochrome P450

dTT = Dilute thrombin time

ECA = Ecarin chromogenic assay

ECT = Ecarin clotting time

FEIBA = Factor eight inhibitor bypass activity

PCC = Prothombin complex concentrate

PT = Prothrombin time

rFVIIa = Recombinant factor VIIa

TT = Thrombin time

CONFLICT OF INTEREST

The authors confirm that they have no conflict of interest to declare for this publication.

ACKNOWLEDGEMENTS

Declared none.

REFERENCES

[1] Holster IL, Valkhoff VE, Kuipers EJ, Tjwa ET. New oral anticoagulants increase risk for gastrointestinal bleeding: a systematic review and meta-analysis. Gastroenterology 2013; 145(1): 105-112.e15.
[http://dx.doi.org/10.1053/j.gastro.2013.02.041] [PMID: 23470618]

[2] Derry S, Loke YK. Risk of gastrointestinal haemorrhage with long term use of aspirin: meta-analysis. BMJ 2000; 321(7270): 1183-7.
[http://dx.doi.org/10.1136/bmj.321.7270.1183] [PMID: 11073508]

[3] Parker DR, Luo X, Jalbert JJ, Assaf AR. Impact of upper and lower gastrointestinal blood loss on healthcare utilization and costs: a systematic review. J Med Econ 2011; 14(3): 279-87.
[http://dx.doi.org/10.3111/13696998.2011.571328] [PMID: 21456948]

[4] Hallas J, Dall M, Andries A, *et al.* Use of single and combined antithrombotic therapy and risk of serious upper gastrointestinal bleeding: population based case-control study. BMJ 2006; 333(7571): 726.
[http://dx.doi.org/10.1136/bmj.38947.697558.AE] [PMID: 16984924]

[5] Bhatt DL, Scheiman J, Abraham NS, *et al.* American College of Cardiology Foundation Task Force on Clinical Expert Consensus Documents. ACCF/ACG/AHA 2008 expert consensus document on reducing the gastrointestinal risks of antiplatelet therapy and NSAID use: a report of the American College of Cardiology Foundation Task Force on Clinical Expert Consensus Documents. Circulation 2008; 118(18): 1894-909.
[http://dx.doi.org/10.1161/CIRCULATIONAHA.108.191087] [PMID: 18836135]

[6] Connolly SJ, Ezekowitz MD, Yusuf S, *et al.* RE-LY Steering Committee and Investigators. Dabigatran

versus warfarin in patients with atrial fibrillation. N Engl J Med 2009; 361(12): 1139-51.
[http://dx.doi.org/10.1056/NEJMoa0905561] [PMID: 19717844]

[7] Patel MR, Mahaffey KW, Garg J, *et al.* ROCKET AF Investigators. Rivaroxaban *versus* warfarin in nonvalvular atrial fibrillation. N Engl J Med 2011; 365(10): 883-91.
[http://dx.doi.org/10.1056/NEJMoa1009638] [PMID: 21830957]

[8] Parekh PJ, Oldfield EC IV, Johnson DA. Current strategies to reduce gastrointestinal bleeding risk associated with antiplatelet agents. Drugs 2015; 75(14): 1613-25.
[http://dx.doi.org/10.1007/s40265-015-0455-1] [PMID: 26330139]

[9] FitzGerald GA, Oates JA, Hawiger J, *et al.* Endogenous biosynthesis of prostacyclin and thromboxane and platelet function during chronic administration of aspirin in man. J Clin Invest 1983; 71(3): 676-88.
[http://dx.doi.org/10.1172/JCI110814] [PMID: 6338043]

[10] Eikelboom JW, Hirsh J, Spencer FA, Baglin TP, Weitz JI. Antiplatelet drugs: Antithrombotic Therapy and Prevention of Thrombosis, 9th ed: American College of Chest Physicians Evidence-Based Clinical Practice Guidelines. Chest. 2012; 141(Suppl. 2): pp. e89S-119S.
[http://dx.doi.org/10.1378/chest.11-2293] [PMID: 22315278]

[11] Parekh PJ, Merrell J, Clary M, Brush JE, Johnson DA. New anticoagulants and antiplatelet agents: a primer for the clinical gastroenterologist. Am J Gastroenterol 2014; 109(1): 9-19.
[http://dx.doi.org/10.1038/ajg.2013.228] [PMID: 24402526]

[12] Kim KA, Park PW, Hong SJ, Park JY. The effect of CYP2C19 polymorphism on the pharmacokinetics and pharmacodynamics of clopidogrel: a possible mechanism for clopidogrel resistance. Clin Pharmacol Ther 2008; 84(2): 236-42.
[http://dx.doi.org/10.1038/clpt.2008.20] [PMID: 18323861]

[13] Taubert D, Kastrati A, Harlfinger S, *et al.* Pharmacokinetics of clopidogrel after administration of a high loading dose. Thromb Haemost 2004; 92(2): 311-6.
[PMID: 15269827]

[14] von Beckerath N, Taubert D, Pogatsa-Murray G, Schömig E, Kastrati A, Schömig A. Absorption, metabolization, and antiplatelet effects of 300-, 600-, and 900-mg loading doses of clopidogrel: results of the ISAR-CHOICE (Intracoronary Stenting and Antithrombotic Regimen: Choose Between 3 High Oral Doses for Immediate Clopidogrel Effect) Trial. Circulation 2005; 112(19): 2946-50.
[PMID: 16260639]

[15] Hagihara K, Kazui M, Kurihara A, *et al.* A possible mechanism for the differences in efficiency and variability of active metabolite formation from thienopyridine antiplatelet agents, prasugrel and clopidogrel. Drug Metab Dispos 2009; 37(11): 2145-52.
[http://dx.doi.org/10.1124/dmd.109.028498] [PMID: 19704027]

[16] Brandt JT, Payne CD, Wiviott SD, *et al.* A comparison of prasugrel and clopidogrel loading doses on platelet function: magnitude of platelet inhibition is related to active metabolite formation. Am Heart J 2007; 153(1): 66.e9-66.e16.
[http://dx.doi.org/10.1016/j.ahj.2006.10.010] [PMID: 17174640]

[17] Jernberg T, Payne CD, Winters KJ, *et al.* Prasugrel achieves greater inhibition of platelet aggregation and a lower rate of non-responders compared with clopidogrel in aspirin-treated patients with stable

coronary artery disease. Eur Heart J 2006; 27(10): 1166-73.
[http://dx.doi.org/10.1093/eurheartj/ehi877] [PMID: 16621870]

[18] Gurbel PA, Bliden KP, Butler K, *et al.* Randomized double-blind assessment of the ONSET and OFFSET of the antiplatelet effects of ticagrelor *versus* clopidogrel in patients with stable coronary artery disease: the ONSET/OFFSET study. Circulation 2009; 120(25): 2577-85.
[http://dx.doi.org/10.1161/CIRCULATIONAHA.109.912550] [PMID: 19923168]

[19] Levine GN, O'Gara PT, Bates ER, *et al.* 2015 ACC/AHA/SCAI Focused Update on Primary Percutaneous Coronary Intervention for Patients With ST-Elevation Myocardial Infarction: An Update of the 2011 ACCF/AHA/SCAI Guideline for Percutaneous Coronary Intervention and the 2013 ACCF/AHA Guideline for the Management of ST-Elevation Myocardial Infarction: A Report of the American College of Cardiology/American Heart Association Task Force on Clinical Practice Guidelines and the Society for Cardiovascular Angiography and Interventions. J Am Coll Cardiol 2015. [Epub ahead of print]
[http://dx.doi.org/10.1002/ccd.26325] [PMID: 26498666]

[20] Huang ES, Strate LL, Ho WW, Lee SS, Chan AT. Long-term use of aspirin and the risk of gastrointestinal bleeding. Am J Med 2011; 124(5): 426-33.
[http://dx.doi.org/10.1016/j.amjmed.2010.12.022] [PMID: 21531232]

[21] Vallurupalli NG, Goldhaber SZ. Gastrointestinal complications of dual antiplatelet therapy. Circulation 2006; 113(12): e655-8.
[http://dx.doi.org/10.1161/CIRCULATIONAHA.105.590612] [PMID: 16567572]

[22] Scheiman JM. NSAIDs, gastrointestinal injury, and cytoprotection. Gastroenterol Clin North Am 1996; 25(2): 279-98.
[http://dx.doi.org/10.1016/S0889-8553(05)70247-8] [PMID: 9229573]

[23] Johnson DA. Upper GI risks of NSAIDs and antiplatelet agents: key issues for the cardiologist. Rev Cardiovasc Med 2005; 6 (Suppl. 4): S15-22.
[PMID: 17710072]

[24] Serebruany VL, Malinin AI, Eisert RM, Sane DC. Risk of bleeding complications with antiplatelet agents: meta-analysis of 338,191 patients enrolled in 50 randomized controlled trials. Am J Hematol 2004; 75(1): 40-7.
[http://dx.doi.org/10.1002/ajh.10451] [PMID: 14695631]

[25] De berardis G, Lucisano G, D'ettorre A, *et al.* Association of aspirin use with major bleeding in patients with and without diabetes. JAMA 2012; 307(21): 2286-94.

[26] Valkhoff VE, Sturkenboom MC, Hill C, Veldhuyzen van Zanten S, Kuipers EJ. Low-dose acetylsalicylic acid use and the risk of upper gastrointestinal bleeding: a meta-analysis of randomized clinical trials and observational studies. Can J Gastroenterol 2013; 27(3): 159-67.
[PMID: 23516680]

[27] McQuaid KR, Laine L. Systematic review and meta-analysis of adverse events of low-dose aspirin and clopidogrel in randomized controlled trials. Am J Med 2006; 119(8): 624-38.
[http://dx.doi.org/10.1016/j.amjmed.2005.10.039] [PMID: 16887404]

[28] Ma L, Elliott SN, Cirino G, Buret A, Ignarro LJ, Wallace JL. Platelets modulate gastric ulcer healing: role of endostatin and vascular endothelial growth factor release. Proc Natl Acad Sci USA 2001;

98(11): 6470-5.
[http://dx.doi.org/10.1073/pnas.111150798] [PMID: 11353854]

[29] Chan FK, Ching JY, Hung LC, *et al.* Clopidogrel *versus* aspirin and esomeprazole to prevent recurrent ulcer bleeding. N Engl J Med 2005; 352(3): 238-44.
[http://dx.doi.org/10.1056/NEJMoa042087] [PMID: 15659723]

[30] Hsu PI, Lai KH, Liu CP. Esomeprazole with clopidogrel reduces peptic ulcer recurrence, compared with clopidogrel alone, in patients with atherosclerosis. Gastroenterology 2011; 140(3): 791-8.
[http://dx.doi.org/10.1053/j.gastro.2010.11.056] [PMID: 21144850]

[31] Lin CC, Hu HY, Luo JC, *et al.* Risk factors of gastrointestinal bleeding in clopidogrel users: a nationwide population-based study. Aliment Pharmacol Ther 2013; 38(9): 1119-28.
[http://dx.doi.org/10.1111/apt.12483] [PMID: 24099473]

[32] Wiviott SD, Braunwald E, McCabe CH, *et al.* TRITON-TIMI 38 Investigators. Prasugrel *versus* clopidogrel in patients with acute coronary syndromes. N Engl J Med 2007; 357(20): 2001-15.
[http://dx.doi.org/10.1056/NEJMoa0706482] [PMID: 17982182]

[33] Wallentin L, Becker RC, Budaj A, *et al.* PLATO Investigators. Ticagrelor *versus* clopidogrel in patients with acute coronary syndromes. N Engl J Med 2009; 361(11): 1045-57.
[http://dx.doi.org/10.1056/NEJMoa0904327] [PMID: 19717846]

[34] García Rodríguez LA, Cattaruzzi C, Troncon MG, Agostinis L. Risk of hospitalization for upper gastrointestinal tract bleeding associated with ketorolac, other nonsteroidal anti-inflammatory drugs, calcium antagonists, and other antihypertensive drugs. Arch Intern Med 1998; 158(1): 33-9.
[http://dx.doi.org/10.1001/archinte.158.1.33] [PMID: 9437376]

[35] Gabriel SE, Jaakkimainen L, Bombardier C. Risk for serious gastrointestinal complications related to use of nonsteroidal anti-inflammatory drugs. A meta-analysis. Ann Intern Med 1991; 115(10): 787-96.
[http://dx.doi.org/10.7326/0003-4819-115-10-787] [PMID: 1834002]

[36] Fries JF, Williams CA, Bloch DA, Michel BA. Nonsteroidal anti-inflammatory drug-associated gastropathy: incidence and risk factor models. Am J Med 1991; 91(3): 213-22.
[http://dx.doi.org/10.1016/0002-9343(91)90118-H] [PMID: 1892140]

[37] Leontiadis GI, Sreedharan A, Dorward S, *et al.* Systematic reviews of the clinical effectiveness and cost-effectiveness of proton pump inhibitors in acute upper gastrointestinal bleeding. Health Technol Assess 2007; 11(51): iii-iv, 1-164.
[http://dx.doi.org/10.3310/hta11510] [PMID: 18021578]

[38] Jankovic SM, Aleksic J, Rakovic S, *et al.* Nonsteroidal antiinflammatory drugs and risk of gastrointestinal bleeding among patients on hemodialysis. J Nephrol 2009; 22(4): 502-7.
[PMID: 19662606]

[39] Van hecken A, Schwartz JI, Depré M, *et al.* Comparative inhibitory activity of rofecoxib, meloxicam, diclofenac, ibuprofen, and naproxen on COX-2 versus COX-1 in healthy volunteers J Clin Pharmacol 2000; 40(10): 1109-20.

[40] Johnsen SP, Sørensen HT, Mellemkjoer L, *et al.* Hospitalisation for upper gastrointestinal bleeding associated with use of oral anticoagulants. Thromb Haemost 2001; 86(2): 563-8.
[PMID: 11522004]

[41] Masclee GM, Valkhoff VE, van Soest EM, *et al.* Cyclo-oxygenase-2 inhibitors or nonselective NSAIDs plus gastroprotective agents: what to prescribe in daily clinical practice? Aliment Pharmacol Ther 2013; 38(2): 178-89.
[http://dx.doi.org/10.1111/apt.12348] [PMID: 23710837]

[42] Goldstein JL, Cryer B. Gastrointestinal injury associated with NSAID use: a case study and review of risk factors and preventative strategies. Drug Healthc Patient Saf 2015; 7: 31-41.
[http://dx.doi.org/10.2147/DHPS.S71976] [PMID: 25653559]

[43] Abraham NS, Hlatky MA, Antman EM, *et al.* ACCF/ACG/AHA. ACCF/ACG/AHA 2010 expert consensus document on the concomitant use of proton pump inhibitors and thienopyridines: a focused update of the ACCF/ACG/AHA 2008 expert consensus document on reducing the gastrointestinal risks of antiplatelet therapy and NSAID use. Am J Gastroenterol 2010; 105(12): 2533-49.
[http://dx.doi.org/10.1038/ajg.2010.445] [PMID: 21131924]

[44] Lanas A, García-Rodríguez LA, Arroyo MT, *et al.* Investigators of the Asociación Española de Gastroenterología (AEG). Effect of antisecretory drugs and nitrates on the risk of ulcer bleeding associated with nonsteroidal anti-inflammatory drugs, antiplatelet agents, and anticoagulants. Am J Gastroenterol 2007; 102(3): 507-15.
[http://dx.doi.org/10.1111/j.1572-0241.2006.01062.x] [PMID: 17338735]

[45] Ng FH, Lam KF, Wong SY, *et al.* Upper gastrointestinal bleeding in patients with aspirin and clopidogrel co-therapy. Digestion 2008; 77(3-4): 173-7.
[http://dx.doi.org/10.1159/000141264] [PMID: 18577887]

[46] Sharma RK, Reddy HK, Sharma RK, *et al.* The interaction between clopidogrel and proton pump inhibitors (PPI): is there any clinical relevance? Clin Pharmacol 2010; 2: 155-62.
[http://dx.doi.org/10.2147/CPAA.S9807] [PMID: 22291500]

[47] Bhatt DL, Cryer BL, Contant CF, *et al.* COGENT Investigators. Clopidogrel with or without omeprazole in coronary artery disease. N Engl J Med 2010; 363(20): 1909-17.
[http://dx.doi.org/10.1056/NEJMoa1007964] [PMID: 20925534]

[48] Fontes-Carvalho R, Albuquerque A, Araújo C, Pimentel-Nunes P, Ribeiro VG. Omeprazole, but not pantoprazole, reduces the antiplatelet effect of clopidogrel: a randomized clinical crossover trial in patients after myocardial infarction evaluating the clopidogrel-PPIs drug interaction. Eur J Gastroenterol Hepatol 2011; 23(5): 396-404.
[http://dx.doi.org/10.1097/MEG.0b013e3283460110] [PMID: 21464720]

[49] Kurata JH, Nogawa AN. Meta-analysis of risk factors for peptic ulcer. Nonsteroidal antiinflammatory drugs, Helicobacter pylori, and smoking. J Clin Gastroenterol 1997; 24(1): 2-17.
[http://dx.doi.org/10.1097/00004836-199701000-00002] [PMID: 9013343]

[50] Huang JQ, Sridhar S, Hunt RH. Role of Helicobacter pylori infection and non-steroidal anti-inflammatory drugs in peptic-ulcer disease: a meta-analysis. Lancet 2002; 359(9300): 14-22.
[http://dx.doi.org/10.1016/S0140-6736(02)07273-2] [PMID: 11809181]

[51] Tang CL, Ye F, Liu W, Pan XL, Qian J, Zhang GX. Eradication of Helicobacter pylori infection reduces the incidence of peptic ulcer disease in patients using nonsteroidal anti-inflammatory drugs: a meta-analysis. Helicobacter 2012; 17(4): 286-96.
[http://dx.doi.org/10.1111/j.1523-5378.2012.00942.x] [PMID: 22759329]

[52] Vergara M, Catalán M, Gisbert JP, Calvet X. Meta-analysis: role of Helicobacter pylori eradication in the prevention of peptic ulcer in NSAID users. Aliment Pharmacol Ther 2005; 21(12): 1411-8. [http://dx.doi.org/10.1111/j.1365-2036.2005.02444.x] [PMID: 15948807]

[53] Malfertheiner P, Megraud F, O'Morain CA, *et al.* European Helicobacter Study Group. Management of Helicobacter pylori infection--the Maastricht IV/ Florence Consensus Report. Gut 2012; 61(5): 646-64. [http://dx.doi.org/10.1136/gutjnl-2012-302084] [PMID: 22491499]

[54] Barkun AN, Bardou M, Kuipers EJ, *et al.* International Consensus Upper Gastrointestinal Bleeding Conference Group. International consensus recommendations on the management of patients with nonvariceal upper gastrointestinal bleeding. Ann Intern Med 2010; 152(2): 101-13. [http://dx.doi.org/10.7326/0003-4819-152-2-201001190-00009] [PMID: 20083829]

[55] Hirsh J, Fuster V, Ansell J, Halperin JL. American Heart Association/American College of Cardiology Foundation. American Heart Association/American College of Cardiology Foundation guide to warfarin therapy. J Am Coll Cardiol 2003; 41(9): 1633-52. [http://dx.doi.org/10.1016/S0735-1097(03)00416-9] [PMID: 12742309]

[56] van Walraven C, Jennings A, Oake N, Fergusson D, Forster AJ. Effect of study setting on anticoagulation control: a systematic review and metaregression. Chest 2006; 129(5): 1155-66. [http://dx.doi.org/10.1378/chest.129.5.1155] [PMID: 16685005]

[57] Liotta EM, Levasseur-Franklin KE, Naidech AM. Reversal of the novel oral anticoagulants dabigatran, rivoraxaban, and apixaban. Curr Opin Crit Care 2015; 21(2): 127-33. [http://dx.doi.org/10.1097/MCC.0000000000000181] [PMID: 25689124]

[58] DeWald TA, Becker RC. The pharmacology of novel oral anticoagulants. J Thromb Thrombolysis 2014; 37(2): 217-33. [http://dx.doi.org/10.1007/s11239-013-0967-z] [PMID: 23860880]

[59] Stangier J. Clinical pharmacokinetics and pharmacodynamics of the oral direct thrombin inhibitor dabigatran etexilate. Clin Pharmacokinet 2008; 47(5): 285-95. [http://dx.doi.org/10.2165/00003088-200847050-00001] [PMID: 18399711]

[60] Wang EH, Bolt JL, Décarie D, Semchuk W, Ensom MH. Stability of Dabigatran Etexilate in Manufacturer's Blister Pack, Unit-Dose Packaging, and Community Pharmacy Blister Pack. Can J Hosp Pharm 2015; 68(1): 16-21. [http://dx.doi.org/10.4212/cjhp.v68i1.1420] [PMID: 25762815]

[61] Abraham NS, Singh S, Alexander GC, *et al.* Comparative risk of gastrointestinal bleeding with dabigatran, rivaroxaban, and warfarin: population based cohort study. BMJ 2015; 350: h1857. [http://dx.doi.org/10.1136/bmj.h1857]

[62] Van ryn J, Stangier J, Haertter S, *et al.* Dabigatran etexilate--a novel, reversible, oral direct thrombin inhibitor: interpretation of coagulation assays and reversal of anticoagulant activity. Thromb Haemost 2010; 103(6): 1116-27.

[63] Gosselin R, Hawes E, Moll S, Adcock D. Performance of various laboratory assays in the measurement of dabigatran in patients receiving therapeutic doses: a prospective study based on peak and trough plasma levels. Am J Clin Pathol 2014; 141(2): 262-7.

[http://dx.doi.org/10.1309/AJCPRNUMI4PVSJ7Q] [PMID: 24436275]

[64] Desai J, Kolb JM, Weitz JI, Aisenberg J. Gastrointestinal bleeding with the new oral anticoagulants--defining the issues and the management strategies. Thromb Haemost 2013; 110(2): 205-12. [http://dx.doi.org/10.1160/TH13-02-0150] [PMID: 23702623]

[65] Granger CB, Alexander JH, McMurray JJ, *et al.* ARISTOTLE Committees and Investigators. Apixaban *versus* warfarin in patients with atrial fibrillation. N Engl J Med 2011; 365(11): 981-92. [http://dx.doi.org/10.1056/NEJMoa1107039] [PMID: 21870978]

[66] Alexander JH, Becker RC, Bhatt DL, *et al.* APPRAISE Steering Committee and Investigators. Apixaban, an oral, direct, selective factor Xa inhibitor, in combination with antiplatelet therapy after acute coronary syndrome: results of the Apixaban for Prevention of Acute Ischemic and Safety Events (APPRAISE) trial. Circulation 2009; 119(22): 2877-85. [http://dx.doi.org/10.1161/CIRCULATIONAHA.108.832139] [PMID: 19470889]

[67] Oldgren J, Budaj A, Granger CB, *et al.* RE-DEEM Investigators. Dabigatran *vs.* placebo in patients with acute coronary syndromes on dual antiplatelet therapy: a randomized, double-blind, phase II trial. Eur Heart J 2011; 32(22): 2781-9. [http://dx.doi.org/10.1093/eurheartj/ehr113] [PMID: 21551462]

[68] Mega JL, Braunwald E, Wiviott SD, *et al.* ATLAS ACS 2–TIMI 51 Investigators. Rivaroxaban in patients with a recent acute coronary syndrome. N Engl J Med 2012; 366(1): 9-19. [http://dx.doi.org/10.1056/NEJMoa1112277] [PMID: 22077192]

[69] Abraham NS. Novel oral anticoagulants and gastrointestinal bleeding: a case for cardiogastroenterology. Clin Gastroenterol Hepatol 2013; 11(4): 324-8. [http://dx.doi.org/10.1016/j.cgh.2012.12.013] [PMID: 23348145]

[70] Graham DJ, Reichman ME, Wernecke M, *et al.* Cardiovascular, bleeding, and mortality risks in elderly Medicare patients treated with dabigatran or warfarin for nonvalvular atrial fibrillation. Circulation 2015; 131(2): 157-64. [http://dx.doi.org/10.1161/CIRCULATIONAHA.114.012061] [PMID: 25359164]

[71] Hernandez I, Baik SH, Piñera A, Zhang Y. Risk of bleeding with dabigatran in atrial fibrillation. JAMA Intern Med 2015; 175(1): 18-24. [http://dx.doi.org/10.1001/jamainternmed.2014.5398] [PMID: 25365537]

[72] Miller CS, Grandi SM, Shimony A, Filion KB, Eisenberg MJ. Meta-analysis of efficacy and safety of new oral anticoagulants (dabigatran, rivaroxaban, apixaban) *versus* warfarin in patients with atrial fibrillation. Am J Cardiol 2012; 110(3): 453-60. [http://dx.doi.org/10.1016/j.amjcard.2012.03.049] [PMID: 22537354]

[73] Chang HY, Zhou M, Tang W, Alexander GC, Singh S. Risk of gastrointestinal bleeding associated with oral anticoagulants: population based retrospective cohort study. BMJ 2015; 350: h1585. [http://dx.doi.org/10.1136/bmj.h1585]

[74] Chai-Adisaksopha C, Crowther M, Isayama T, Lim W. The impact of bleeding complications in patients receiving target-specific oral anticoagulants: a systematic review and meta-analysis. Blood 2014; 124(15): 2450-8. [http://dx.doi.org/10.1182/blood-2014-07-590323] [PMID: 25150296]

[75] Levi M, Hovingh GK, Cannegieter SC, Vermeulen M, Büller HR, Rosendaal FR. Bleeding in patients receiving vitamin K antagonists who would have been excluded from trials on which the indication for anticoagulation was based. Blood 2008; 111(9): 4471-6. [http://dx.doi.org/10.1182/blood-2007-11-123711] [PMID: 18316627]

[76] Eikelboom JW, Wallentin L, Connolly SJ, *et al.* Risk of bleeding with 2 doses of dabigatran compared with warfarin in older and younger patients with atrial fibrillation: an analysis of the randomized evaluation of long-term anticoagulant therapy (RE-LY) trial. Circulation 2011; 123(21): 2363-72. [http://dx.doi.org/10.1161/CIRCULATIONAHA.110.004747] [PMID: 21576658]

[77] Camm AJ, Lip GY, De Caterina R, *et al.* ESC Committee for Practice Guidelines-CPG, Document Reviewers. 2012 focused update of the ESC Guidelines for the management of atrial fibrillation: an update of the 2010 ESC Guidelines for the management of atrial fibrillation--developed with the special contribution of the European Heart Rhythm Association. Europace 2012; 14(10): 1385-413. [http://dx.doi.org/10.1093/europace/eus305] [PMID: 22923145]

[78] Larsen TB, Rasmussen LH, Skjøth F, *et al.* Efficacy and safety of dabigatran etexilate and warfarin in "real-world" patients with atrial fibrillation: a prospective nationwide cohort study. J Am Coll Cardiol 2013; 61(22): 2264-73. [http://dx.doi.org/10.1016/j.jacc.2013.03.020] [PMID: 23562920]

[79] Hylek EM, Evans-Molina C, Shea C, Henault LE, Regan S. Major hemorrhage and tolerability of warfarin in the first year of therapy among elderly patients with atrial fibrillation. Circulation 2007; 115(21): 2689-96. [http://dx.doi.org/10.1161/CIRCULATIONAHA.106.653048] [PMID: 17515465]

[80] Dager WE, Gosselin RC, Kitchen S, Dwyre D. Dabigatran effects on the international normalized ratio, activated partial thromboplastin time, thrombin time, and fibrinogen: a multicenter, *in vitro* study. Ann Pharmacother 2012; 46(12): 1627-36. [http://dx.doi.org/10.1345/aph.1R179] [PMID: 23232017]

[81] Winkler AM, Tormey CA. Education Committee of the Academy of Clinical Laboratory Physicians and Scientists. Pathology consultation on monitoring direct thrombin inhibitors and overcoming their effects in bleeding patients. Am J Clin Pathol 2013; 140(5): 610-22. [http://dx.doi.org/10.1309/AJCP9VJS6KUKNCHW] [PMID: 24124139]

[82] Gehrie E, Tormey C. Novel oral anticoagulants: efficacy, laboratory measurement, and approaches to emergent reversal. Arch Pathol Lab Med 2015; 139(5): 687-92. [http://dx.doi.org/10.5858/arpa.2013-0677-RS] [PMID: 25927153]

[83] Harenberg J, Marx S, Erdle S, Krämer R. Determination of the anticoagulant effects of new oral anticoagulants: an unmet need. Expert Rev Hematol 2012; 5(1): 107-13. [http://dx.doi.org/10.1586/ehm.11.79] [PMID: 22272710]

[84] Garcia D, Barrett YC, Ramacciotti E, Weitz JI. Laboratory assessment of the anticoagulant effects of the next generation of oral anticoagulants. J Thromb Haemost 2013; 11(2): 245-52. [http://dx.doi.org/10.1111/jth.12096] [PMID: 23216682]

[85] Barrett YC, Wang Z, Frost C, Shenker A. Clinical laboratory measurement of direct factor Xa inhibitors: anti-Xa assay is preferable to prothrombin time assay. Thromb Haemost 2010; 104(6): 1263-71.

[86] Tran HA, Chunilal SD, Harper PL, Tran H, Wood EM, Gallus AS. Australasian Society of Thrombosis and Haemostasis (ASTH). An update of consensus guidelines for warfarin reversal. Med J Aust 2013; 198(4): 198-9.
[http://dx.doi.org/10.5694/mja12.10614] [PMID: 23451962]

[87] Siegal DM. Managing target-specific oral anticoagulant associated bleeding including an update on pharmacological reversal agents. J Thromb Thrombolysis 2015; 39(3): 395-402.
[http://dx.doi.org/10.1007/s11239-015-1167-9] [PMID: 25586208]

[88] Glund S, Moschetti V, Norris S, *et al.* A randomised study in healthy volunteers to investigate the safety, tolerability and pharmacokinetics of idarucizumab, a specific antidote to dabigatran. Thromb Haemost 2015; 113(5): 943-51.
[http://dx.doi.org/10.1160/TH14-12-1080] [PMID: 25789661]

[89] Pollack CV Jr, Reilly PA, Eikelboom J, *et al.* Idarucizumab for Dabigatran Reversal. N Engl J Med 2015; 373(6): 511-20.
[http://dx.doi.org/10.1056/NEJMoa1502000] [PMID: 26095746]

[90] Winkler AM, Tormey CA. Education Committee of the Academy of Clinical Laboratory Physicians and Scientists. Pathology consultation on monitoring direct thrombin inhibitors and overcoming their effects in bleeding patients. Am J Clin Pathol 2013; 140(5): 610-22.

[91] Woo JS, Kapadia N, Phanco SE, Lynch CA. Positive outcome after intentional overdose of dabigatran. J Med Toxicol 2013; 9(2): 192-5.
[http://dx.doi.org/10.1007/s13181-012-0276-5] [PMID: 23212788]

[92] Pragst I, Zeitler SH, Doerr B, *et al.* Reversal of dabigatran anticoagulation by prothrombin complex concentrate (Beriplex P/N) in a rabbit model. J Thromb Haemost 2012; 10(9): 1841-8.
[http://dx.doi.org/10.1111/j.1538-7836.2012.04859.x] [PMID: 22812619]

[93] Eerenberg ES, Kamphuisen PW, Sijpkens MK, Meijers JC, Buller HR, Levi M. Reversal of rivaroxaban and dabigatran by prothrombin complex concentrate: a randomized, placebo-controlled, crossover study in healthy subjects. Circulation 2011; 124(14): 1573-9.
[http://dx.doi.org/10.1161/CIRCULATIONAHA.111.029017] [PMID: 21900088]

[94] Moll S. Letter by Moll regarding article, “Hemostatic therapy in experimental intracerebral hemorrhage associated with the direct thrombin inhibitor dabigatran”. Stroke 2012; 43(2): e24.
[http://dx.doi.org/10.1161/STROKEAHA.111.643247] [PMID: 22267830]

[95] Körber MK, Langer E, Ziemer S, Perzborn E, Gericke C, Heymann Cv. Measurement and reversal of prophylactic and therapeutic peak levels of rivaroxaban: an *in vitro* study. Clin Appl Thromb Hemost 2014; 20(7): 735-40.
[http://dx.doi.org/10.1177/1076029613494468] [PMID: 23832064]

[96] Lu G, DeGuzman FR, Hollenbach SJ, *et al.* A specific antidote for reversal of anticoagulation by direct and indirect inhibitors of coagulation factor Xa. Nat Med 2013; 19(4): 446-51.
[http://dx.doi.org/10.1038/nm.3102] [PMID: 23455714]

[97] Siegal DM, Curnutte JT, Connolly SJ, *et al.* Andexanet Alfa for the Reversal of Factor Xa Inhibitor Activity. N Engl J Med 2015; 373(25): 2413-24.
[http://dx.doi.org/10.1056/NEJMoa1510991] [PMID: 26559317]

SUBJECT INDEX

Atta-ur-Rahman & M. Iqbal Choudhary (Eds.)

L

M

P

T

U

V

W

Made in United States
North Haven, CT
04 November 2026

21719582R00226